DON'T FENCE ME IN

BY THE SAME AUTHOR

Stories from the Dole Queue (*with Joe Kenyon*)
In Limbo: The Story of Stanley's Rear Column
Inside Outsider: The Life and Times of Colin MacInnes
Death in Chile: A Memoir and a Journey
A Summer Plague: Polio and Its Survivors
Imperial Warriors: Britain and the Gurkhas

DON'T FENCE ME IN

Leprosy in Modern Times

TONY GOULD

BLOOMSBURY

For permission to reprint extracts from copyright material the author and publishers gratefully acknowledge the following: the Orion Publishing Group for *The Mask of a Lion* by A. T. W. Simeons, published by Victor Gollancz; the Random House Publishing Group for *Young Man in the Sun* and *The Painted Leopard* by Peter Greave, published by Eyre & Spottiswoode; the German Leprosy and TB Relief Association for the English translation of *Memories & Reflections* by G. Armauer Hansen; *The Star* and La Societé des Quarante Hommes et Huit Chevaux for *Alone No Longer* by Stanley Stein; HarperCollins Publishers Inc for *Pain: The Gift Nobody Wants* by Paul Brand and Philip Yancy; and Dr Fujio Ohtani for *The Walls Crumble*. Full details of all works quoted are given in the references and bibliography.

First published 2005

Bloomsbury Publishing Plc, 38 Soho Square, London W1D 3HB

A CIP catalogue record for this book
is available from the British Library

ISBN 0 7475 7510 X

10 9 8 7 6 5 4 3 2 1

Typeset by Hewer Text Ltd, Edinburgh
Printed by Clays Ltd, St Ives plc

All papers used by Bloomsbury are natural,
recyclable products made from wood grown in well-managed
forests. The manufacturing processes conform to the
environmental regulations of the country of origin.

www.bloomsbury.com/tonygould

For J.P. CROSS
and
in memory of my father-in-law, DENNIS A. COWELL

CONTENTS

ACKNOWLEDGEMENTS

The credit for thinking that leprosy would make a suitable subject for a non-specialist readership should go to Rosemary Davidson, my editor at Bloomsbury. When my agent, Gill Coleridge (who has been wonderfully supportive over the years), first conveyed Rosemary's idea to me, I wasn't at all sure about it. I hesitated for two reasons. The obvious one was that the little I knew – or thought I knew – about the disease made me nervous of seeking a closer acquaintance with it, even if much of my research would be done in libraries rather than hospitals or 'leprosaria'. The other reason was to do with my instinctive aversion to being categorised as a certain type of writer. The half-dozen books I have written have little in common apart from the fact that they are all non-fiction. The genres include reportage (contemporary and historical), biography and autobiography, medical and military history. I've tried to avoid repeating myself, though I'm aware that this is professionally self-defeating, and now I was being invited to do something similar for leprosy to what I had already done for my own disease – polio – in *A Summer Plague*: weave together the many different strands of the disease and produce a narrative history. So I prevaricated, but once I started to study the subject its intrinsic fascination gripped me and my doubts fell away.

My biggest material debt is to the Society of Authors (as it has been more than once before) and to the assessors of the Authors' Foundation in 2000 – Orlando Figes, Shena Mackay, Douglas Matthews, Jilly Paver and Jo Shapcott – who considered my project worthy of support and made a travel award that enabled me to spend several weeks during the following year in the United States, as well as in Nepal. My old comradein-arms in the 1st battalion, 7th Gurkha Rifles, Lt Col John Cross (joint dedicatee of this book), generously paid my air fare to Nepal, where he – along with his surrogate son Buddhiman Gurung and family – was my host during the ten busy and pleasurable days I spent in Pokhara.

John put me in touch with Eileen Lodge, a missionary nurse who became a Nepali citizen and is the doyenne of leprosy workers in Nepal. Eileen organised my visit so that I got to see several places concerned with leprosy, from an old-fashioned state leprosarium in the Kathmandu valley to a fairly new and very busy leprosy hospital in the Terai – the southern plain adjacent to India. In charge of the latter at that time was Dr Hugh Cross, a podiatrist (and no relation to John Cross), who showed me much and taught me more during my all-too-brief stay at Lalgadh. Dr Friedbert Herm welcomed me to Green Pastures in Pokhara, which was once but is no longer exclusively concerned with leprosy, and there my main guide and mentor was the very experienced physiotherapist Wim Brandsma. Among the leprosy patients and ex-patients I met I would mention two in particular, both of whom had become members of staff at Green Pastures: Shankar Pantha and Shobhakher Thapa. The life stories of these two gentle and courageous men were deeply moving.

Other people who contributed to my visit to Nepal include Bidur Basnet and Dr R.K. Shrestha of the Nepal Leprosy Relief Association, Sharmila Shrestha and Sher Thapa of the United Mission to Nepal, Kamal Shrestha of the Nepal Leprosy Trust, visiting consultant Virginia Bond and Chitra Bahadur KC of New SADLE (Skill and Development Learning Experience) and the Sewa Kendra Leprosy Station in Kathmandu, and my ex-Gurkha friends Maniprasad Rai, Robin Marsden and Kit Spencer.

Professor Gilla Kaplan from New York stimulated my curiosity about scientific research into leprosy and provided me with names of other doctors and researchers, one of whom, Dr James L. Krahenbuhl, was my initial contact with Carville in Louisiana. When my wife and I spent ten days at the only leprosarium ever to be built on the mainland of the United States, we were well looked after by Tanya Thomassie of the US Public Health Service, by Sister Francis de Sales, Mary-Ruth Daigle (both now dead) and Willie Kikuchi, in particular. I also benefited from conversations with the Editor of the *Star*, Emanuel Faria (who also died recently), and a former Carville resident, Tom K. Sue Renault of the American Leprosy Missions in Greenville, South Carolina, pulled out all the stops to make our one-day stay there as productive as possible (a special thank-you to Diane for all the photocopying!). In West Virginia, Anwei Skinsnes Law, International Co-ordinator of IDEA (International Association for Integration, Dignity and Economic Advancement), gave us the run of her superb private leprosy archive – and her husband Henry gave us an expert guided tour of the National Park there. While at the National Library of Medicine in Bethesda, Maryland, I received help from the PHS historian John Parascandola. Thanks, too, to American friends Abby Collins, John Dyck and Beth Hardesty.

Closer to home, I am especially indebted to the British leprologist Dr Diana Lockwood, who acted as a kind of unofficial consultant, allowing me to draw on her expertise whenever I needed to, reading and commenting on a draft of this book, and introducing me to a number of former leprosy patients in this country. Though several of these patients prefer to remain anonymous, I am particularly grateful to one, Les Parker, for telling me about his life at St Giles in Essex and his friendship with the writer Peter Greave.

Carole Rawcliffe, Professor of Medieval History at the University of East Anglia, provided useful seminars on medieval leprosy over enjoyable lunches and also read and commented on parts of my typescript. Dr Shubhada Pandya, leprosy historian and neurophysiologist from Mumbai in India, not only provided me with much interesting material, but also read and commented on my chapter on nineteenth-century India and empire. Michel Lechat, Emeritus Professor at the University of Louvain, was a lively and entertaining correspondent on a wide range of topics, including his friendship with the novelist Graham Greene in what was then the Belgian Congo. The podiatrist Barbara Wall sparked off my interest in the nineteenth-century nurse and intrepid traveller, Kate Marsden, and provided me with the newspaper cutting that was absolutely crucial to making sense of her story.

Joyce Missing and all the staff of The Leprosy Mission International in Brentford and Irene Allen of LEPRA (The British Leprosy Relief Association) in Colchester gave me unlimited access to their archival material. So did Sarah Strong of the Royal Geographical Society, in relation to my research on Kate Marsden, and the staffs of the British Library (Oriental and India Office Collections), the Public Record Office, the School of Oriental and African Studies library and, most significantly, the Wellcome Library and Centre for the History of Medicine were invariably helpful and courteous.

I would also like to thank the following individuals, who helped me in various ways: Helga Brömmelhaus, Piers Burton-Page, the late Jo Colston, Roger and Elizabeth Cozens, Dr Tim Dudgeon, Zoe Heming, Vanessa Lee and Steve Miller, Dorothy Pirkis, Lt Col L.D. Ponnaiya and his daughter Ruth Khanna, Sir Richard Posnett, Julia Sheppard, Paul Sommerfeld and Dr Yo Yuasa. To my wife Jenny, who accompanied me to America and threw herself into the research there with her customary energy and read and reread each chapter as I wrote and rewrote it, my debt is incalculable.

INTRODUCTION

> Leprosy is dreaded most of all diseases, not because it kills, but because it leaves alive; not for its pain – though painful at times, the loss of pain and tactile sensation is dreaded more. Mask face, unclosing eyes, slavering mouth, claw-hands and limping feet; or, even worse, beetling brows, stuffed nose, ulcerating legs, and painful eyes drawing on towards blindness – such is the picture conjured up in the mind of the patient when the physician after making his examination pronounces the word – *leprosy* . . .[1]
>
> Dr Ernest Muir (1948)

For westerners of my generation (born 1938) the word leprosy evokes images of grotesquely deformed, poverty-stricken black or brown people cared for by missionaries. On collecting boxes and in mission literature these leprosy sufferers used to be represented in postures of supplication, leaning on rough-hewn staves, lacking digits, or hands, or feet, or noses, or sight, their faces transformed into grimacing yet expressionless masks. They were the stuff of nightmares; but at the same time there was something cartoonish, almost unreal, in their extremity. Well-fed, well brought-up Christian children were encouraged to correspond with 'leper' pen friends in exotic places, whose stamps at least were worth collecting. Leprosy happened elsewhere, in another country, almost – it seemed – in another time. It was a primeval relic and the people who suffered from it, so strangely *in*human did they seem, existed in some kind of time warp. It was not a threat as, say, polio was; it was hardly even a disease; like the poverty from which it seemed to arise, it was more a condition of life. Hence, one supposed, its attraction for missionaries.

Yet the period of the late 1940s and early 1950s, when leprosy first impinged upon my consciousness, was one of great optimism for people affected by this baffling disease. At long last there was a drug, or class of drugs, that could actually cure it if caught in the early stages and arrest it even in advanced cases. Suddenly there was light at the end of the tunnel for those undergoing what had been until then a life sentence without hope of remission; people who had been shut away for years in institutions across the world were getting their first whiff of freedom. No wonder that the inmates of the only leprosarium on the mainland of the United States, at Carville, Louisiana, latched on to a contemporary popular song, 'Don't Fence Me In', and made it their own.

From the middle of the nineteenth century, when doctors began to take a scientific interest in leprosy, until after the Second World War (and even longer in some countries) the unsightliness of the disease in its advanced stages, combined with the lack of an effective treatment, condemned its sufferers to an outcast existence, exile and/or incarceration. Before the sulphone drugs were tried out in the 1940s, the only treatment of any repute was chaulmoogra oil, an Asian remedy so ancient that it features in Hindu legend dating from before the time of Buddha. Rama, the king of Benares, is stricken with leprosy and flees to the jungle, leaving the throne to his son. He lives on wild fruits, and those of the chaulmoogra tree cure him of his disease. As is the way of legends, he rescues a damsel in distress (threatened by a tiger) who turns out to be suffering from leprosy herself, but also just happens to be a princess. Like the story of Adam and Eve in reverse, Rama gives Piya the fruit of the chaulmoogra tree; her health and beauty are restored; they marry and enter paradise, returning to Benares, 'where their joyful reception gave birth to the "Festival of the Lamps"'.[2] However ancient treatment with chaulmoogra oil was – and a reference to it can be found in the *Sushruta Samhita*, a compilation of ancient Indian medical writing dating from around 600 BC[3] – it was so unpalatable that its therapeutic potential was not taken seriously by western doctors until early in the twentieth century, when they began to experiment with ways of injecting it.

The detailed and accurate descriptions of leprosy provided in the *Sushruta Samhita* bear witness to the antiquity of the disease in the Far East at least. Yet despite several references to leprosy and 'lepers' in the Old Testament, to the best of our knowledge the disease did not exist in the Middle East in the time of Moses; it may have been around in

Palestine during Christ's lifetime, but even that is debatable. Far from being the most ancient of diseases, as the biblical references led our forebears to believe, it is now considered a relatively recent arrival in the lands around the Mediterranean, probably brought there by Alexander the Great's troops returning from India in about 300 BC – though Lucretius (99–44 BC) claimed that it emanated from Africa: 'High up the Nile midst Egypt's central plain/Springs the dread leprosy, and there alone.'

So why did Moses say things like, 'And the leper in whom the plague *is*, his clothes shall be rent, and his head bare, and he shall put a covering upon his upper lip, and shall cry, Unclean, unclean . . .' and, 'Command the children of Israel, that they put out of the camp every leper . . .'?[4] On top of everything else, it seems leprosy sufferers are the victims of mistranslation. The Hebrew word *tsara'ath*, translated as *lepra* in Latin and Greek, conveys the notion of one who is stricken or defiled, insofar as the concept is at all translatable into a modern idiom; it certainly does not mean leprosy, as we understand it. It is generally taken to be a generic term covering a range of dermatological diseases: leukoderma, vitiligo and psoriasis are among the most frequently cited.

When the novelist John Updike published a story called 'From the Journal of a Leper' in the 1970s, there were mutterings from the more articulate patients at Carville. Their mouthpiece, the *Star*, had been conducting a long and largely successful campaign to outlaw the L-word, whose biblical associations, they felt, contributed so greatly to their stigmatisation; and here it was again, emblazoned in the title of a story. The fact that Updike wasn't even referring to leprosy, but to his own disease, psoriasis, hardly mitigated his offence in their eyes. His narrator explains:

> Leprosy is not exactly what I have, but what in the Bible is called leprosy (see Leviticus 13, Exodus 4:6, Luke 5:12–13) was probably this thing, which has a twisty Greek name it pains me to write. The form of the disease is as follows: spots, plaques, and avalanches of excess skin, manufactured by the dermis through some trifling but persistent error in its metabolic instructions, expand and slowly migrate across the body like lichen on a tombstone. I am silvery, scaly. Puddles of flakes form wherever I rest my flesh. Each morning, I vacuum my bed. My torture is skin deep: there is no pain, not even itching; we lepers live a long time,

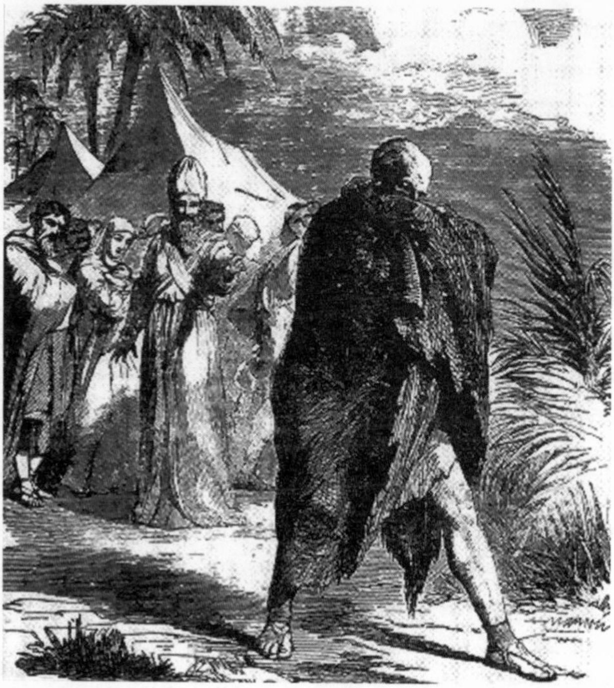

(Illustrert Bibelleksikon)

The priest expels the 'leper', *Leviticus* 13, 45–46, engraving by Gustave Doré

> and are ironically healthy in other respects. Lusty, though we are loathsome to love. Keen-sighted, though we hate to look upon ourselves. The name of the disease, spiritually speaking, is Humiliation.[5]

The disease so graphically described by Updike bears little resemblance to true leprosy, in which the 'torture' – loss of sensation resulting from damage to the peripheral nerves – is much more than 'skin deep'. But if we do as he suggests and look up Exodus 4:6, for example, we find God demonstrating His power to Moses with a couple of instant miracles, the second of which involves afflicting him with 'leprosy': 'And the Lord said furthermore unto him, Put now thine hand into thy bosom. And he put his hand into his bosom: and when he took it out, behold, his hand was leprous as snow.' In the next verse, God undoes the damage: when Moses removes his hand from his bosom the second time, 'behold, it was turned again as his *other* flesh' – i.e., smooth and luscious as opposed to white and scaly.

The New Testament example cited by Updike contains no description of leprosy whatsoever; the only hint that it is different in kind from other diseases comes from the language employed: where the sick are 'healed', so-called lepers are 'cleansed'. This, too, fits a dermatological condition like psoriasis much better than a disease with neurological involvement such as leprosy. Updike's protagonist bemoans the 'avalanche of excess skin' and the 'puddles of flakes' that oblige him to vacuum his bed every morning, but he is 'healthy in other respects'. In other words, his disease sets him apart, not as unwell, but as unclean.

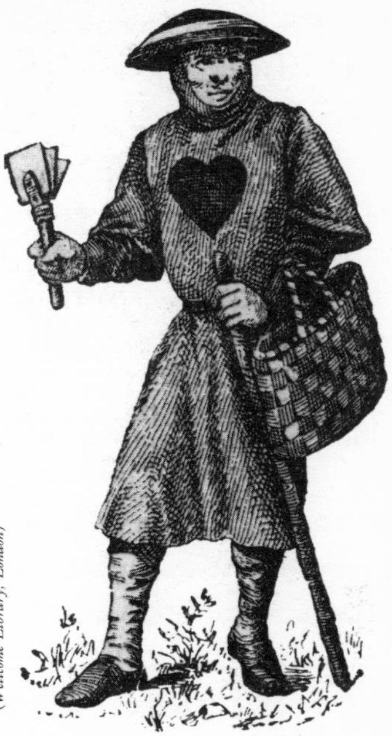
(Wellcome Library, London)

Nineteenth-century image of medieval 'leper' with clapper and basket

The idea of compelling psoriatics like Updike, or the late playwright Dennis Potter, to dwell 'without the camp' because they are 'unclean' is patently absurd. Yet this was the fate of true leprosy sufferers in both medieval and modern societies. Indeed, medical writers in the nineteenth and early twentieth century can be said to have reconstructed the Middle Ages in such a way as to provide historical justification for their own practice of segregating leprosy sufferers.

The popular image of a medieval 'leper' is of a hooded, cloaked and gloved figure with clapper and cop – a rattle (or bell) to announce his presence and a dish to solicit alms – standing downwind of other folk and crying out by way of warning, 'Unclean, unclean!' An image, in other words, of an outcast and beggar, someone to be avoided, at best an object of charity. According to this version of history, for about three centuries – from the eleventh until the middle of the fourteenth century when bubonic plague, in the form of the Black Death, struck – leprosy was the most feared disease in Europe and the 'loathsome leper' (an alliteration irresistible even to Marlowe and Shakespeare, who between them used the identical line, 'I am no loathsome leper, look on me', in three different plays[6]) the most despised creature, subject to a special 'leper's mass' that pronounced him 'dead among the living'.

Present-day medieval historians, who have steeped themselves in contemporary sources, paint a rather different picture, in which those afflicted with leprosy are represented as 'Christ's poor', *pauperes Christi* – and, by extension, even as Our Lord Himself, *Christus quasi leprosus* – persons whose earthly purgatory guaranteed them on their decease exemption from that particular staging post en route to heaven. We know that their plight attracted the attention of the great and holy such as Saint Louis (Louis IX of France) and Henry I's wife, Queen Matilda, who described washing their ulcerous feet as 'better than kissing the lips of a mortal king'.[7] For some of these good people, leprosy represented a religious vocation rather than an affliction and they prayed that they might manifest in their own bodies such a sign of divine favour (a tradition far from extinct in the nineteenth century, as the sequel will show). From this perspective, the lazar houses, or leprosaria, that sprang up all over Europe in the eleventh, twelfth and thirteenth centuries, were not so much prisons, segregating and incarcerating unfortunates for the crime of leprosy, as monasteries, religious houses to which it was a privilege rather than a penance to belong.[8] Hence the most serious punishment a disobedient inmate of some lazar houses might incur was not further incarceration or confinement in a prison within the prison, as in latter-day leprosaria, but . . . expulsion.

As for the 'leper's mass', at which the leprosy sufferer was ritually buried alive – and in some instances, allegedly, obliged to stand in a coffin – while the priest intoned the 'ten commandments' consigning him to outer darkness, this was largely a sixteenth-century concoction and in England, at least, was never performed. When nineteenth-century commentators cited the rules of the various lazar houses – at St Magdalen in Exeter, for instance, 'no brother or sister shall go or pass out of the house beyond the bridge, without the gate of the said hospital, without the license of the Warden or his deputy, upon

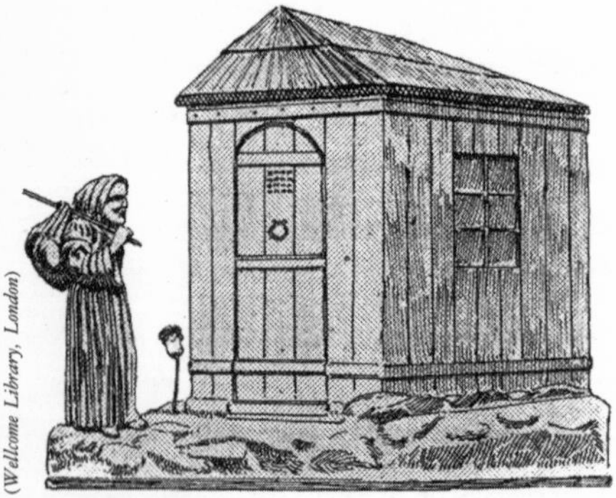
(Wellcome Library, London)

A fifteenth-century 'leper's' retreat

pain to be put into the stocks, and to have but bread and water for a day'[9] – as evidence of the practice of segregation, they omitted to point out that such rules were not exclusive to leprosy patients but applied to *all* patients in *all* hospitals. The idea of segregation as a public health measure would have baffled our medieval forebears; insofar as leprosy patients were segregated (and their visibility at fairs and markets suggests this wasn't very far) it was from fear of pollution rather than contagion.

The extent of true leprosy in the Middle Ages is another contentious issue, as the Belgian doctor, Michel-François Lechat, who played host in Africa to Graham Greene when the latter was researching the background for his novel *A Burnt-out Case*, points out: 'it is impossible to even hazard a guess about its actual prevalence, its distribution or its relative frequency in towns as compared to the countryside . . . more is known about the epidemiology of the lazarets than about the epidemiology of the disease itself!'[10]

The nineteenth-century pioneer of medical history, Charles Creighton, alleged that in medieval England:

> the village leper may have been about as common as the village fool; while in the larger towns or cities such as London, Norwich, York, Bristol, and Lincoln, true lepers can hardly have been so numerous as the friars themselves, who are supposed to have found a large part of their occupation in ministering to their wants.[11]

His suspicions about the activities of friars may not have been misplaced, if Chaucer's Friar – who, in contrast to St Francis, prefers the company of innkeepers and barmaids to that of 'lazars'[12] – is anything to go by, but modern archaeological evidence refutes his scepticism about the extent of true leprosy. Many of the skeletons excavated from the graveyards of leprosaria such as St Mary's, Chichester, bear unmistakable evidence of the ravages of the disease and thus confirm what most recent historians claim: that the priest-physicians of the Middle Ages were quite sophisticated enough to be able to make an accurate diagnosis of leprosy. There is not much doubt that medieval leprosy, unlike biblical 'leprosy', is the disease that we know by that name today.

The rapid decline of leprosy in the late Middle Ages has been attributed to several possible causes, of which the most commonly held are: the segregation of sufferers in leprosaria, the Black Death itself, an improvement in people's diet and living conditions, and the rise of tuberculosis. The first of these, as we've seen, is highly improbable: even in the nineteenth century some advocates of segregation had to admit that in medieval times it had been 'very lax, careless, and therefore useless' and that 'no one can carefully read the detailed accounts of the various leper hospitals in England and feel assured that they acted as "arresters" of the spread of the disease'.[13] The theory that the Black Death killed off already weakened leprosy sufferers is equally unconvincing, since leprosy was on the decline *before* the plague struck. And given that leprosy and tuberculosis alike flourish in conditions of poverty and malnutrition, any improvement in people's living conditions should theoretically see the decline of *both diseases* simultaneously. But could the decline of one and the rise of the other be more than coincidental?

Charles Mercier, lecturing at the Royal College of Physicians in London in 1914, thought so: 'The disease of tuberculosis resembles the disease of leprosy in many respects . . . An hereditary susceptibility is without doubt an important factor in both diseases.'[14] The theory of some kind of cross-immunity, based on the similarity of the bacilli causing the two diseases, has been strengthened by the discovery, much later in the twentieth century, that the BCG vaccine for tuberculosis is effective against leprosy in some parts of the world, if not in others. A recent writer sees 'the rise in prevalence of pulmonary tuberculosis and the associated immune relationship between the Mycobacterial diseases' as the most probable explanation of the decline and virtual disappearance of leprosy in late medieval Europe.[15] Another puts it even more strongly: 'tuberculosis won an edge over leprosy in the struggle to find a niche in the human body. It is a case of ecological competition, with *M. tuberculosis* winning.'[16]

The tendency of modern patients (such as the group at Carville that put out the *Star*) to blame the Bible for the stigmatisation of leprosy ignores the fact that its sufferers have been treated just as badly, or worse, in many non-Judaeo-Christian societies where, in the words of one writer, 'it became a curse of the gods, because its nature made it an ideal scapegoat for fear, disgust and superstition'.[17] In China, for example, victims of the disease were routinely cast out of towns and villages and herded into walled enclaves that were so squalid that some preferred to take their own lives rather than enter one. They were also subject to periodical massacres. In the nineteenth century, a mandarin invited all the people with leprosy in his region to a feast and, when they were gathered under one roof, closed the doors and set fire to the place.[18] And at the end of 1912, outside the city of Nan-ning in southern China:

> . . . the lepers occupying a wretched village of their own were surrounded by soldiers, and at the point of the bayonet, driven to an already prepared pit. They were shot down like vermin, and dead and wounded, including women and children, were cast into the trench and burned. Fifty-three at least perished in this abominable massacre, and perhaps the saddest feature about it is that it was done by official direction and met with public approval.[19]

The same thing happened again on Easter Day 1937 at the leprosy settlement at Yeung-Kong in southern Kwangtung (Guang-dong). The military authorities who had been threatening to shoot any of the

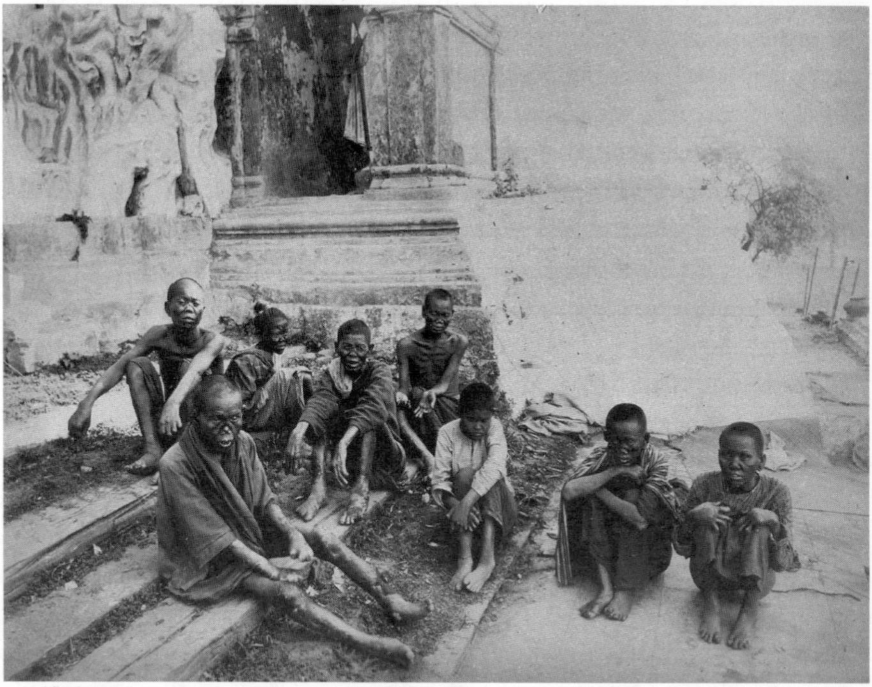

(Wellcome Library, London)

Leprosy sufferers on the steps of a Chinese pagoda

inmates they came across appeared to have a sudden change of heart and announced that leprosy sufferers would receive a daily allowance of ten cents. This turned out to be nothing more than a ruse to ensure that all were present when the soldiers moved in, tied them up and dragged them out to be shot. After the execution of more than fifty people, a third of whom were women, the soldiers returned to plunder the village and set it alight. Missionaries were preparing to hold an Easter service when they heard about the massacre. One wrote:

> I simply couldn't believe it. We all jumped into the car and went out. Sure enough as we neared we saw the smoke pouring from the village and a hundred soldiers marching away. We got out of the car and ran to the village. Police were at the entrance and wouldn't let us in. They pointed over the hill and we went and looked. There in a row lay the lepers, all shot. If I live to be a hundred this day will follow me. There lay the best friends I had in China. I still can't believe it.[20]

In countries like China, of course, the presence of Christian missionaries was itself seen as a provocation, a kind of foreign invasion, however benign in intent. The victims of the Kwangtung massacre, having been rejected by their own society, readily embraced the beliefs of the only people ever to make them feel welcome, and who's to say that the soldiers – in this instance acting in defiance of the civil authorities – were not punishing them for apostasy as well as for leprosy?

The Carville patient and founding editor of the *Star*, Stanley Stein, wrote of the 'tropistic attraction of leprosy for organized religions', both Protestant and Roman Catholic, and one of the themes of this book is the missionary involvement with this particular disease. After all, as Stein goes on to say, there is 'no Mission to the Tubercular, no Mission to the Diabetics, no Mission to the Syphilitics . . . There seems to be some special reward for working with "lepers"'.[21] An influential British missionary doctor, the late Stanley G. Browne, argues that the misidentification of biblical 'leprosy' has not been 'an unrelieved misfortune', since at a time 'when nobody else cared or bothered, Christians did, and their example still inspires those of other faiths and of no faith'. This is certainly true, but it has not been an unalloyed blessing either. The ambivalence of the biblical message – punitive in the Old Testament, compassionate in the New – has been reflected in the treatment of leprosy patients throughout the history of the disease. Even Browne admits, 'it cannot be denied that serious prejudice against leprosy sufferers has in historical times been reinforced by the wholesale transfer of the corpus of *ṣāra'ath* beliefs to the perfectly innocent victims of a myco-bacterial disease'.[22]

Leprosy is certainly not the only disease to have a moral dimension equating illness with punishment for sins committed in this or past lives, but its symbiotic relationship with Christianity in both medieval and modern times has exacerbated that general tendency and transformed a physical ailment into a moral condition. This has meant that, arguing backwards from effect to cause rather than vice versa, leprosy has been frequently characterised as 'dirty' and 'venereal'.[23] Here is the earliest nineteenth-century description of the disease I have been able to discover, written not by a doctor but by a retired indigo planter in a book called *Sketches in India*; that this farrago of fantasy and observation was thought worthy of quotation in the pages of the recently founded scientific medical journal, *The Lancet*, is telling:

> A person attacked with the species of leprosy prevalent in India, is bloated in his face; his forehead, nose, lips, and ears, swell out; his nostrils expand; his eyes appear sunk, and very fiery; the tone of his voice is altered to a loud and somewhat nasal sound; no eruptions appear upon his body, but his skin is hard, parched, and dry, having entirely lost its softness and moisture. About the shoulders he appears tight and contracted; his knees are stiff, and his motions constrained; the hairs fall off him, or are seen in their stunted stalks, dried up from want of wholesome nourishment; his breath is foetid, his perspiration stopped, or, if it flows at all, is rank and stinking; he complains of excessive internal heat, cannot bear exposure to the sun, and is irregular in his discharges, the digestive organs performing their functions very imperfectly; there is a certain numbness seizes all his faculties, so that his sensations of pleasure and pain are considerably impaired; and lepers of this kind have no excessive propensity to venery after the disease appears, although they may have had it before. It is a common opinion, that people seized with this malady are of a warm and amorous temperament; but, when a person is seized with leprosy, the pleasure derived from such indulgencies, and the capacity for them, are in a great measure annulled. After these primary symptoms, when the disease has become inveterate, the leper's fingers are gradually eaten

> away, and drop off at the joints; his toes are affected in a similar manner, sores break out about his ankles and wrists. During the progress of these cancerous attacks, no pain is endured by the leper, owing to that numbness which I have already stated as pervading his system, whilst the disease gradually proceeds ulcerating his flesh, and dissolving his joints, till the vitals become affected. In the last stage his flesh gapes with long sores, his mouth, nose, and brain, dissolve before the leprous poison, till death happily relieves him from such accumulated miseries.[24]

Even people who should know better have held that leprosy was a venereal disease, as the superintendent of the Sungei Buloh settlement in Malaya before and during the Second World War, Dr Gordon Ryrie, relates:

> The writer recently saw a highly educated leprosy worker who had developed a small tuberculoid lesion on the inner side of the right arm. The patient's unsolicited commentary was 'You needn't think I got this sitting embracing a native woman.' Here we have a well-educated worker, experienced and trained in modern ideas about leprosy. The presence of a tuberculoid lesion, however, had flared up the guilt and punishment complex with an instinctive reversion to the lay concepts of leprosy being dirty, infectious and venereal. Leprosy work frequently attracts doctors and workers who have a religious outlook and it is precisely such people who tend to have the guilt and punishment complex most deeply.[25]

Leprosy formed no part of the standard medical school curriculum and on the whole doctors who were not fired with evangelical zeal did not want to know about it. The medical missionary Dr Ernest Muir, who spent most of his working life in British India, wrote:

> In most endemic countries leprosy was for long considered to be a subject for charitable organisations or, failing them, for the police. It is only in recent years that it has been classed with other infective diseases as a responsibility of the public health authorities. In India in 1925 leprosy was classed with insanity, blindness and deafness as an 'infirmity' – not a disease.[26]

It doesn't require a great deal of imagination to see that if you treat a person as a suitable case for charity or, worse, as an offender, that person will behave accordingly. Individual sufferers who were aware of what the early symptoms of leprosy – seemingly harmless patches of numbness and discoloration of skin – portended would conceal them for as long as possible; when unsightly ulcers developed and concealment ceased to be an option, they'd generally be ejected from their community, would lose employment, husband or wife and family; then they had no alternative but to seek refuge in an asylum, or leprosarium, thus acknowledging others' discrediting valuation of them, or to live as outcasts and beggars, importuning the very people who wished them out of sight. The literature of leprosy is replete with studies with titles such as 'Stigma and the Leprosy Phenomenon: The Social History of a Disease in the Nineteenth and Twentieth Centuries' and 'Learning to Be a Leper: A Case Study in the Social Construction of Illness'. In different societies, leprosy patients might react in different ways, some passively, some aggressively, but a common factor is the stigmatisation of their disease.

To define leprosy as 'a chronic infectious disease which attacks the skin, peripheral nerves and mucous membranes (eyes, respiratory tract)'[27] is to disregard not just the fact that throughout its history it has been a social as well as a physical disease but also that its *sui generis* characteristics, such as 'its low toxicity, its long latent period, its insidious onset and long duration'[28] continue to puzzle medical scientists. Though *Mycobacterium leprae* was among the first bacilli to be discovered (in 1873 by a Norwegian, Gerhard Henrik Armauer Hansen), another century would pass before it was successfully transmitted to an experimental animal (in this case, the nine-banded armadillo) and it has yet to be cultivated *in vitro*. There is no vaccine specific to leprosy and its exact mode of transmission remains a mystery. As early as 1906 an eminent English surgeon, Jonathan Hutchinson, was writing:

> The problem of leprosy is not for the idle-minded. It is full of intricacy and difficulty . . . However repulsive the disease itself in some of its phases may be, there is nothing whatever of that nature about its study. It is a sort of aristocrat among diseases . . .[29]

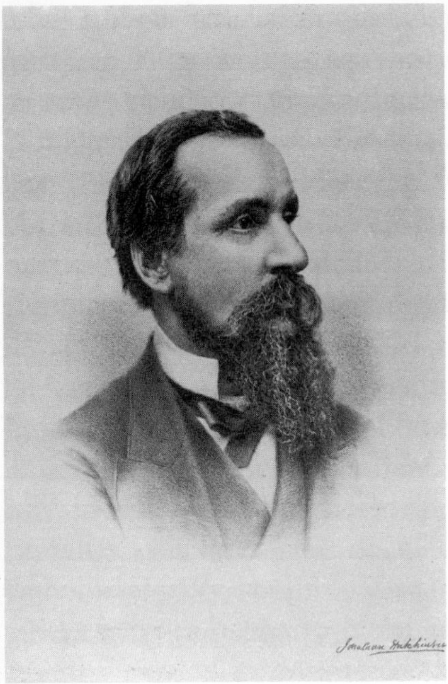

(Wellcome Library, London)

Sir Jonathan Hutchinson – lithograph

On the Indian subcontinent one of its names is *Maha rog*, the Great disease. It is an awe-inspiring disease, which has yet to yield up many of its secrets.

So how do you contract leprosy? Despite the myths that still abound, you do not get it by sharing food or drink, or by shaking hands with an infectious leprosy patient; it is not spread by touch; *M. leprae* doesn't seem to have the enzymes it would need to penetrate intact skin, though it's possible it can enter abraded or broken skin. It is a very hardy micro-organism and experiments have shown it can survive in the dust of India for up to five months. What seems to happen is that untreated leprosy sufferers cough and sneeze the bacteria into the environment and other, unsuspecting people breathe them in; they settle on the lining of the nose and enter the body via the nasal mucosa. That's when the body's immune response kicks in and either protects it from the bacilli or allows them to spread and settle in the skin and nerves, causing one or other form of the disease.[30]

Leprosy is notoriously difficult to diagnose in its early stages. Its onset is insidious, it mimics a whole range of other, unrelated skin diseases and presents itself in so many different ways – 'ranging from a small solitary hazy macule to widespread multiple shiny nodules'[31] – that it's hard to believe that they can all be the product of a single micro-organism. The nature of the immune response (cell-mediated immunity) to the incursion of *M. leprae* determines not only whether or not an individual gets the disease, but also what type of leprosy is involved. If the immune system goes into overdrive to repel the microscopic invader, the resulting infirmity is called tuberculoid, or paucibacillary (PB), leprosy; if, on the other hand, it offers nugatory or no defence at all, the result will be lepromatous, or multibacillary (MB), leprosy. These are the two ends of the spectrum; in the middle there is borderline leprosy which, if left untreated, may develop into lepromatous leprosy.

From both the individual's and the public health point of view, a diagnosis of tuberculoid leprosy is the 'least worst' option. It is regarded as 'relatively benign' in the sense that it produces few bacteria (hence 'paucibacillary') in comparison with 'multibacillary' lepromatous leprosy and is therefore less infectious, or even noninfectious – though nerve damage can still be severe if it's allowed to run its course. For reasons that are probably genetic but have yet to be fully understood, Indians and Africans tend to get the tuberculoid form of leprosy, while Europeans, Anglo-Indians, Parsees, Burmese, Chinese and Japanese are more prone to the lepromatous type.[32]

The initial diagnosis will often be of 'indeterminate leprosy', which may either develop into one or other of the 'determinate' types (PB, borderline or MB) or be 'self-limiting' – i.e., heal spontaneously without recourse to drugs, as may also happen in some cases of tuberculoid leprosy. Signs of indeterminate leprosy may be hard to detect, usually amounting to one or more discoloured but 'symptomless' (non-itchy) patches of skin. Since sensation in these patches may be unimpaired and the peripheral nerves normal, there is nothing to distinguish this from many other possible, and harmless, skin diseases. The only way to be sure it is leprosy is to keep a watching brief and perhaps perform a skin biopsy. It is curious how a disease that in its advanced stages is so grotesquely noticeable is in its initial phases so difficult to discover. Yet early diagnosis is vital if irreversible nerve damage is to be avoided. By the time the three 'cardinal signs' – sensory impairment, enlargement of peripheral nerves and evidence of *M. leprae* bacilli – are apparent, the process is already under way.[33]

'Once a leper, always a leper' – a dreadful truism a hundred years ago – mercifully no longer applies. The most important drug used in the treatment of leprosy is also the cheapest – the sulphone known as dapsone or DDS, an expensive derivative of which, Promin, was first used at Carville (intravenously) in 1941. Dr Robert Cochrane in India was the first to use dapsone itself in 1946; he experimented with it in an (intramuscularly) injectable form. The first doctor to try it out in an oral form was John Lowe in Nigeria in 1947.[34] Dapsone kills dividing bacteria and so reduces the overall load. It also reduces the inflammation and redness of existing skin lesions and prevents new ones appearing.

Where the skin has been thick and heavily infiltrated with bacilli it becomes much softer; favoured sites for the bacteria such as earlobes shrink dramatically, the swelling being replaced by fine wrinkling of the skin. Dapsone also reduces the bacterial load in the eyes and noses of patients with lepromatous leprosy.[35]

Today it is one of the three drugs that constitute multiple drug therapy (MDT) promoted by the World Health Organization. The second is rifampicin, which – in contrast to dapsone, a bacteriostatic (or weakly bactericidal) drug – is strongly bactericidal: 'A single dose as low as 600mg will kill the great majority (99.9%) of leprosy bacilli within a few days, so rendering the patient with multibacillary leprosy non-infectious.'[36] The third, clofazimine, is another bacteriostatic drug like dapsone and is also anti-inflammatory. The British leprologist Dr Diana Lockwood admits, 'We don't know how it works.'[37] But it is particularly useful in the treatment of ENL (erythema nodosum leprosum) reactions in patients with lepromatous leprosy.

There are two types of reaction. Type 1, known as reversal reaction, is confined to skin and nerves and is to do with cell-mediated immunity; it causes painful neuritis and is treated with steroids. (In paucibacillary patients, reversal reactions are almost indistinguishable from relapses; often the only way a doctor can tell the difference is to prescribe steroids and see what happens: if they work, it's a reaction; if they don't, it's a relapse![38]) Type 2, or ENL, reactions are caused by the antigens and antibodies coming up against each other and can affect everything including the eyes. Thalidomide, despite its scary reputation, has proved an effective drug in controlling ENL reactions. Both sorts of reaction are acute episodes that may occur in all types of leprosy before, during and after MDT. Skin lesions and nerves become inflamed and tender: 'Acute neuritis may cripple patients with borderline leprosy overnight, while acute iritis may rapidly result in blindness.'[39] Because they are painful episodes in a disease characterised by painlessness, or insensitivity, reactions are often what makes a patient seek medical help in the first place.

In the nineteenth century the medical debate focused on whether leprosy was hereditary or contagious, a debate which even Hansen's discovery of the bacillus failed to settle completely. Sceptics such as Jonathan Hutchinson conceded that Hansen's bacillus might 'be counted as the

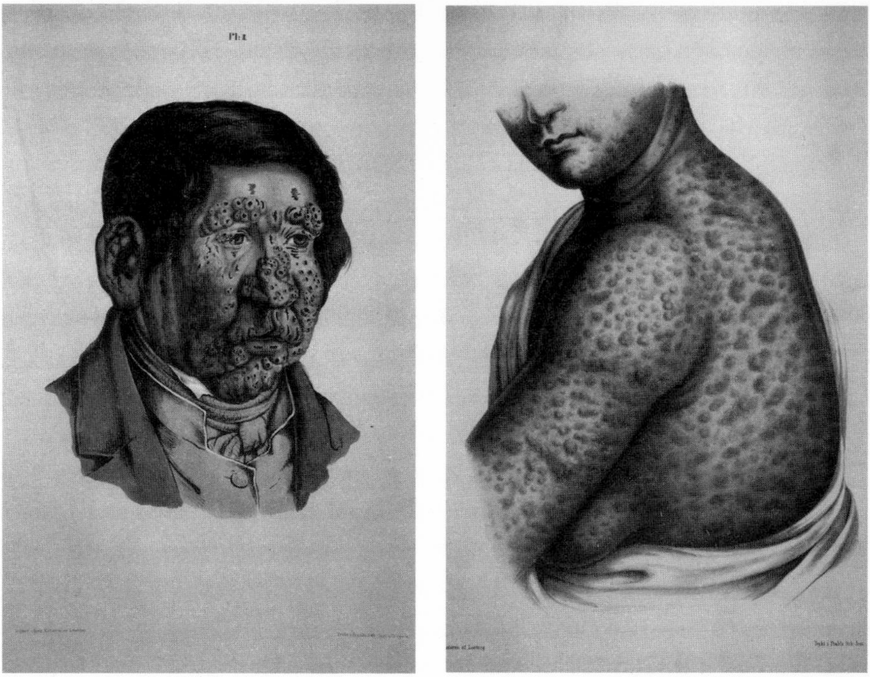

(Wellcome Library, London)

Illustrations from Danielssen & Boeck's *Atlas of Leprosy*, 1848

cause of leprosy', but did not consider that ended the argument: 'The question remains, what is the cause of the bacillus, and how does it gain access?'[40] From the leprosy patients' point of view, this debate was anything but academic, for their fate depended upon its outcome: if it was decided that the disease was hereditary, and therefore no risk to public health, there was little to be gained by segregating them from the rest of society; but if the contagionists won the day, then the pressure to isolate them would become irresistible. From the scientific point of view, Norway made all the running, providing the chief protagonists for both camps in Daniel Cornelius Danielssen, the 'father of leprology', and his son-in-law Hansen, who challenged Danielssen's anti-contagionist position.

Hansen's discovery of the leprosy bacillus might be the most significant scientific event in relation to the disease in the nineteenth century, but in terms of public impact it paled beside the life and, more particularly, death of the Belgian Catholic missionary, Joseph de Veuster, better known as Father Damien. The fact that Damien arrived at the Hawaiian leprosy settlement on the island of Molokai in 1873, the same year that Hansen made his discovery, is a nice historical coincidence. But whereas Hansen remained largely unknown outside Norway and the medical community, Damien's sixteen-year struggle with the authorities, with the more recalcitrant members of his chosen congregation and with the disease that eventually claimed him, too, made him an international celebrity.

His example inspired other would-be martyrs and raised public awareness of leprosy throughout the world, particularly in Britain, whose empire contained many countries where leprosy was rife; and his death induced a measure of panic, since it seemed to offer conclusive proof that the disease was indeed contagious. Leprosy became an 'imperial danger'; with easier travel and the wholesale movement of peoples brought about by colonial activity the fear was that it would return to its old European haunts via the back door. For Britain the main focus of anxiety was India, 'the jewel in the crown', where the sheer number of people affected by leprosy made segregation financially impracticable, however desirable it might otherwise be.

While the government of British India temporised, doing little more than calling on the missionaries to help clear the streets of leprosy-affected beggars, the American authorities in Hawaii and then in the Philippines pursued the policy of segregation to its logical conclusion, hunting out everyone they suspected of having leprosy and despatching them to state-of-the-art leprosaria on remote island sites.

By the 1920s, however, the medical authorities in a number of countries had begun to doubt the efficacy of the policy of compulsory segregation. It was no coincidence that the practice of isolation fell out of favour as soon as there was a treatment that to begin with, at least, looked promising (chaulmoogra in an injectable form); or that the individual who did most to develop this treatment, Sir Leonard Rogers of the Indian Medical Service, should become the leading advocate of phasing out the leprosaria. His treatment was only effective if applied in the initial phases of the disease, but early cases were the hardest to find since the policy of segregation deterred people with leprosy from seeking treatment for fear of being ostracised. Rogers was not the first to argue that isolating advanced cases of leprosy in order to prevent contagion was equivalent to closing the stable door after the horse had bolted – Jonathan Hutchinson had made the same point at the turn of the century – but as the co-founder and driving force behind the British Empire Leprosy Relief

Association (BELRA) he had the means to get his message across to a wide constituency.

By the 1940s, when experimentation with the sulphone drugs that would render chaulmoogra obsolete began, there were already alternatives to leprosaria in many parts of the world, particularly in Africa, where BELRA's message had been heeded. Local clinics and resettlement villages provided a more open form of leprosy control than the now discredited policy of mandatory segregation. But the new treatment of choice, while it enabled many people with leprosy to live in their communities again, did not immediately do away with the need for asylums. During the second half of the twentieth century these institutions still housed a number of people whose leprosy was too far advanced for the sulphones to provide more than relief; these drugs could not reverse the damage already done. In addition, some inmates had over the years become too institutionalised to be able to cope with living in an open society where prejudice against them was still strong. So the better institutions changed with the times and became places of refuge rather than incarceration. Leprosy patients had struggled so long for freedom; now, in the era of multiple drug therapy and the 'horizontal' – as opposed to 'vertical' – model of health care, they have achieved it, but at a cost. The danger they now face is neglect.

The attempt to secularise leprosy and bring it into the medical fold, to change its status from 'a disease apart' to 'a disease like any other', has been so successful that specialists in the field now worry that their patients' needs will be ignored, since their disease is neither life-threatening nor acute. In recent years, the World Health Organization has campaigned intensively to eliminate leprosy and, while such campaigns are valuable for the focus they bring to a disease and the funds they provide for its treatment, for those very reasons they cannot be maintained indefinitely. The WHO's latest deadline for achieving 'elimination' (the inverted commas are necessary because in WHO-speak elimination means less than 1 case per 10,000 population in all endemic countries) is the year 2005. Since nobody believes that leprosy will be eradicated by the end of this year – the signs are that it will not even be 'eliminated', except by statistical sleight of hand – the question concerning leprosy workers is: what now?

This book spans nearly two centuries of the history of leprosy. It cannot claim to be comprehensive: many events, even countries where leprosy has been rife, are omitted or mentioned only in passing. The literature on the subject is vast and I've had to be highly selective to avoid making the book as unpalatable as chaulmoogra oil. My approach has been biographical, to tell the story as far as possible through the lives of individual men and women – doctors, missionaries and, above all, patients. This has been a rewarding experience, since many of these lives are so extraordinary; none more so than that of Stanley Stein, the Jewish pharmacist from Texas whom leprosy transformed into a campaigning editor and writer of such courage and persistence that at times he, like David in the Bible, took on the Goliath of the US Public Health Service almost single-handedly – and won.

Then there is Peter Greave, a refugee from riot-torn, post-war and post-Partition Calcutta whose arrival in England was heralded by the *News of the World* with the headline 'Leper at Large on Liner'; he survived this notoriety and became a writer and broadcaster, whose last book, *The Seventh Gate* – about his unconventional childhood and youth in India, terminated by leprosy – is a minor masterpiece.

Among the missionaries and doctors, Paul Brand, who also had an Indian childhood, stands out for his originality, inventiveness and imaginative sympathy; he too (with his co-author, Philip Yancey) wrote a memorable book, but of a very different kind, called *Pain: The Gift Nobody Wants*. And for sheer strangeness the story of the late nineteenth-century nurse, Kate Marsden, takes some beating: her mission of mercy took her across Russia 'on sledge and horseback' (as she entitled her account of it) into the depths of the Siberian forest; on her return she was fêted by Russian and British royalty and honoured by the Royal Geographical Society, only to have the rest of her – long – life undermined by innuendo, suspicion and penury.

A NOTE ON NOMENCLATURE: With apologies to the ghost of Stanley Stein (and to his heirs on the *Star*), I can't go along with his campaign to outlaw the name 'leprosy' and substitute the morally neutral 'Hansen's disease', though I am at one with him about the other, and much more odious L-word, *leper*. The latter inevitably crops up frequently in historical, and even contemporary, writings and cannot be avoided in quotations. If, for one reason or another, I have felt obliged to use it in the body of the text, I have quarantined it like a computer virus by putting it in inverted commas. It is a word whose metaphorical use and pejorative meaning have so far overtaken its original application that it's now impossible to use it of a person with leprosy without giving offence. This does not seem to me the case with the word *leprosy*, which, being the name of the disease rather than the afflicted person, remains *im*personal, though it, too, can be used metaphorically in a pejorative sense. I know that in some countries – Brazil, for example – the stigma attached to both was so great that it was found necessary to change both. But a change of name does not necessarily bring about a change in public attitude, and once it becomes known that Hansen's disease is what used to be called leprosy the same old prejudices attach themselves to the new name. I have nothing against *Hansen's disease* as a name and have used it more or less interchangeably with *leprosy* in describing, say, Carville, in modern times, but because by no means everyone knows what it is I have for the most part stuck with leprosy.

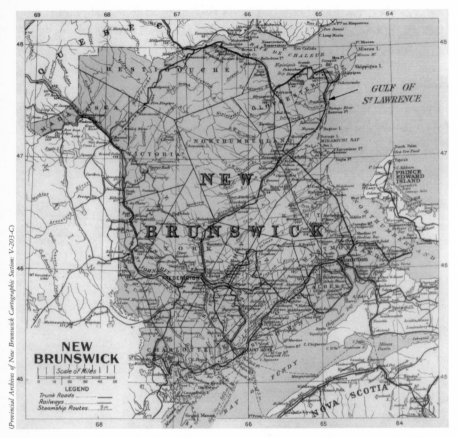

(Provincial Archives of New Brunswick Cartographic Section: V-203-C)

The Province of New Brunswick, Canada, c. 1915 –
arrow marks the coastal village of Tracadie

Chapter 1

A NEW DISEASE IN NEW BRUNSWICK

Leprosy is generally categorised as a tropical disease. But this is one of the many misconceptions about this most mysterious of maladies. Though a map showing the prevalence of leprosy in the world today would be overwhelmingly equatorial, in the mid-nineteenth century one of the main focal points of the disease was coastal Norway. Another was New Brunswick in Canada, where our story begins.

At about the time when the armies of Napoleon and Wellington were confronting one another for the final showdown at Waterloo, on the other side of the Atlantic in the English-sounding counties of Gloucester and Northumberland – where the vast majority of the inhabitants were French – two women, Ursule Benoit and Mary Gardiner, presented the first, ominous signs of an unrecognised disease. By the time of their deaths, in 1828 and 1829 respectively, or shortly after, it had spread to many of their intimates and been identified as leprosy. Joseph Benoit, the husband of the deceased Ursule, as well as her two sisters, Isabelle and Françoise, and one of the pallbearers at her funeral, François Sonier (who claimed that he had been contaminated with fluid oozing out of the decomposing body of the corpse when the sharp edge of the coffin had cut into his shoulder[1]), had all developed the disease, as had two of the sons and a friend of the family with whom Mary Gardiner had lodged.

The communities of northern New Brunswick, such as Tracadie and its neighbours – whence nearly all the early victims came, from five interconnected families – were unflatteringly described in a local doctor's reply to a leprosy questionnaire circulated by the Royal College of Physicians in London in the 1860s:

> The disease is entirely confined to the poor, who live in rude log huts, hardly sufficient to protect themselves from the inclemency of the weather. Usually there is but one room, which is occupied by pigs, poultry, &c., as well as by the family. They are poorly clad, and all around them betokens the most abject poverty. Their habits are indolent, improvident, and extremely unclean. In the winter months their diet consists solely of salt herrings, salt and dried codfish, and potatoes, at times salt pork; in summer they live on fresh fish; they have very little bread. They are chiefly employed in fishing, farming, and lumbering.[2]

Social problems, as a more recent writer puts it, were 'washed away with a generous dose of Jamaica rum'.[3] There were no amenities for the sufferers, whose sickness provoked alarm rather than pity among their neighbours. According to the Provincial Grand Jury:

> The people . . . generally shun the afflicted and have hitherto been in the habit of confining, in some instances, the Leper in a log enclosure constructed for the purpose and handing his food to him through an opening in the logs until he can no longer receive it when of course he dies. A practice most revolting to humanity and discreditable to the country in which it is permitted.[4]

By the mid-1840s the disease, as well as the alarm, had spread sufficiently to demand action on the part of the authorities. Appeals from the local doctor and priest prompted the Lieutenant Governor of New Brunswick, Sir William Colebrooke, to recommend that 'provision should be made for the due care of sufferers, and with a view to prevent the spread of this distemper'.[5] A commission of investigation (the first of many), consisting of three doctors and the local priest, traced the two dozen or so cases they found back to a single source, Ursule Benoit; but they could not say how she had acquired the disease.

No country or people likes to assume responsibility for an outbreak of disease – particularly a disease as 'frightful and loathsome' as leprosy[6] – so the possibility that it may be home grown has to be dismissed and other explanations sought. The trick is to focus on individual immigrants (in this case, hypothetical escapees from lazarettos in Trinidad or Norway), or racial groups thought to be especially susceptible to the malady: in the late nineteenth century on the west coast of the United States, in

Hawaii and the south Pacific, as well as in south-east Asia and Australia, the Chinese fitted this bill to perfection. If there are no obvious candidates for blame, then another scenario is fleeting contact with an alien source of contamination. So here the story got about that Ursule had contracted the disease as a result of washing the clothes of infected sailors belonging to a Mediterranean ship. But Ursule's aged mother, when she was interviewed in the later 1840s, denied that any of the sailors her daughter had befriended had had leprosy. It was also surmised that the disease had been imported from the French West Indies, which sent emigrants to Canada, or even from the Normandy district of France itself, where immigrants had been coming from since the end of the seventeenth century.

The commission identified the New Brunswick disease as Greek elephantiasis, 'the contagious "Leprosy of the Middle Ages"', and recommended a suitably 'medieval' solution to the problem – the erection of a lazaretto and the strict seclusion of all those affected with leprosy within its confines.[7]

In April 1844 the newly formed Board of Health, the first of its kind in the province of New Brunswick, acquired the location for a lazaretto at a peppercorn rent; this was the abandoned island of Sheldrake in the mouth of the Miramichi River, not far from the town of Chatham. The island had been a quarantine station housing cholera victims as late as 1832, and the old quarantine sheds were still standing, though in a dilapidated state.[8] Minimal repairs were undertaken and the priest at Tracadie, Father Lafrance, backed by Dr Alexander Key, set about convincing the afflicted members of his flock of the advantages to be had from allowing themselves to be removed to Sheldrake Island – comfortable accommodation, medical treatment, spiritual succour and, from time to time, family visits. He represented it as a place of refuge rather than imprisonment.

The reality was very different. The accommodation was basic: a kind of barracks divided into two dormitories, one for males and the other females, with no consideration of differences in age or severity of affliction; the rooms were dark and airless; the beds were wooden planks covered with palliasses and there was only one blanket per person; the washhouse was in a separate building and the latrines outside. The majority of leprosy sufferers had not been persuaded to leave their families and had either concealed their affliction or hidden from the authorities who sought to remove them to Sheldrake. But those who did go along – just over thirty in all – reacted angrily when they discovered what awaited them. Apart from the lack of amenities, there was no treatment worthy of the name and visits from the doctor and priest were few and far between.[9] The only staff on the island were a man and his wife who had been hired to act as caretakers. The newcomers found they were expected to work – the women at domestic tasks such as cooking and cleaning, and the men on the land, cultivating crops or cutting down trees. From the start they refused to co-operate, spurning the pittance offered in return for their labour.

As far as the authorities were concerned, they were obstructive and ungrateful for all that was being done for them on the island. For the inmates themselves – exiled from their homes and families and everything they held dear – there was only misery and more misery in 'that dreadful pest-house'.[10] The ones who accepted their fate became lethargic, dispirited and depressed; they neglected to look after themselves and ceased to care whether they lived or died. The more rebellious among them, however, concentrated on escape, turning logs into makeshift rafts in an effort to reach the mainland. At least one is believed to have died in the attempt.

The authorities condemned these escapes, or 'desertions' as they preferred to call them.[11] The Board would send one of its members, accompanied by a constable, to apprehend those on the run, and this proved costly in time and money. They might succeed in catching one fugitive but the others would disperse into the depths of the forest, where they would remain hidden until they got word that the search party had moved on. Bernard Savoy was one of the unlucky ones: he was at home when the Board member and constable came. They trussed him up and were about to take him away when his father intervened, so they threatened the older man with a pistol.[12] Not only had leprosy become a criminal offence, it seems; harbouring a 'leper', even if he were your own flesh and blood, amounted to aiding and abetting.

In February 1845, George Kerr, secretary-treasurer of the Board of Health, admitted in a report to the provincial government, 'There have been frequent desertions from the island', and sought the authority to lock up the offenders or punish them in some other way for their 'improper conduct'.[13] Kerr conveniently overlooked the fact that it was the action of the Board of Health in ostracising them in the first place that was responsible for transforming law-abiding if stricken individuals into outlaws. It was a vicious circle. The House of Assembly inevitably gave the Board of Health the further powers it requested, and the inmates of Sheldrake were no longer allowed to wander about the island as they pleased, but were confined to the main building of the lazaretto and only let out for exercise at specified times. Armed guards were employed to prevent further escapes, and visitors were not allowed on the island without the written permission of a Board member.[14] If it had not been a penitentiary from the beginning, Sheldrake was fast becoming one.

One night in the middle of October 1845, even before the new regulations had come into force, the lazaretto was destroyed by fire. Despite the hour of the blaze, between four and five in the morning, all the inmates managed to escape along with their meagre bedding and clothes, so there was no doubt who'd started it. This act of arson prompted a yet more draconian response from the authorities. A new building that was cheaper to heat went up in November; the yard was surrounded by a high picket fence and at night the gate was locked to prevent escape. As Drs Robert Bayard and William Wilson, two New Brunswick doctors who opposed the Board of Health's policy of locking up the afflicted, wrote in 1847: 'The building is not well suited for the purposes of a hospital.'[15] But by this time all pretence that Sheldrake Island was any kind of refuge for sufferers from leprosy had been abandoned.

Unlike Dr Key, who believed that leprosy was contagious, Bayard and Wilson thought it was hereditary. In their 1848 report, they recommended as an alternative to the lazaretto that victims of the disease be maintained at home, as there was no likelihood of infection and families often became destitute when the breadwinner was sent away. (But being hereditarians they also recommended as a prophylactic measure that intermarriage in families where it prevailed should be forbidden; quite how this was to be achieved without preventive detention is hard to imagine.) For his part Dr Key did not deny that there might be a hereditary factor that predisposed certain people to get leprosy, but he argued that the fact that the disease ran in families was hardly conclusive evidence of heredity, the close proximity of the afflicted being far more suggestive of contagion.[16]

A measure of the provincial government's uncertainty over how to handle the problem was the number of commissions of investigation held between 1844 and 1858. There were no less than nine in just fourteen years, six of them taking place in the critical three years between 1848 and 1851, when the failure of Sheldrake either to provide protection for the healthy community or to alleviate the sufferings of the afflicted was recognised. But in the face of conflicting medical advice the provincial authorities did nothing – until Father Lafrance successfully petitioned on behalf of his parishioners to have the lazaretto relocated at Tracadie, 'within sight of their Chapel and within hearing of its Bell', and a new Board of Health was created to run it.[17]

Tracadie was home to the patients, and when the new lazaretto opened in September 1849 they were glad to find a bigger and airier building and better facilities than had been provided on Sheldrake Island. The new Board of Health was intent on pursuing a more liberal policy than its predecessor and allowed frequent visits from family and friends, so to begin with all went well. Hopes soared among the patients when Father Lafrance introduced an ex-surgeon of the French navy, Dr Charles La Billois, into the lazaretto. La Billois's first impressions were unpromising:

> I must frankly state that I never saw a spectacle more calculated to harrow the feelings of humanity. The stench was so intolerable from putrefaction, that it required the greatest determination even to undertake the treatment of the unfortunate so situated, and so far advanced in the disease . . .[18]

But during his relatively brief, unauthorised spell there, La Billois became extremely popular with patients and their families alike; not only did he talk confidently of curing the disease, he also took a personal interest in the afflicted. It is true, he treated leprosy as though it were 'inveterate syphilis' (a common misapprehension in those days, as we shall see); but that did not deter the patients or prevent other sufferers in search of a cure from volunteering, for the first time ever, to enter the lazaretto.

Treatment with mercury, whatever it did for syphilis, had an adverse effect on leprosy, as Dr Key had earlier discovered when a patient died under his ministrations. But hope itself can do wonders, at least in the short run, and La Billois's confidence rubbed off on his patients, who felt better for having him around. Unfortunately, the good doctor overreached himself, claiming unlikely cures. Exposure inevitably followed: it turned out that La Billois had been admitting people with negative symptoms in order to release them again as cured. To the distress of his devoted patients, this 'self-styled miracle worker' was dismissed in 1852 and the government added insult to injury by refusing to pay him for his services.[19]

For this and other reasons, the honeymoon period at Tracadie did not last. Family visits made the inmates restless, and the proximity to home had encouraged another round of escapes; on top of which, visitors had taken advantage of the more lenient regime to indulge in petty pilfering. The Board of Health cracked down: a new twelve-foot fence was erected. The inmates threw stones at the workers who were sealing them off from the outside world; and the authorities brought in guards to protect the workers. Visits were severely curtailed: to twice a year instead of once a month. Special dispensations to visit at any other time required the written authority of the priest. One patient, incensed by the lack of access to his children, protested bitterly and demanded the dismissal of the caretaker, who, he maintained, had 'insulted' his children and treated them 'like criminals'.[20]

Once again the inmates resorted to arson. In the early hours of 5 September 1852 the lazaretto was razed to the ground. Instead of building a new one immediately, the authorities herded the inmates into what had previously served as a jail. Cramped into a suffocatingly small space, no less than eight of the thirty-eight inmates died that winter, a higher than usual rate of mortality. And when the new building went up the following summer, iron bars over the windows made the intentions of the Board of Health plain for all to see. They put spikes on top of the fence, too, and the inmates were locked up every night as soon as darkness descended.

Father Gauvreau, who had replaced Father Lafrance as priest and also served on the Board of Health, acted as liaison officer between the authorities and the patients during the 1850s. In person he was unimpressive, being short and podgy, but he did what he could for his charges, whose situation was now so bad that on one occasion he had to step over a corpse left on the floor to reach a dying girl to whom he'd been summoned to administer last rites.[21] Throughout this grim decade, while the lazaretto stagnated, Father Gauvreau repeatedly petitioned the government to appoint a resident physician (there was a 'visiting physician', but he lived some seventy miles away and might as well have been on another planet). When the government continued to ignore him, the priest resigned from the Board of Health and went public with his story. In a series of articles published in two newspapers between May and July 1861, Gauvreau exposed the conditions at the lazaretto and succeeded with the pen where he had failed in person: the following March a resident physician was duly appointed.[22]

In the course of an official tour in the summer of 1862 the new Lieutenant Governor, Arthur H. Gordon, visited Tracadie. He described the lazaretto in a despatch he sent to the Duke of Newcastle, Secretary of State for the Colonies, in London the following April:

> Its situation is dreary in the extreme, and the view which it commands embraces no object calculated to please, or indeed to arrest the eye. On the one side is a shallow, turbid sea, which at the time of my visit was unenlivened by a single sail; on the other lies a monotonous stretch of bare, flat, cleared land, only relieved by the ugly church and mean wooden houses of a North American village.[23]

Gordon was moved by the plight of the people – particularly the younger people – forced to spend their entire lives in such surroundings:

> There is something almost appalling in the thought that from the time of his arrival until his death, a period of perhaps many long years, a man, though endowed with the capacities, the passions, and the desires of other men, is condemned to pass from youth to middle life to old age, with no society but that of his fellow sufferers, no employment, no amusement, no resource, with nothing to mark his hours but the arrival of some fresh victim, with nothing to do except watch his companions slowly dying round him. No provision seemed to be made to provide them with any occupation either bodily or mental, and under these circumstances I was not surprised to learn that in the later stages of the disease the mind generally became greatly enfeebled.[24]

So the newly appointed doctor, James Nicholson, could count on the support of the Lieutenant Governor in his attempts to raise the morale of the twenty-two patients he found at Tracadie. He removed some of the outward and visible signs of their incarceration, including most of the bars on the windows; he encouraged them to take exercise and he organised games for their physical and mental well-being; he even arranged for them to have a boat, in which they could go sailing and fishing. He regarded the building as 'well adapted for a hospital', though he referred to the twelve-foot-high picket fence disparagingly:

> This was deemed necessary at one time, to prevent the escape of the lepers during the night. Outside this fence is the keeper's house, in which their food is prepared; likewise a small prison for the confinement of the refractory. The whole is surrounded by a common fence inclosing an area of six acres, within which inclosure the patients may go about for exercise and amusement.[25]

Unfortunately, Dr Nicholson died within two years of arriving at Tracadie and in 1865 a protégé of his, Dr Alfred C. Smith, took up the post left vacant by his untimely death. For the next forty-four years (with one long gap), in various capacities, the aloof, paternalistic and – in the grand Victorian manner – eccentric Dr Smith presided over the

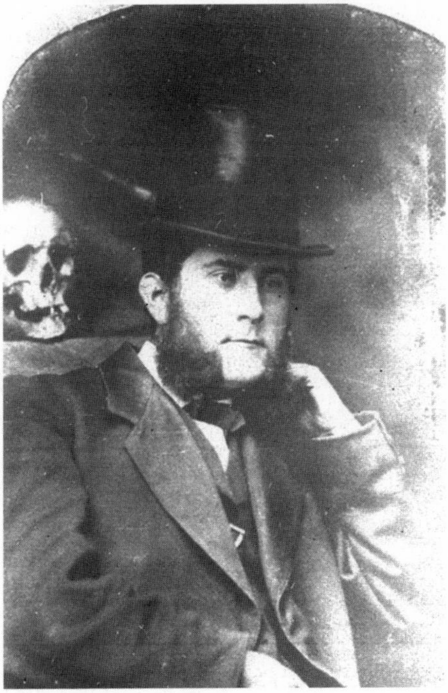

(Provincial Archives of New Brunswick, Nicholas Denys Historical Society Photographs – P20–262)

Dr Alfred C. Smith as a young man, with *memento mori*

lazaretto. (He had such an obsession with privacy that when he was practising medicine in the town of Newcastle in the 1870s, he put up a high fence to screen his movements between home and office from the public gaze,[26] so perhaps the enclosed world of the lazaretto suited some psychological need in him.) His passionate scientific engagement with the disease was never in doubt, but his distant manner with patients and ruthless enforcement of segregation did not immediately endear him to the inmates of Tracadie. He once confided in a letter to the American Dr Albert Ashmead, who held hysterical and racist views about leprosy, that the victims of the disease in New Brunswick were 'degenerated French' – a comment that Ashmead promptly published in an article in the *Journal of the American Medical Association*.[27] But by the time of his death in 1909, he had become a respected, even revered, father figure.

After little more than three years, Dr Smith's contract as resident physician was terminated – for reasons of economy. During his tenure, the temporal and spiritual authorities of New Brunswick had hit upon the idea of inviting a religious order of nursing sisters to run the lazaretto, a pattern that would be repeated over the years in many other parts of the world. The beauty of the idea, from the point of view of the authorities, was that it combined cheapness with efficiency: the nuns would provide a professional and devoted service at a low cost. Since there was no effective treatment for leprosy anyway, why bother with doctors when nurses could do all that was medically necessary and maintain order into the bargain?

In September 1868, the first seven sisters from the Roman Catholic order of Les Hospitalières de Saint-Joseph arrived from Montreal, ready to dedicate their lives to the care of the 'lepers'. Father Gauvreau described the 'abject misery' of the inmates immediately before the coming of the nuns: 'discord, revolt and insubordination toward the government, divisions and quarrels among themselves, made the history of their daily lives. The walls rang with horrible blasphemies, and the hospital seemed like a den of thieves.'[28] The sisters set to work with a will, cleaning up the place physically and morally. In the beginning they encountered resistance, especially when they enforced segregation of the sexes, which had become lax in recent times. But the losses in personal liberty experienced by the patients under the strict regime imposed by the nuns were offset by the gains in diet, regularity of meals, comfort and

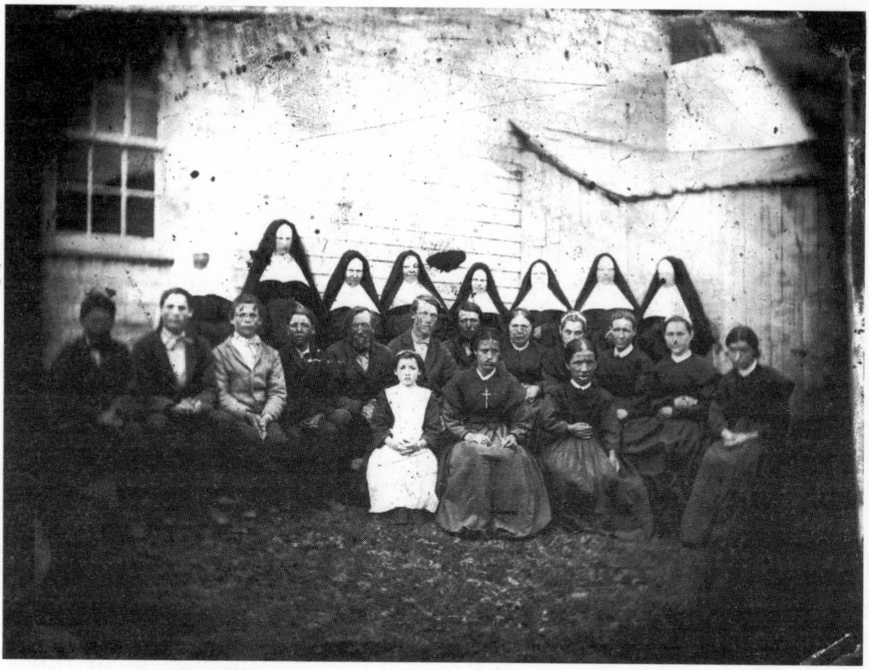

(Provincial Archives of New Brunswick, Tracadie Lazaretto Photographs – P67-3)

Sisters of the Order of Saint Joseph with their patients at Tracadie, c. 1890

cheerfulness of surroundings – one of the first things the sisters did was to cultivate a garden – the encouragement of recreation and the replacement of the atmosphere of a prison with that of a convent or monastery. There might be more regimentation under the sisters, but at least it was benign in intent.

Spiritually, the nuns had fertile soil in which to work. The patients' predicament as outcasts of society made them peculiarly susceptible to the consolations of religion: spurned by their fellow human beings, they could still see themselves as children of God and, given the extreme nature of their trials in this life, might justifiably look for some reward in the next. The young in particular responded to the religious instruction provided by the sisters, whose first Christmas at Tracadie was brightened by the number of patients – nine in all, most of them children – who received their first communion then.[29]

But what most of the patients clamoured for was effective treatment, a cure for their terrible and disfiguring disease, and here the sisters had no more success than the doctors before them, though one of their number, Soeur St Jean de Goto, came with a reputation for healing. She opened a pharmacy and tried out a number of remedies, but was disappointed to find – as many before and since have done – that seemingly miraculous recoveries were almost invariably followed by a return of the illness in an even more virulent form. However, it was not the lack of medical success, but the misdiagnosis of leprosy in certain cases that led to the recall of Dr Smith as 'consulting physician' in October 1878, almost a decade after he had been ousted as resident physician. At the same time it was made clear to him that he would have no authority within the lazaretto; the sisters remained very much in charge.[30]

Although Dr Smith forbore to come down on one side or the other of the heredity versus contagion debate – at least until the beginning of the twentieth century – he was a firm believer in segregation, and he and the sisters were united in their resolve to enforce it. Their aim was to achieve 'segregation without coercion',[31] but the methods adopted by the doctor when he went leprosy 'hunting', as he called it, were not without an element of coercion. 'When I declare an individual leprous,' he remarked, 'his nearest friends avoid him; he is refused employment, and he soon finds a resting place in the home for such unfortunates.' In other words, Dr Smith let it be known that a person had leprosy and popular prejudice did the rest. But he also had the power to reprieve those wrongly suspected of having the disease by certifying them free from leprosy.[32]

In 1889 the Canadian government gave him the grand title of 'Inspector of Leprosy for the Dominion' (but paid him a pittance). His tours of inspection inevitably aroused mixed feelings. He was subjected to verbal abuse and, on occasion, threatened with physical violence; he reported having had 'guns fired near me in a menacing manner'.[33] But nothing deterred Dr Smith from his appointed task and he could claim considerable success in carrying it out. In 1895, he was able to report of Tracadie, 'There is not one case of leprosy (outside the hospital) in this village. None have been admitted to the lazaretto from this parish for many years; newcomers are invariably from outlying districts.' In New Brunswick generally the disease was in decline – from thirty-seven known cases in 1853 to a mere twenty in 1897.[34]

Despite the decreasing need for it – and against Dr Smith's advice – the Canadian government enacted further repressive legislation in the early twentieth century. The disease continued to decline, though the

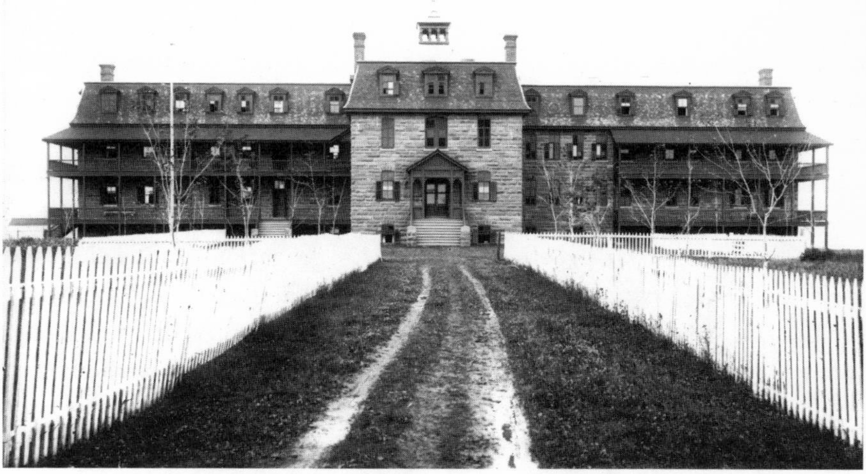

(Provincial Archives of New Brunswick, Ole Larsen Photographs – P6–43)

The rebuilt Tracadie Lazaretto in the 1890s

lazaretto in Tracadie, which had been rebuilt as an imposing stone structure in the 1890s, did not finally close until 1965.

If the treatment of people afflicted with leprosy in nineteenth-century New Brunswick harks back to the Middle Ages (or to the version of that period propagated in Victorian times), the attitude of the patients themselves, in one important respect at least, looks forward to the mid-twentieth century when the issue of stigmatising language became critical. An article on 'Les Lepreux de Tracadie' in *Le Moniteur Acadien* of 7 September 1882 noted that 'they are particularly sensitive to the word "leprosy" and we avoid using it within their hearing. They speak of the disease as "la maladie", the sickness.'[35] Stanley Stein and the staff of the *Star* would have approved of this early attack on the 'odious word'.

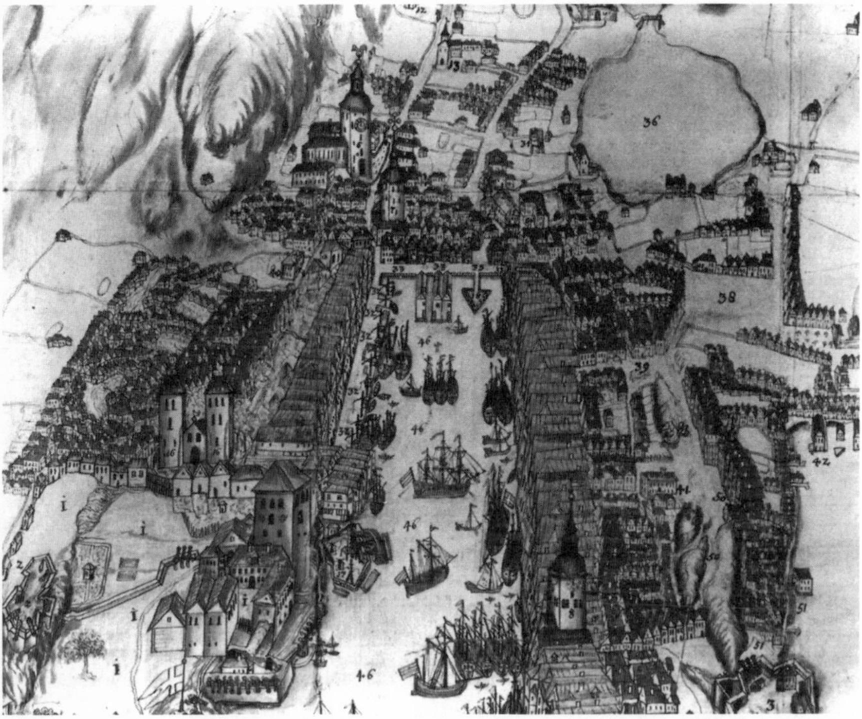

(Photography section, Bergen Museum)

Bergen in the 1740s –
St Jørgens Hospital is at the top of the map, marked No. 13

Chapter 2

THE FATHER OF LEPROLOGY – AND HIS SON-IN-LAW

Bergen, the oldest city in the Norwegian kingdom, has been called 'the cradle of modern leprology' and one of its native sons, the physician Daniel Cornelius Danielssen, 'the father of leprology'. With the help of his colleague from Christiania (Oslo), Carl Wilhelm Boeck, Danielssen became the first doctor to map out in a scientific way precisely what was, and what wasn't, leprosy. Their book *Om Spedalskhed (On Leprosy)* was first published in 1847, but it was the French translation, published in 1848, the year of revolutions in Europe, that brought about a revolution in thinking about leprosy and marks the beginning of the modern, scientific era in the approach to – and treatment of – this disease. Danielssen's son-in-law, Gerhard Henrik Armauer Hansen, has an even greater claim to fame as the discoverer of the leprosy bacillus, *Mycobacterium leprae*, in 1873. Both were part of the nineteenth-century artistic and scientific renaissance – whose cultural centre was Bergen, home of Ibsen, Greig (a close friend of Hansen), as well as the poet Bjornson and the explorer Nansen – that accompanied Norway's burgeoning nationalism and would culminate in complete independence from neighbouring Sweden in 1905.[1] And though they opposed one another on the critical question of whether leprosy was a hereditary or a contagious disease, Danielssen and Hansen were united in their determination to rid Norway of the affliction.

Leprosy in Norway, as in most of Europe, dates back to early medieval times. The predatory Vikings are said to have had a special fondness for Irish maidens and may have imported the disease along with their captive women. It is known to have been prevalent in Ireland as early as the tenth century and had probably taken root in Norway by the year 1000. By the beginning of the nineteenth century, when leprosy had died out in much of Europe, it lingered on in some of the remote fringes of the continent and was particularly rife in pockets along the west coast of Norway. At the start of the twentieth century, the English doctor Jonathan Hutchinson wrote that:

> the prevalence of leprosy in Norway during the last century, and probably for much longer, has been somewhat peculiar. It has been strictly limited . . . to the labouring part of the community; to the fishermen, boatmen and peasants. None of the middle-class inhabitants of Bergen or Trondhjem ever feared to contract the disease, although its victims sat about in their streets and sold their wares without restriction. . .[2]

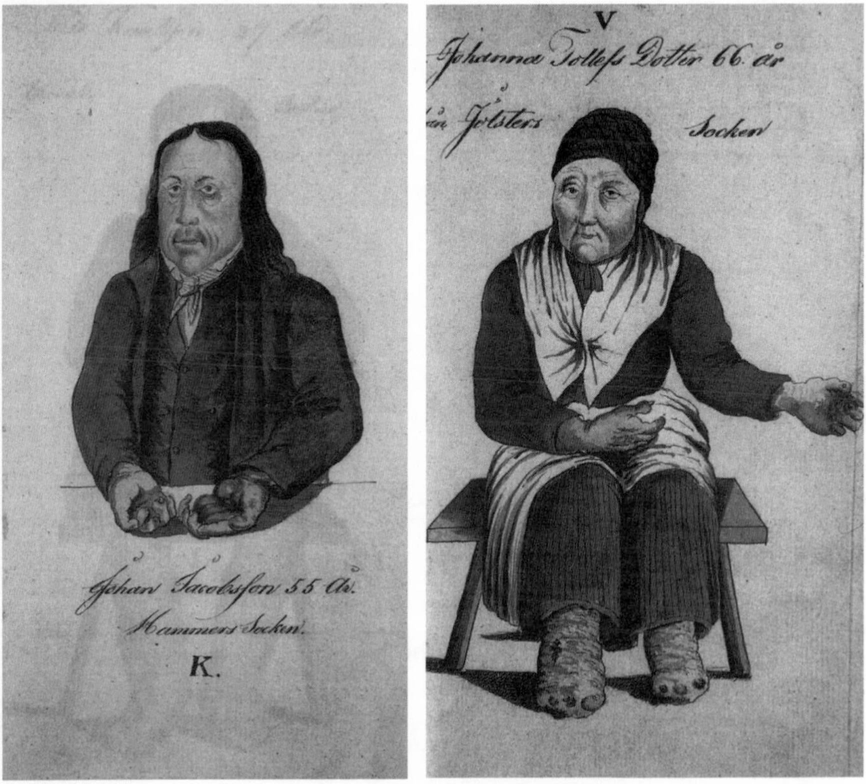

(The Hagströmer Medico-Historical Library, Swedish Society of Medicine – Karolinska Institutet, Stockholm)

Two denizens of St Jørgens in 1816:
a) Johan Jacobsen, aged 55 and b) Johanne Tollefsdotter, who had been admitted in 1780

St Jørgens (St George's) Hospital in Bergen housed about 150 sufferers. Conditions there were so appalling that in 1816 the pastor Johan Ernst Welhaven described it as 'a sort of graveyard for the living',[3] and drawings of several of the inmates were made with the intention of awakening the conscience of the medical authorities. A year later, St Jørgens did acquire a doctor, the first to be appointed to a leprosy hospital in Scandinavia. Up to that time the only recourse open to leprosy sufferers was to hope for a miracle. The more desperate among them might seek out an unscrupulous 'witch' such as Lucia Pytter who claimed she could cure the disease, as two girls from St Jørgens did in 1804. History does not record what sort of treatment they received at her hands, only that both were dead within a year.[4]

In 1832 Dr J.J. Hjort made a tour of leprosy districts in western Norway and wrote a report that drew attention to the terrible living conditions of people with leprosy and their lack of nursing care. (Surprisingly, he maintained that the disease was curable. Seventy years later, Dr H.P. Lie wrote, 'in the great majority of cases leprosy runs its regular course in spite of all treatment; but for my own part I have never seen any case in which I was convinced that the treatment had done harm. I must add, however, that neither have I seen many cases in which the treatment had been of any great use.'[5]) Representations of the plight of leprosy sufferers sparked off what one writer has called 'the great crusade against leprosy in Norway which lasted throughout the nineteenth century'.[6]

There were three strands to this crusade: epidemiological, pathological and clinical. From the epidemiological perspective, the first census aimed at discovering the extent of leprosy in Norway was undertaken in 1836, soon after Hjort's tour; another took place in 1845; but neither of these was particularly accurate: the first had been conducted by parish ministers and the second as part of a national census to determine population. It wasn't until 1852 that a census was carried out by medical officials. The district health officers then came up with 1,782 cases – or 11 per 10,000 of the population – a much higher figure than had previously been discovered. In 1854, a Chief Medical Officer (CMO) for Leprosy was appointed. Two years later, on 30 July 1856, a National Leprosy Registry was set up by royal decree – said to be the first of its kind to be created for a specific disease anywhere in the world – and local

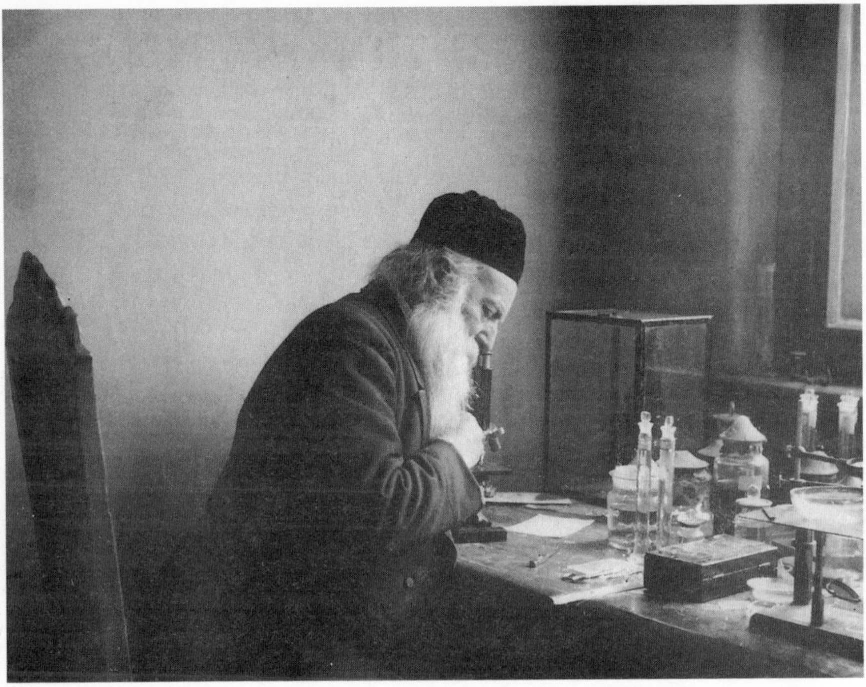
(The Leprosy Museum, St Jørgens Hospital, Bergen)

The 'father of leprology', Daniel Cornelius Danielssen, in old age

boards of health were established in leprosy districts.[7] The total number of cases registered that year was 2,858, over 20 per 10,000 of the population. And in the Bergen district the ratio was more than twelve times higher than that.[8] Dr O.G. Høegh, the first CMO for leprosy in Norway, regarded the data provided by the leprosy registry as evidence that the disease was spread by contagion.[9] This challenged the prevailing view, most firmly – not to say dogmatically – held by the father of leprology, D.C. Danielssen, himself.

From the pathological point of view, Danielssen was the pioneer. He was born in Bergen in 1815, the son of a watchmaker. To become a doctor he had to triumph over considerable adversity. His parents were poor and he became apprenticed to a pharmacist at the age of thirteen. When he was seventeen, he contracted tuberculosis of the hip; he was bedridden for a year and a half and for the rest of his life walked with a limp. But he persevered with his studies and in Christiania in 1832 distinguished himself by passing top in a medical exam (though this exam was pitched at a lower level than the standard medical degree). In 1839 he returned to Bergen, where he became a physician at St Jørgens

Hospital.[10] His work with his colleague C.W. Boeck, who had been awarded a travel grant to study leprosy in other parts of Europe, soon bore fruit. The publication of their joint productions, *On Leprosy* and the illustrated *Atlas of Leprosy*, in the prize-winning French edition of 1848 established its authors as *the* authorities on the disease. The German doyen of pathologists, the great Rudolf Virchow, described the work as 'the beginning of the biologic knowledge of leprosy'.[11]

Combining clinical studies with post-mortem findings, Danielssen and Boeck classified leprosy into two main types, the tubercular, or 'nodular', and the anaesthetic, or 'smooth' (these names are confusing, since over time they have more or less been reversed: we now call the anaesthetic, smooth type tuberculoid and the tubercular, nodular type lepromatous or, indeed, anaesthetic!). Though certain aspects of this typology have been disputed, it has stood the test of time and is still basic to the science of leprology. Their second significant contribution was on the transmission of leprosy. They argued that, for the most part, the disease was inherited, though it could on occasion occur 'spontaneously' – i.e., in some mysterious manner arise directly out of adverse living conditions. Danielssen several times inoculated himself and others with leprous matter to test the contagion thesis and, failing to transmit the disease in that way, concluded that, since it ran in families, it must be hereditary. A 'hereditary dyscrasia' was what he and Boeck called it.[12] (Webster's dictionary defines *dyscrasia* as 'an imbalance of physiologic or constitutional elements, especially of the blood', tracing its origin to the Greek, meaning 'mixture of the humours in bad proportion'. This conveys just the right combination of ancient and modern, of the archaic and the scientific, given that these Norwegian doctors were living and working on the threshold of the bacteriological revolution in medicine.)

The third aspect of the Norwegian leprosy crusade, the clinical, also owed much to Danielssen and Boeck. Their research reports in the early 1840s led to the foundation of a clinical and research centre for leprosy in Bergen, Lungegaard Hospital, which could accommodate ninety patients. A wooden building was completed in 1849, and Danielssen was appointed chief physician of the hospital, a post he held until his death in 1894. (On Christmas night 1853 it burned down – as a result of an accident, not arson in this case – and six patients and one member of staff died in the fire; it was rebuilt in stone.[13]) By 1861, three more leprosy hospitals had been built. An early foreign visitor, the British Surgeon-

Major Henry Vandyke Carter, a leprosy specialist from the Bombay Presidency in India, described these asylums in a report to the Under-Secretary of State for India in 1874:

> There are rules applying to the conduct of the inmates; the sexes are strictly separated; egress is permitted only at stated intervals, and so visits of friends; certain parts of their clothing are provided by the patients themselves; and inmates of both sexes are made to work at profitable or useful occupations. Their diet is doubtless better than their food at home: meat broth is allowed four days a week; fish is given three times; potatoes, bread, and farinaceous food; milk, tea, seldom ale. Milk and fish may be taken together . . .[14]

Carter was deeply impressed by 'the liberality of so enlightened a government as the Norwegian, which out of a revenue of about

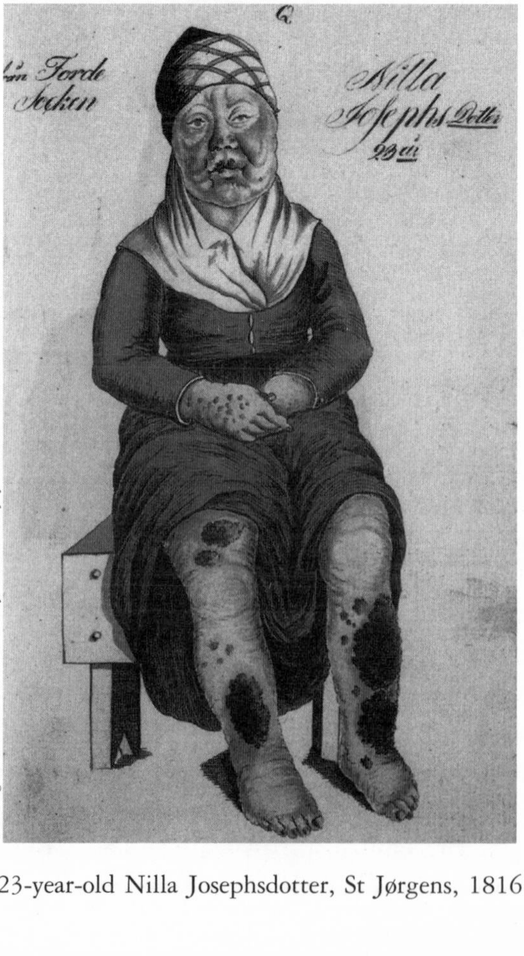

(The Hagströmer Medico-Historical Library, Swedish Society of Medicine – Karolinska Institutet, Stockholm)

23-year-old Nilla Josephsdotter, St Jørgens, 1816

1,000,000*l* expends, I suppose, near 20,000*l*, if not more, on the single object of ameliorating the condition of the leprous poor'.[15] You can almost hear him sighing: if only the government of British India were half so generous.

Between 1816, when the indignant Pastor Welhaven had characterised St Jørgens Hospital as a graveyard for the living, and 1861, when that hospital was but one of five devoted to leprosy, Norway had come a long way. As one modern scholar writes, it 'had already conducted four nationwide leprosy censuses, established a permanent leprosy registry, funded a research center for clinical study at Lungegaard Hospital . . . put into operation a national leprosy control scheme, and formulated an acceptable theory of the pathogenesis of the disease.' Not bad for 'a small, impoverished, but forward-looking country'.[16] And in 1861 Gerhard Henrik Armauer Hansen was not yet twenty-one, still in the early stages of his medical studies.

Armauer Hansen was the eighth child in a family of fifteen, ten of whom were boys. Part of his early childhood was spent in the idyllic surroundings of an estate belonging to his aunt and uncle on an island near Bergen. At the age of seven he returned to the mainland to go to a school where his father Claus was one of the teachers (this was in addition to Claus's other work as a businessman – wholesale merchant – and bank cashier, a job he had taken on in 1841, the year of Armauer's birth, perhaps as a consequence of having so many children). Though he was an apt pupil, Armauer's academic record at school was not outstanding; he enjoyed sport and took part in the rough-and-tumble of teenage gang life on the streets.[17]

When Claus's business collapsed and he was declared bankrupt in 1851, Armauer Hansen followed his elder brothers' example and earned a little money by giving Sunday school lessons and private tuition. In 1859 he went to the University of Christiania to study medicine. Over the next few years he supported himself in a variety of ways – as private tutor to a boy four years younger than himself whose parents were rich; as a teacher of natural sciences in a girls' school, where he was teased by the older girls for his habit of beginning sentences with the phrase 'Now then . . .'; and most satisfactorily as, first, prosector, then tutor of anatomy within the university itself.[18] Despite all these extra-curricular activities, he passed his medical exams with honours in the autumn of 1866 and, after a period of internship in Christiania, became physician to the fishing fleet at Lofoten, where he gained useful experience of the kind of patients he would get to know better when he turned to leprosy.

On 1 January 1868, Hansen was appointed physician at one of the new leprosy hospitals in Bergen. Towards the end of his life, he recalled his early experience there:

> I suffered terribly. I had never seen so much misery concentrated in one place. Gradually, though, as I commenced handling the patients, my aversion disappeared and was replaced by a great desire to learn the illness in detail. As I commenced *post mortems* my interest grew deeper. Pathological anatomy was my greatest interest in life and here I discovered many things about it I had never seen before. I suspected that some were entirely new to medical science. The result was that after a few months I eagerly looked forward to dealing with my ravaged patients.[19]

If, for the sake of convenience, doctors may be divided into those who practise the art of medicine and those who explore its scientific frontiers, this passage clearly shows into which category Hansen fell.

His biographer retails a story about the first meeting between the young Hansen and the fifty-three-year-old Daniel Cornelius Danielssen that he admits is 'perhaps too good to be true'. It is taken from an obituary written by Hansen's future brother-in-law, Professor Gerhard Gran, in 1912. The tyro was paying a duty visit to the sage and had only been in Danielssen's presence a few minutes when he blurted out '. . . and I may as well tell you that in my opinion your views on leprosy are altogether wrong. You think the disease is hereditary and not contagious, whereas the truth is that it is contagious and not hereditary.' A furious Danielssen promptly showed the young man the door. But the next day he called Hansen back and told him he'd been considering what he'd said and, while of course he was wrong, he should have every opportunity to follow his hunch. He, Danielssen, would make it his business to ensure that Hansen had a laboratory and all the books and equipment he needed to pursue his research.[20]

Like many an apocryphal or 'improved' tale, this one catches something of the essence of both men: Danielssen's fundamental shrewdness and generosity, which was to some extent masked by his bluster, a tendency to jump to conclusions – 'his only weakness', according to Hansen[21] – and dogmatic adherence to his own views; Hansen's con-

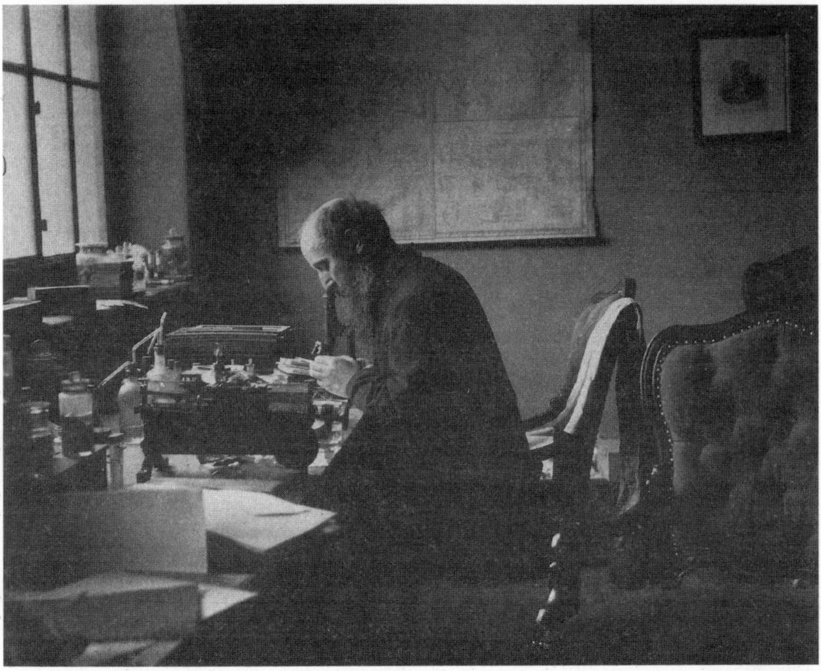

(The Leprosy Museum, St Jørgens Hospital, Bergen)

The discoverer of *M. leprae*, G. Armauer Hansen, in the 1880s

fidence in his own judgement and readiness to challenge even the highest authorities if he thought they were wrong. What it does not reveal about Hansen is his sense of rectitude – a favourite saying of his as a child was, 'Right is right' – and his phenomenal patience in pursuit of scientific goals.

His first scientific paper, for which he won a prize, was on lymph nodes. Like Danielssen before him, he observed in the lymph nodes of leprosy cases 'yellowish granular masses' which he also found in nodules in other organs affected by leprosy. In their book on leprosy, Danielssen and Boeck had called these 'brown bodies', and over the years Danielssen had come to regard them as specific to leprosy. But Rudolf Virchow, when he'd visited Bergen in 1859 and Danielssen had showed him his collection of diseased organs, had denied this, saying they might also be found in syphilis and lupus. Virchow had dismissed them as 'fat-degenerated cells' and Danielssen had meekly taken his word for it.

Hansen, when he came to look for the causative agent of the disease, was not prepared to bow to Virchow's or anyone else's authority and, examining these 'brown bodies' under the microscope, he perceived that they were not degenerated cells, but contained 'rod-shaped bodies' which might or might not turn out to be bacteria. He concluded that whatever these 'manifestations' were, they spoke to 'the specificity of leprosy'.[22] Thus, with proper scientific caution, Hansen described the first-ever sighting of *Mycobacterium leprae* almost a decade before the discovery of the tuberculosis bacillus (1882) and a decade or more before that of typhoid (1883), diphtheria and cholera (1884), and tetanus (1886).[23]

Hansen had every reason to be cautious. On the one hand, if his 'rod-shaped bodies' proved to be the causal agent of leprosy, then his finding would discredit the work of the man who, at the beginning of the year of his great discovery, 1873, had become his father-in-law (Hansen's marriage to the twenty-seven-year-old Stephanie, or 'Fanny', Danielssen, was sadly short-lived; Fanny died of pulmonary tuberculosis, an ailment to which the family was particularly prone, later that same year; and in 1875 Hansen married again, acquiring two step-children and fathering a son of his own[24]). On the other hand, in order to establish that the bacteria, if that was what they were, were indeed the cause of the disease, he had to satisfy Jacob Henle's principles of 1840 (which would become better known as 'Koch's postulates') that the micro-organisms should not only be present in all patients suffering from the disease, but should also be cultivable outside the human or animal organism – in other words, *in vitro* – and induce a similar disease in an inoculated animal.[25]

Well, it would be almost another hundred years before the American medical scientist Charles Shepard succeeded in inoculating mouse footpads with *M. leprae*, thereby enabling the experimentation with drugs that led to today's treatment of choice, MDT or multiple drug therapy, to happen; and even now there are only two other animals known to be susceptible to 'experimental' (i.e., artificially induced) leprosy, the nine-banded armadillo and the sooty mangabey monkey – neither exactly a household name. As for cultivating the bacillus in the test tube, we still await that breakthrough.

Another problem for Hansen was the inadequacy of available methods of staining the bacilli, the better to observe their pattern of activity. New staining methods were being developed in Germany, but Hansen had not succeeded in applying these. So he welcomed the arrival in Bergen of the young Albert Neisser, a pupil of Robert Koch, in 1879. Hansen showed Neisser his rod-shaped bodies, and together they tried to stain them in the latest German fashion – but without success. Hansen was happy to let

Neisser take away leprosy-infected material for further experimentation, but he was not so happy when Neisser, who on his return to Breslau had succeeded in staining the bacilli so that they could at last be clearly seen, published a paper in which, though he paid tribute to Hansen, he seemed to be putting himself forward as the real discoverer of the causative agent of leprosy. He said about Hansen that 'he does not seem to have been able to reach the conclusion that he had found the germ of leprosy'. Hansen lost no time in publishing a paper, in German and English as well as Norwegian, asserting his prior claim. This drew a huffy response from Neisser who, while conceding priority to Hansen, sought to belittle him in other ways, saying that he was ignored by his colleagues and mocked by Danielssen for his obsession with 'his bacteria'.[26]

Now Danielssen, too, was upset. When Hansen came to write his mostly unrevealing memoirs, he had achieved the recognition he deserved and could afford to recollect his earlier emotions in tranquillity. So he played down this spat with the excitable German (whose major claim to fame as a microbe hunter was his discovery of the causal agent of gonorrhoea), and wrote:

> I didn't think there was any particular hurry to publish my discovery since I felt there was still a great deal to be done before one could claim that the bacillus was definitely the origin of the disease. Not so Neisser. He published immediately, though honestly reporting what I had demonstrated to him. Unfortunately he also recorded a conversation with Danielssen in which my chief had asked him, 'ironically' – according to Neisser – if I had shown him my bacillus . . .
>
> Danielssen was absolutely furious, though, especially over Neisser's description of his attitude towards my bacillus. He told me off severely for my indolent concern over the matter since, in his opinion, there was a definite and deliberate attempt to steal my finding. Under the circumstances I felt it prudent to have my observations printed in a German publication . . .[27]

In fact, the sequence of events wasn't quite as Hansen chose to recall it in old age. Hansen had published his paper establishing his priority *before* Neisser, stung by the implication of theft to which Hansen has Danielssen allude, reported his conversation with the sceptical Danielssen in a second article in 1881. It's impossible to say if this was simply a case of failing memory or a deliberate attempt by Hansen to edit the record in order to minimise his own pique at Neisser's sharp practice and convey an impression of Olympian detachment suitable to a great scientist.

In his memoirs he passes in silence over another event from the same period of his life that reflects badly on him, and this time it can hardly have been unintentional.

Case No. 99/1880 was heard at the City of Bergen Law Courts on 31 May 1880 and concerned 'Legal Proceedings against Gerhard Henrik Armauer Hansen'.[28] Since Hansen is generally considered to have been a model of rectitude, how did he end up as defendant in a court of law at the age of thirty-eight and at the peak of his career, when he had already been Chief Medical Officer for Leprosy in Norway for five years?

This is the story the court was told. On 3 November 1879, Hansen sent for a thirty-three-year-old female patient suffering from the anaesthetic (i.e., tuberculoid) form of leprosy, who had been in the hospital where he was physician since she was sixteen. The woman, whose name was Kari Nielsdatter, found two other doctors waiting for her in Hansen's office; she took fright and burst into tears. Hansen called her up to the table where they were gathered, but when she caught sight of the sharp instrument he was about to apply to her eye she fended him off with one arm and raised the other to protect her face. Another doctor calmed her and persuaded her to sit down, so that the operation might continue.

This time Hansen succeeded in inoculating her eye with leprous material taken from a patient with nodular (lepromatous) leprosy. Nielsdatter claimed that she had been inoculated twice, once in each eye, but the doctors denied this. They also argued that, given the degree of insensitivity in her eye, she should not have suffered the sleep-disturbing pain she claimed she had experienced for the next seven weeks as a result of the inoculation. One of the doctors present, an ophthalmologist, 'was of the opinion that the operation is so harmless that it would not have caused any considerable amount of pain even in a healthy eye, but added that the pain might be aggravated in such a nervous and hysterical subject as the deponent, due to her imagination'.

While his colleagues gave him their full support, Hansen himself admitted that he 'was not justified in carrying out the operation as he had neither obtained her permission in advance, nor told her of his aim in doing it'. His explanation of why he had failed to do so was disarmingly frank. He told the court he could not 'presuppose that the patient would regard the experiment from the same point of view as I myself did'.[29] His aim had been to prove the infectiousness of the disease: if he had succeeded in inducing nodular leprosy in a patient suffering from the anaesthetic type of the disease, it would have been an important step forward in the scientific understanding of leprosy. As for the patient, since she'd had leprosy for many years, it was not as though she were being exposed to a new disease. In any case, Hansen was confident that, had the inoculation taken (which it did not), he could have removed the resulting nodule without difficulty, as he had done in several other cases where he had saved the patient's eyesight.

The Chief Magistrate, who'd brought the case against Hansen, had proposed a charge of occasioning actual bodily harm to an innocent party, since Hansen's stated aim had been to inflict on the patient 'a more malignant form' of leprosy than the one she already had. The case had been submitted to the Director-General of the Norwegian Health Directorate, who took the line that no further action was called for than 'to administer a severe reprimand to Hansen, who undertook the experiment in order to discover the answer to a question of the greatest importance in the interests not only of science and the nation, but also of the leprosy patient's own environment, and who, in my opinion, has already performed vital services in seeking the answer to this question'.[30] As far as the poor patient was concerned, the Director-General, in his eagerness to exonerate Hansen from all but token blame, resorted to sophistry, asserting that although she had not given her permission for the operation, she had not actively opposed it.

The case was regarded as such an important one that it was referred to the Ministry of Justice, which came up with a formula worthy of Solomon. Hansen, the judiciary argued, held two distinct posts: CMO for Leprosy and resident physician at the leprosy hospital. It was only in his capacity as a doctor that he could be said to have misbehaved. Therefore he should be dismissed from his hospital post while remaining CMO for Leprosy in Norway. Such a judgement may well be questioned, in that it is based on an artificial and ultimately unsustainable distinction, but it offered an eminently practical way out of a tricky legal situation; even the prosecutor advocated it and the court in Bergen was only too happy to accept it. Hansen forfeited his position as physician at the leprosy hospital and had to pay costs amounting to ninety kroner.

Hansen's defence, insofar as he offered one, was that earlier inoculations of a similar sort had been practised on patients without giving rise to complaints. Danielssen had inoculated hospital staff and patients, as well as himself, on more than one occasion, but he was protected by his popularity among patients, whereas they regarded Hansen with some suspicion – unsurprisingly, given his constant reiteration of the need to isolate them to minimise the danger of infection and his freely expressed opinion that 'one was oneself to blame' if one contracted leprosy. Even so, the case would never have got off the ground had it not been for the intervention of the pastor at the hospital, whose name was Grönvold. Without his support, Kari Nielsdatter might have complained till kingdom come without hope of redress. Patient rights did not feature in the medical ethics of that era and the reason Hansen was so ready to admit what he had done may have been that he did not feel he had done anything very wrong – except, perhaps, in not obtaining the patient's consent before he attempted to inoculate her. In his view – and that of many in his time, if not in ours – the end more than justified the means.

Since Hansen didn't record his feelings about the trial, there is a limit to how far we can carry our speculations. One thing is certain, however. It did nothing to soften his stance on the need to isolate leprosy patients. During his time as CMO for Leprosy, two important Acts were passed by the Norwegian parliament. The first, in May 1877, denied people with leprosy the right of *lagd*, the time-honoured Norwegian system of communal relief for the poor, which allowed them to wander from farm to farm, staying some weeks at each at the farmer's expense. Since leprosy sufferers were entitled to public assistance, it was argued, they must now either go into hospital or be isolated in one of the official homes for the poor; they were no longer permitted to lead the kind of vagrant existence that would promote the spread of their disease.[31] Perhaps because it only affected the very poor, the passage of this Act was not seriously opposed.

Eight years later, in May 1885, a second, stricter law was passed. This applied to all leprosy sufferers, not just the poor. If they did not want to be hospitalised they could be isolated at home provided they satisfied the health authorities that they represented no risk to other home dwellers; in practice this meant having a room of their own (married couples were permitted go on living together if that was their wish). If they did not, or could not, comply with the rules for home isolation the police could forcibly remove them to hospital. A number of doctors protested against 'this last drop in the cup of suffering of the leprosy patients'. Hansen was unmoved. As he recalled:

> There was an emotional outburst and strong opposition to this, the cry going up that such treatment of human beings was cruel; that it was a case of punishing them because they had an illness which either fate or the Almighty had wished on them. I maintained that healthy people must have the same humane treatment as the sick. If the fit found that the diseased could be a danger to them and consequently to the community as a whole, they had the right and duty to isolate them as long as it was done compassionately . . .[32]

The isolation of leprosy patients did not, of course, begin with Hansen. As he put it, 'I only happened to be fortunate enough to discover the cause [of the disease] and to prove that safeguards previous to my time had been correct and beneficial'. His 'accomplishment' was to have 'widen[ed] them on the strength of having found the starting place of the affliction'.[33] But in 1885 this 'starting place' was still disputed, and not just by Danielssen, who continued to doubt that the disease was infectious. The revered 'father of leprology' might be warmly regarded by the patients, but he had earlier proposed a far more draconian measure than any sponsored by his son-in-law: on the assumption that leprosy was hereditary and that the only way to control it was to prevent its victims from reproducing, he and Boeck had advocated a ban on marriage for all sufferers from the disease and their descendants 'in the first and second degree'. The permanent medical committee at the Ministry of the Interior had endorsed this proposal in 1851, but the Norwegian parliament refused to ratify it.[34] This was by no means the last attempt to prevent people with leprosy from marrying and having children, and the attitude of some governments would be considerably less enlightened than Norway's.

The outcry against the 1885 Act soon died down, mainly because it was humanely applied and people found they had little to fear. Only a proportion of leprosy sufferers were in hospital at any one time, and several of these were allowed to return home on leave, sometimes for weeks at a stretch. The Norwegian model of isolation did not mean being locked up twenty-four hours a day; in the daytime people could come and go as they pleased; they were obliged only to spend their nights in hospital. And it worked – or so it seemed. Certainly the number of leprosy cases declined rapidly in the second half of the nineteenth century: in 1856, as we have seen, there were 2,858 registered cases; by 1875, before the two Leprosy Acts, the number had already dropped to 1,752; and by the end of the century it was a mere 577 (fifty years later, it was just seven and the CMO for Leprosy declared himself redundant).[35] The decline was unmistakeable; but the reasons for it were from the beginning a matter of contention.

An English public health doctor, W.J. Collins, who visited Norway in 1889, opined in *The Lancet* that it would be 'entirely erroneous' to attribute it to compulsory isolation, since such a provision could hardly be said to exist: 'it would be impossible without further accommodation to segregate even the reduced number of lepers in Norway at the present time'. No, he concluded, it was not segregation that was stamping out leprosy in Norway, but 'the increased material prosperity of the people . . . and the opportunities . . . for better and more varied subsistence'.[36]

In 1906 Jonathan Hutchinson, who had an obsession about fish eating being the cause of leprosy but was otherwise a knowledgeable and trenchant commentator, maintained that 'the attempt to isolate lepers always has been, and always will be, illusory'. He went on:

> In no part of the world is it more utterly illusory and further removed from completeness than in Norway, where it is held to be succeeding. The wise men of Gotham attempted to confine the cuckoo by building a wall to surround him, and when the bird flew over, regretfully admitted that they had not built high enough. So will it ever be with attempts to exterminate leprosy by isolation measures. How can you adequately isolate a malady which takes years to declare itself and of which at the same time the contagious influence is so insidious, so obscure and so slightly powerful that husband and wife hardly ever suffer together?[37]

This question raised by Hutchinson would be rehearsed many times over in the succeeding half-century.

Hansen's successor as CMO for Leprosy, H.P. Lie, writing in 1929 on 'Why Is Leprosy Decreasing in Norway?', argued that the decline was due both to 'progress . . . not least in hygiene and sanitation' and to the policy of isolation, which 'also . . . played a considerable role'.[38] More recently, Professor Lorentz M. Irgens, of the University of Bergen's Institute of Hygiene and Social Medicine, examined the data provided by the National Leprosy Registry and concluded that it all depended on which phase of the 'epidemic' one was looking at as to whether or not isolation could be said to have been effective. Taking his cue from other researchers he argues that leprosy may be transmitted in two different ways, which he terms 'infection in the household' and 'infection in the community'.

> Thus, in an epidemiological situation characterized by a high relative importance of infection in the household, i.e. when a high number of households is affected and prevalence rates are high, isolation may cause a fall in subsequent incidence rates. However, when prevalence rates are low, and the relative importance of infection in the community is higher, due to a lower occurrence of infection in the household, the effects of isolation may be low . . . Accordingly, physical isolation in Norway of infectious patients in special leprosy hospitals is considered an important cause of the initial decline in incidence rates during the observation period.[39]

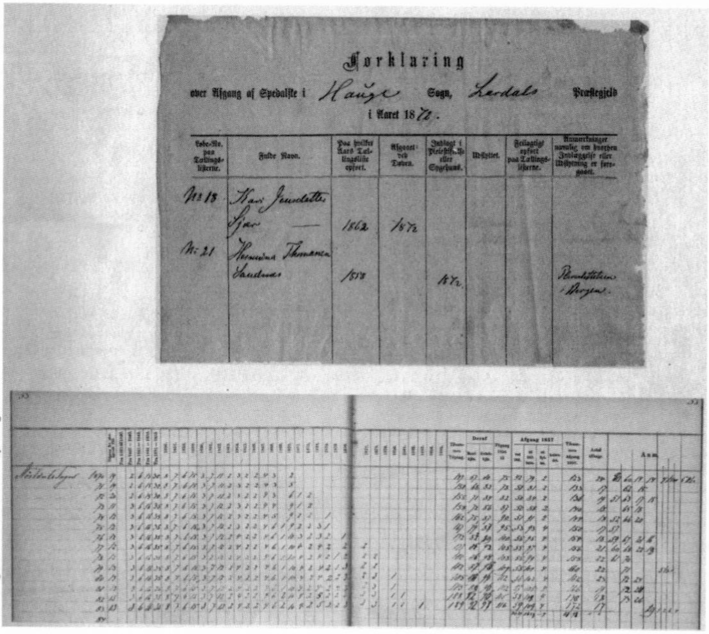
Forklaring
over Afgang af Spedalske i Hauge Sogn, Lærdals Præstegjeld
i Aaret 1872.

(The Regional State Archives of Bergen)

Local and central registrations –
the Norwegian National Leprosy Registry of 1856 is said to be the first of its kind to be created for a specific disease anywhere in the world

If Irgens is right about there being two distinct ways in which leprosy may be transmitted and only one of these can be forestalled by isolation, the irony is that at the very moment Hansen was pushing for legislation to promote the segregation of leprosy sufferers, the policy of isolation had already done its work and would no longer be so effective. Nevertheless, Irgens puts *physical isolation* top of his list of three 'important causes of the decline'; the other two are (improved) *nutritional conditions* and *selective emigration* to the United States.[40]

(Incidentally, in 1887 Hansen became the third leading Norwegian leprologist to visit the Upper Mississippi Valley to study the implications of the spread – or, more accurately, non-spread – of leprosy among Norwegian immigrants there. The first, J.A. Holmboe in 1863, believed in spontaneous outbreaks of the disease; the next, C.W. Boeck in 1869, was, like his co-worker Danielssen, a confirmed hereditarian; and Hansen, of course, was a contagionist.[41] Each returned home convinced that the North American experience proved the validity of his particular theory of causation – an example of how easy it is to find evidence to support whatever it is you are looking for in the first place.)

Another explanation put forward for the dramatic decline of leprosy in Norway in the late nineteenth and early twentieth century is that, partly at least, it was brought about by the concurrent rise in tuberculosis. As early as 1867, a Norwegian district medical officer, Christian Homann, observed that in districts were leprosy was rooted, tuberculosis was rare, and vice versa. These two endemic diseases, he suggested, 'in some way behaved as if they antagonized or replaced one another'.[42] A century or so later tangible evidence of this sort of cross immunity was provided when it was found that in some parts of the world, though not in others, the BCG vaccine provided a measure of protection against leprosy. It all depended on which form of the disease predominated, the theory being that the tuberculoid type results from an over-reaction of the immune system to the invading bacteria, and the lepromatous sort from an under-reaction or no reaction at all. BCG might protect people from developing tuberculoid leprosy, but it would be powerless to prevent lepromatous leprosy. This helps to explain why the theory is not necessarily disproved by the fact that some 30 per cent of Norwegian leprosy sufferers in the latter half of the nineteenth century died of tuberculosis.

The tuberculosis hypothesis casts into doubt the theory that improved hygiene, nutrition and living standards were responsible for the decline of leprosy. Since both leprosy and tuberculosis are often described as diseases of poverty, arising out of poor diet, overcrowded housing and generally adverse social conditions, how can it be that in the supposedly improved situation of the second half of the nineteenth century in Norway one was waxing while the other waned? As in the later Middle Ages, if standards had really improved, then both diseases should have been on the decrease. Whatever the explanation, the Lungegaard Hospital in Bergen ceased to be a leprosy hospital in 1895 for lack of new cases; and in 1912 – the year of Hansen's death – it was turned into a hospital for tuberculosis. Hansen's only son, Daniel Cornelius (named after Danielssen), became Chief Physician for tuberculosis there in 1929.

Hansen's biographer records a conversation the doctor once had with a peasant farmer. Hansen remarked that if he lived long enough he hoped to see the day when leprosy would be a thing of the past in Norway. The farmer exclaimed, 'What a fool you are! How would you make your living then?'[43] Hansen loved such anecdotes. In his memoirs he relates that he had just returned from a year abroad, 1870–1, which – he admits – had turned him into 'what, in Norway, was referred to as a European – a somewhat snobbish world citizen who had developed a distaste for his countrymen's spiritual development and cultural point of view', when he met the poet Bjornson for the first time. Bjornson took him to task for his 'rather disparaging judgment of the Norwegian peasant'. At that time, Hansen remarks, Bjornson's romanticism was still 'burning brightly'.[44] Later, it would give way to a realism that somehow diminished his work and he never 'rediscovered the hope and promise still inherent in the simple people who made him a poet in the first place'.[45] Hansen implies that he himself made the journey in the opposite direction, discovering that 'what is commonly referred to as peasant cunning is, I am satisfied, simply people using their heads . . .'[46] He was personally modest, but was a strong nationalist, proud to be Norwegian. When he reflected on his great discovery, it was with satisfaction that 'my life has been of some use and that I have faithfully served my country'.[47]

Yet he was also a European – not just in the Norwegian sense of the word. His year abroad, in Bonn and Vienna, had broadened his mind in the way travel is supposed to do but so rarely does. His time in Bonn coincided with the start of the Franco–Prussian War in 1870. The disruption it caused affected even Hansen in his laboratory; telling his friends he hoped the Germans would be initially rebuffed 'so that they would not be too arrogant and sure of themselves when they finally won', he acquired a Red Cross armband and took a Rhine steamer to the front at Saarbrucken.[48] He arrived the day after the battle and visited the battlefield, where the 'sight of the dead horses, lying on their backs with their guts spilled out and all four legs raised stiffly made a far worse impression on him than did seeing the dead soldiers'.[49] He did not linger there, but made his way to Vienna, where a revelation awaited him in the form of the discovery of Charles Darwin. Darwin's works became, as he wrote in his memoirs, 'the foundation of my outlook on life'. He made it his mission to 'bring the scientist and his teachings to the attention of the Norwegian people'.[50] For Hansen, this amounted almost to a Damascene conversion. Darwinism became his religion.

Like Danielssen before him, Hansen had wide scientific interests. Both were keen zoologists and served on the board of directors of the Bergen Museum. After Danielssen's death Hansen took over as chairman of the board and was also chair of its natural history department. In his public life he achieved all he could possibly wish for; he was the Norwegian delegate to the first International Congress of Leprology, held in Berlin in 1897, and was elected honorary chairman of the conference that formally recognised that leprosy was a contagious disease and endorsed not just his discovery but also the Norwegian model of leprosy control, which owed so much to him. And the fact that twelve years later, in 1909, the second International Congress of Leprology was staged in Bergen, was itself a tribute to Hansen's pre-eminence in the field, and he was made its President (which Virchow had been at the Berlin conference). Only in his private life, after the premature death of his first wife Fanny, was there any cause for dissatisfaction.

His second marriage, to Johanne ('Hanne') Margrethe Tidemand, née Gran, was not a happy one, even though they had a son together. Hanne soon felt neglected by Armauer who, she maintained, was 'more interested in his research than in his home'. She became increasingly shrewish and her own family took Hansen's side against her, inviting him, but not her, to parties. As Hansen's biographer puts it in his rather po-faced way, 'This did not improve their relationship'.[51] The composer Edvard Grieg and his wife Nina remained friends of both, but few other people were intimate with them as a couple. In their old age, though, when Hansen

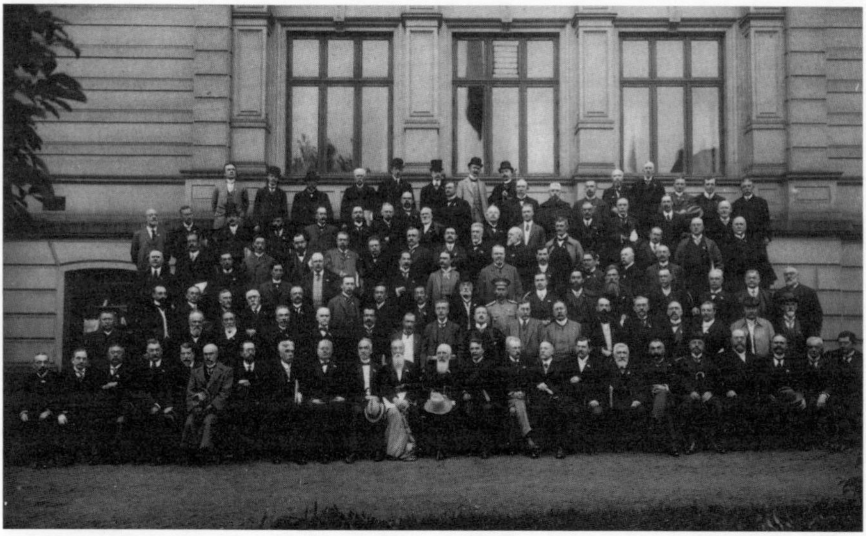

(*The Leprosy Museum, St Jørgens Hospital, Bergen*)

The 1909 International Congress of Leprology in Bergen with the white-bearded Hansen (*centre*, *front row*) as its President. The other greybeard seated to his right is his successor as Chief Medical Officer for Leprosy in Norway, H. P. Lie

was no longer quite so obsessed with his work, they grew more affectionate again.

Hansen died in bed and in harness, as it were. He was on his annual tour of inspection of the districts north of Bergen when his heart gave out while he was staying overnight in a friend's house. It was a good death for a man who, despite the blemish on his career of his treatment of the leprosy patient Kari Nielsdatter, had lived an honourable and useful life and is forever commemorated in the nomenclature of the disease to which he'd dedicated that life.

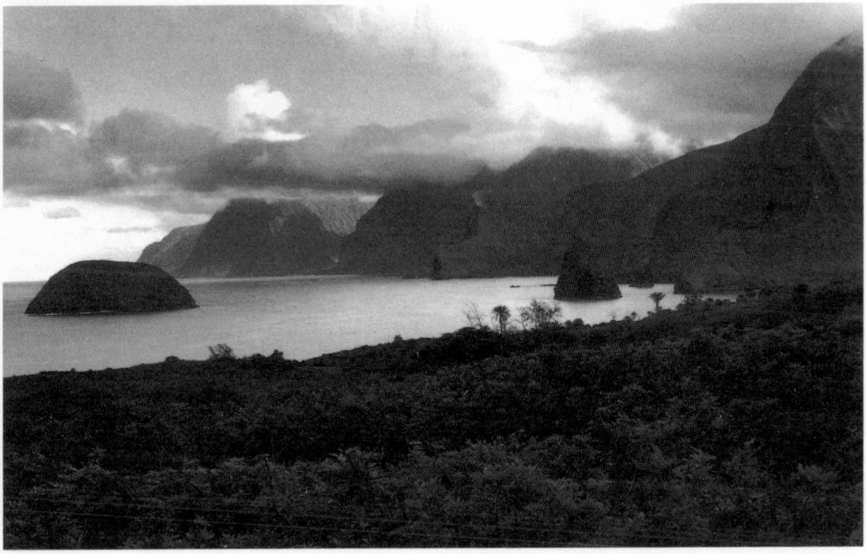

(Wayne Levin Photography)

The north shore of Molokai seen from Kalawao (now part of the Kalaupapa National Historical Park), photographed by Wayne Levin in 1984

Chapter 3

THE MARTYR OF MOLOKAI

In retrospect 1873 may be regarded as leprosy's *annus mirabilis*, but at the time neither of the events that make it so caused much of a stir in the world at large. Hansen's reluctance to trumpet abroad his discovery of the leprosy bacillus meant (as we've seen) that the credit for it almost went to another microbe-hunter; while on the other side of the world, in what were then known as the Sandwich Islands, the departure that year of a young Belgian Roman Catholic priest to the island of Molokai was only of local interest, a kind of ten-day wonder in the Honolulu press. Yet Father Damien's death, sixteen years later, from the 'separating sickness' – as Hawaiians, with good reason, came to call leprosy – had an impact of seismic proportions throughout the world. Damien did not actively seek publicity, but the example of this stubborn, self-sacrificing peasant-priest who identified with his chosen congregation to such an extent that he addressed them as 'We lepers' long before he himself showed any sign of the disease (and not, as some of his hagiographers have asserted, as a dramatic way of announcing that he'd become one of them) drew public attention to the plight of leprosy sufferers everywhere.[1]

In his 1959 blockbuster *Hawaii*, the popular novelist James A. Michener gives a highly coloured account of the 'epidemic' of leprosy that overtook the Hawaiian archipelago in the second half of the nineteenth century and endorses the prevalent but unproven assertion that its origins were Chinese: hence *Mai Pake*, or 'Chinese sickness', the designation of the disease in Hawaii that preceded 'separating sickness'. But if Michener is guilty of pandering to popular prejudice in his sensationalist treatment of the disease in his novel, he does at least provide a detailed historical context. Leprosy in Hawaii was far more than a disease; it was a political, as much as a medical, phenomenon; and the way it was handled by the authorities and experienced by the – mostly – Hawaiian victims furnishes crucial evidence of a racial and cultural conflict that went far beyond contagionist and anti-contagionist arguments about the nature of the malady and was more about controlling undesirable 'deviants' than treating – let alone attempting to cure – ordinary people who happened to be suffering from a debilitating and disfiguring disease.

The Hawaiians proved to be their own worst enemy. They were a hospitable people and warmly welcomed to their beautiful islands foreigners who would cuckoo them out of their nests. Acquisitive westerners took over land that had previously been communally held and gained power over their hosts by encouraging them – or their rulers – to become indebted and ultimately, therefore, dependent. The process, though gradual, was inexorable. The indigenous Polynesian monarchy might achieve formal recognition as the Kingdom of Hawaii in 1840 but this was not, as the innocent might imagine, a guarantee of independence, ensuring the future of Hawaii for the Hawaiians; it was rather a means of preventing any one of the Western powers that were casting covetous eyes on this enchanting, strategically and commercially well-placed archipelago from stealing a march on its rivals and excluding them from a share of the spoils. In the event, the American influence soon became predominant and, though Hawaii did not become a United States Territory until the turn of the century (or acquire statehood until 1959), the charade of kingship ended in 1894 when a Republic of Hawaii was proclaimed. The *haole* – as whites were called – now felt confident enough to step out from behind their puppet rulers to govern the country themselves.

From the early 1820s the islands had been linked with New England through two disparate activities – whaling and missionary work. What the Hawaiians made of the contrasting ethics of hedonistic ship's crews, who regarded the islands as a paradisiacal playground in which there were any number of willing Eves, and puritanical New England pastors, for whom this paradise was full of serpents, is anybody's guess. But each set of invaders – and the traders in sandalwood and sugar plantation owners who followed in their wake – had their own agenda, which for better or worse involved the transformation of the land and the people. In the words of one commentator, 'Hawaii supplied the land and the climate. Western nations provided money, management skills, and expertise in agricultural technology'.[2] And there was a third element: labour. For this essential function Hawaiians were regarded by westerners as unsuitable, too pleasure-loving and lazy. So the colonisers looked to Asia for their worker bees: first to China and later Japan. With the influx of both westerners and Asians in the latter part of the nineteenth century the population of Hawaii expanded, but at the expense of the Hawaiians themselves. Even before the arrival, or explosion, of leprosy, the diseases that foreigners brought, venereal or otherwise, were decimating native Hawaiians who had little or no resistance to them. But leprosy was different: it did not merely kill off expendable Hawaiians; it threatened westerners too, and unlike the Hawaiians, who saw no reason to break up the family if one or more of its members contracted the disease, these foreigners were very, very frightened of it.

Dr Arthur A. St Maur Mouritz, who was physician to the leprosy settlement on Molokai for three years during Father Damien's sojourn there, wrote a quirky historical account of the disease in Hawaii in which he offered 'the following facts about the Hawaiian race (the chief victims of leprosy)':

1. Healthy Hawaiians will eat, drink, sleep, and live with a leper voluntarily, and without fear.
2. A healthy Hawaiian man or woman will marry a leper, although there are plenty of well men and women in sight.
3. In order to lead a lazy, free from care existence, many *kokuas*, or helpers, are willing to become lepers at the Molokai Reservation; try to imitate the signs of leprosy by burning their skins, rubbing in irritating substances, and by other traumatic means, desire to be placed on the list as lepers in order to get their daily food free.
4. In spite of the fact that the main race affected with leprosy are themselves, the Hawaiians view with ignorant contempt the fears of the foreigners, and appear to think that the law of segregation is a special device aimed at them only to cause trouble, injustice, and break up their homes. The Hawaiians mostly view the segregation of their lepers as a tyrannical act, and wholly unnecessary, and cannot for the life of them perceive that the said law is the only means to prevent their possible extermination.

5. It has been said in my presence by Hawaiians of the better class, 'Hawaii is our country, it belongs to us, or at least it did until the *haole* got possession of most of it. If the *haole* is afraid of leprosy let him go back to where he came from.'[3]

Given Mouritz's views, it is not surprising to find that the Hawaiians on the Molokai 'reservation' (the *mot juste*) reciprocated his feelings about them and thought him lazy and unenthusiastic about his work. This may have been because, although he had come out from England to 'work with lepers' after hearing about Father Damien, he had been sent from Honolulu to Molokai against his wishes and couldn't wait to get away from the place.

In the heyday of imperialism the racial superiority of the whites who constituted the ruling clique was, of course, taken for granted: that was their justification for taking power in the first place; theirs was a civilising mission. The authorities who disciplined you and deprived you of your liberty had your own best interests at heart. Thus the segregation law in Hawaii – 'An Act to Prevent the Spread of Leprosy, 1865' – was designed not to protect enlightened but frightened foreigners from contamination *but as the only means to prevent Hawaiians themselves from being exterminated*. In view of which it might seem strange that no sooner had the German surgeon at the Queen's Hospital in Honolulu, Dr W. Hillebrand, reported that *Mai Pake* was 'the genuine Oriental leprosy' and called for the isolation of its victims than he was despatched to China to recruit labour to work on Hawaiian plantations. Admittedly, his mission was also to learn as much as he could about 'Chinese leprosy' while he was there.[4] But to swamp the islands with the very people who were regarded as the source of a disease requiring special legislation to check its spread was a peculiar way of preserving the Hawaiian race from extinction.

Following the passage of the segregation law in January 1865, the Board of Health reported that it had come up with a suitable site for a settlement, the northern end of the island of Molokai, full of valleys 'which were by nature favourably located for the purpose, containing hundreds of acres of cultivable land, abundance of water, separated from other parts of the island by steep *palis* [precipices, cliffs], and the landings on the sea shore difficult to approach so as to insure the seclusion desired'.[5] The authorities had a vision of a self-sustaining community of

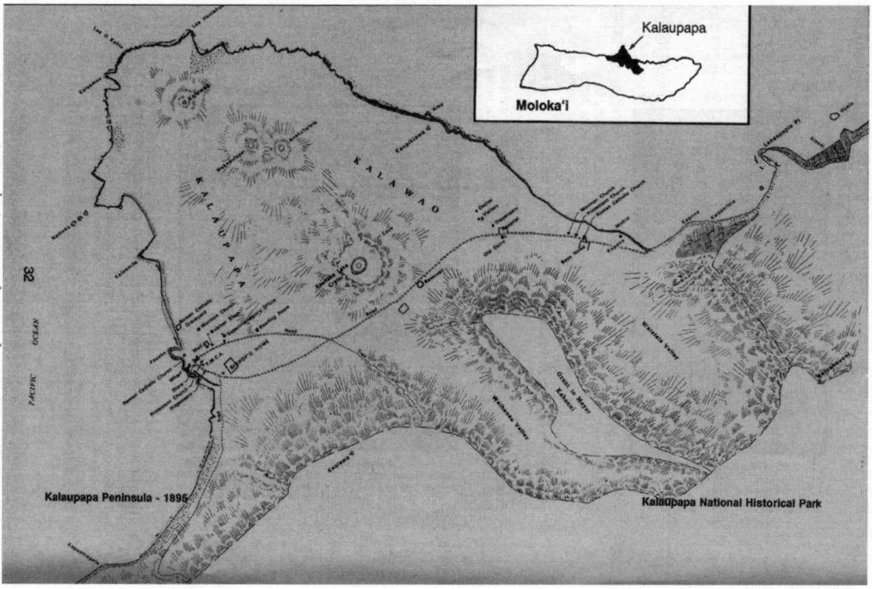

Kalaupapa Peninsula, 1895

of Kalaupapa Settlement, 1865 to the Present' by Linda W. Greene, Denver Service Center, National Park Service, Department of the Interior, Sept 1985)

leprosy-affected people, all happily working together in idyllic surroundings, the strong supporting the weak – just the kind of cut-price utopia Dr Hillebrand had envisaged back in April 1863 when he'd stated that it would be 'the duty of the next legislature to devise and carry out some efficient, and at the same time, humane measure, by which the isolation of those affected with this disease can be accomplished'.[6]

The first Board of Health report following the establishment of the settlement at Molokai and its staging post, the Kalihi Hospital and Detention Station outside Honolulu, was decidedly upbeat:

> It is gratifying to be able to state . . . that the condition of these poor people has been improved in every respect by their having been transferred to the care of the Government . . . We are informed that those sent to Molokai have settled contentedly on the place, and those able to work have commenced to erect new houses and cultivate the land, feeling that they are permanent settlers there . . .[7]

But less than two years later, in 1868, the rosy vision had already begun to fade as 'the obstacles met with have exceeded even the anticipations of the Board', and the corner-stone of its policy, the establishment of a self-supporting group that would not subject 'the resources at the disposal of the Board . . . to a regular and constant drain', was proving unviable:

> . . . the terrible disease which afflicts the Lepers seems to cause among them as great a change in their moral and mental organization as in their physical constitution; so far from aiding their weaker brethren, the strong took possession of everything, devoured and destroyed the large quantity of food on the lands, and altogether refused to replant anything; indeed, they had no compunction in taking from those who were disabled and dying, the material supplies of clothes and food which were dispensed by the Superintendent for the use of the latter; they exhibited the most thorough indifference to the sufferings, and the most utter absence of consideration for the wants, to which many of them were destined to be themselves exposed in perhaps a few weeks; in fact, the most of those in whom the disease had progressed considerably, showed the greatest thoughtlessness and heartlessness.[8]

As if that weren't bad enough, 'Drunkenness, pilferings, immorality and general insubordination were very prevalent; ki-root beer was manufactured and drunk in very large quantities, and great orgies took place'. But the Board flattered itself that it had solved the disciplinary problem with the appointment of a magistrate for the peninsula and by making constables out of the husbands of diseased women. Its main concern now was the 'embarrassment' caused by the separation of families. To some, this separation might come as a relief, but to others – the Board was surprised to discover – it was 'a great grievance' and these families tried to counter it by hiding their sick loved ones. There had been two absconders from Kalihi Hospital, 'and all enquiries have failed to elicit the places of their concealment'. As a matter of policy, the Board, to begin with at least, felt obliged to allow husbands, wives, or parents to accompany their relatives to their place of exile and become their *kokuas* – assistants or nurses. But in a throwback to the Middle Ages, it solemnly proposed that the Legislature might care to consider 'whether divorces should not be granted to the wife or husband of a leper, if the said leper has been certified as having the disease – whether, in fact, the party afflicted should not be regarded by the Court as "civilly dead".'[9] (And sure enough an Act of 1870, Relating to Divorce, sanctioned divorce 'when it is shown to the satisfaction of the Court that either party has contracted the disease known as Chinese leprosy, and is incapable of cure'.[10])

Hawaiian husbands and wives of leprosy sufferers were not clamouring for divorce, however. Many of them, far from seeking a legal separation, unaccountably resented and, in some cases, actively resisted the legislation that divided them. The 1870 Board of Health report acknowledged that its 'delicate and difficult' duty, 'the forcible separation of individuals from their friends and the world, although necessary for the welfare of society at large, must appear harsh to many of those afflicted, and even to many persons not personally interested in the matter', especially those who doubted leprosy's contagiousness. Nevertheless – and one can sense here a collective stiffening of resolve – 'the Board have no hesitation in reasserting the opinion made in their last report that "the disease is contagious".' Yet it continued to bother them that, despite the acquiescence of the majority of the afflicted, 'most painful scenes are sometimes experienced on the forcible separation of husbands and wives, parents and children'.[11]

Dr Mouritz described the enforcement of segregation as a 'political football'.[12] It all depended on who was in charge at any given time: if the royal party was in the ascendancy and Hawaiians were influential it tended to be lax; but when foreigners gained power and curbed the royal prerogative, an effort was made to round up all the leprosy suspects in the islands and ship them off to Molokai, regardless of the wailing and gnashing of teeth this caused – and despite the cost. For the control of leprosy was proving a costly business. In 1872, out of a total budget of $51,000 for expenditure on health, $31,000 – well over half – was spent on leprosy. By 1874 the amount spent on leprosy alone had risen to $55,000. It continued to rise, but at the same time the proportion of the total health budget that went to leprosy decreased.[13]

It wasn't until 1873 that the first really determined attempt to apply the segregation act took place. In that year alone there were as many victims of the disease apprehended and exiled to Kalaupapa (or rather to the adjacent Kalawao, where the original settlement was) as there had been in the previous seven years of its existence. At the same time, in an effort to make segregation more effective and to reduce the opportunities for what the Board of Health regarded as freeloading, the privilege of being accompanied by husbands or wives or other relatives who would act as *kokuas* was withdrawn, giving rise to a further bout of concealment of leprosy sufferers by their families.

So the arrival of Father Damien on 10 May 1873 was timely. As he would recall, 'A great many lepers had lately arrived from the different islands; they numbered 816 [in all]. Some of them were old acquaintances of mine from Hawaii [Island], where I was previously stationed as a missionary priest; to the majority I was a stranger.'[14] Though he had volunteered to go to Molokai – indeed, insisted that he should be the one chosen by his Catholic order for this tough assignment – what he found at the Kalawao settlement appalled him. The people were huddled together in makeshift huts, constructed out of branches of castor oil trees and covered with leaves.

> Under such primitive roofs were living pell-mell, without distinction of ages or sex, old or new cases, all more or less strangers to one another, those unfortunate outcasts of society. They passed their time with playing cards, hula (native dances), drinking fermented ki-root beer, home-made alcohol, and with the sequels of all this. Their clothes were far from being clean and decent on account of the scarcity of water, which had to be brought at that time from a great distance.[15]

Damien himself preferred to sleep in the open, under a pandanus tree, than in the damp and filthy hovels occupied by his flock. It took him some time to adjust: the 'smell of their bodies, mixed with exhalation from their sores was simply disgusting and unbearable to a newcomer'. On entering a hut he would often have to hold his breath to prevent nausea and, when that failed, rush out into the fresh air and breathe deeply before returning. He took up pipe smoking in order to counteract the foul odours that assailed him on every side and attached themselves to his clothes. A large number of the people sent to Molokai were in advanced stages of the disease and, likely as not, the conditions there would finish them off. Kalawao was full of the dead and dying, and not for nothing had it (like St Jørgens in Bergen in 1816) acquired 'the name of a living graveyard'.[16] Before Damien's arrival, burials were performed in the most perfunctory manner, coffins were a luxury, and corpses frequently interred so shallowly that scavenging dogs and wild pigs soon exposed their putrid flesh.[17] There was plenty of work of a practical and a spiritual nature for an energetic priest, and Damien set to with a will.

Damien was the son of a prosperous farmer. Born on 3 January 1840 in Tremeloo, near Louvain in the Flemish speaking part of Belgium, Joseph de Veuster was the seventh child in a family of eight. He enjoyed having the run of his father's farm, but chafed at the disciplinary restraints imposed by his quick-tempered, not to say violent, mother. Anne-Catherine Wouters, or Cato, as she was known, was – according to a recent biographer – 'no God-fearing farmer's wife, gathering her eight children around her every evening by the hearth to read from the big book of lives of the saints. She did so occasionally, but in general she was a harpy, a shrew or – as it was whispered in Tremeloo – a "witch"'.[18] Joseph – Jef for short – was not the only member of his family to be drawn to the religious life. His elder brother Auguste, who took the name of Pamphile as Joseph would select the religious name of Damien, had already joined the order of the Sacred Hearts, whose headquarters was in rue de Picpus in Paris – hence their common designation, Picpus Fathers – when Damien followed in his footsteps. The two brothers remained close, though there was a strong element of rivalry in their relationship. Pamphile was the one originally selected to go as a missionary to the Sandwich Islands, but he had to pull out through ill health and Damien begged to be allowed to go in his place, despite the fact that he had not yet been ordained. He got his way by defying his immediate superiors and petitioning a higher authority, but then, as a teacher of his observed, 'Damien was one of those who try to storm heaven and risk breaking their bones in the process'.[19]

The voyage to Hawaii in those days included the fearful passage round Cape Horn, but Damien took such things in his stride. He disembarked at Honolulu on 19 March 1864, at the time when the Hawaiian authorities were becoming preoccupied with the burgeoning leprosy on the islands, though that was not his immediate concern. He had to prepare himself for ordination two months later in Honolulu Cathedral and then familiarise himself with the Hawaiian language and people so that he could perform his duties as a parish priest in a remote and volcanic district of the island of Hawaii. There, as his letters to his brother Pamphile and his favourite sister Pauline reveal, he became caught up in the rivalry between Roman Catholic and Protestant missionaries in attracting converts among the ever-diminishing *kanaka* (native Hawaiian) population. 'At present,' he told his sister, 'there are 60,000 natives in our group of islands [there had been an estimated 400,000 at the time of

Captain Cook's arrival in 1778] . . . We do our best to hold our own against the Protestants. Our Sisters beat them with their girls' schools; but as regards the education of boys they beat us . . .'[20]

In his isolation, Damien wrestled with his demons and yearned for a brother to keep him company. As he wrote to his superiors, 'a missionary needs the "constant" help of a fellow-priest in order to dispel the black thoughts that arise as a result of daily contact with a sinful world and that give rise to an intolerable kind of melancholy'.[21] Throughout his time in the islands, and even after his death, there would be rumours of relationships with women, sexual liaisons, which Damien himself firmly denied. Such whispers probably arose out of his carelessness in maintaining the proprieties in his dealings with Hawaiians; rather than keeping a distance, he adapted to their easygoing ways in order that he might use his influence for the good, as he saw it. But there can be little doubt that in the process he was exposed to sexual temptation that tried him to the limit of his endurance and gave rise to those 'black thoughts' and moods he struggled to transcend.

Damien had encountered leprosy before he went to Molokai. He wrote to his parents, 'Leprosy is beginning to be very prevalent here. There are many men covered with it. It does not cause death at once, but it is very rarely cured. The disease is very dangerous, because it is highly contagious . . . ' Along with his parishioners he read the notice posted in his village, announcing in no uncertain terms that 'ALL LEPERS ARE REQUIRED TO REPORT THEMSELVES TO THE GOVERNMENT HEALTH AUTHORITIES WITHIN FOURTEEN DAYS FROM THIS DATE FOR INSPECTION AND FINAL BANISHMENT TO MOLOKAI'.[22] He visited leprosy sufferers who went into hiding to avoid such a fate; he thought it no more than his Christian duty to hear the confessions of these poor souls living in fear of forced separation from their loved ones. But he did not question the need to segregate the afflicted.

So when one of the more colourful characters to step on to the Hawaiian stage in the mid-nineteenth century, Walter Murray Gibson, a Mormon missionary turned journalist turned politician, future President of the Board of Health and Prime Minister to King Kalakaua, wrote of the outcasts on Molokai, 'Were a noble Christian priest or pastor to find the inspiration to offer his life to comfort the poor wretches, that noble soul would shine forever on a throne constituted of human love', Damien was eager to take up the challenge.[23] And he wasn't the only one. Several priests volunteered, and the bishop's original intention was to rotate four of them, giving Damien the first go. As it transpired, none of the others got a turn and Damien was to remain on Molokai for the rest of his life, with very few breaks. (It is often forgotten, however, that during his fifteen years or so on Molokai, other priests did come and go; and one in particular, Father André Burgerman, who was jealous of Damien's position and claimed that he, too, had leprosy, tried hard to oust him.)

'Picture to yourself a collection of huts with 800 lepers,' Damien wrote to his brother Pamphile after six months on Molokai. 'No doctor: in fact, as there is no cure, there seems no place for a doctor's skill. A white man who is a leper, and your humble servant, do all the doctoring work.'[24] There was a hospital of sorts, a building at least, and this was William Williamson's domain; he was British and had been a nurse at the Queen's Hospital in Honolulu, where he had contracted the disease. At Kalihi Hospital he had acquired enough medical knowledge working as an assistant to the doctors to be placed in charge of what passed for a hospital

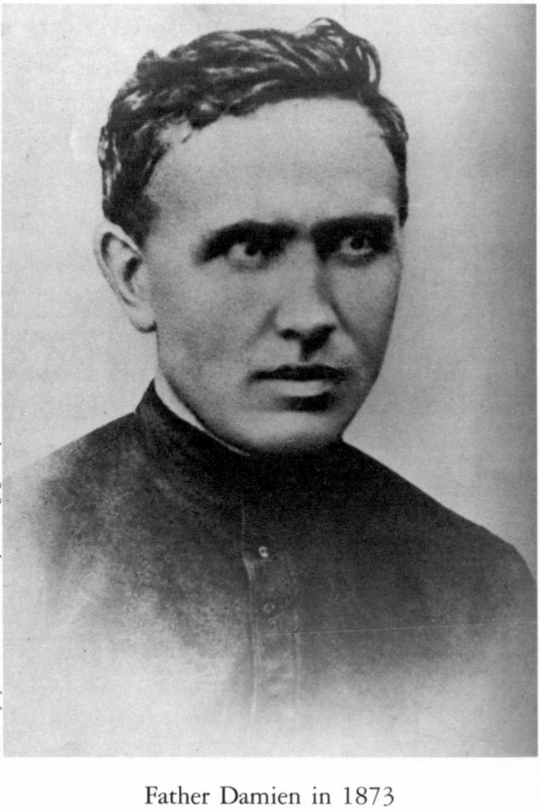

(Courtesy of the General Archives of the Congregation of the Sacred Hearts – Rome)

Father Damien in 1873

on Molokai. He showed Damien around when the priest first arrived. He told him, 'We have no enemies here save scabies, vomit, fleas and lice.' There was one tiny hut Williamson might have preferred not to show Damien, but as they were passing it someone with a cloth over his nose pushed a wheelbarrow into the doorway and tipped a bundle of rags on to the floor. The bundle emitted a groan and turned out to be a person, whose feet had to be shoved further into the hut before the door could be closed. This squalid little hut was known as the 'dying-shed' and was, in Williamson's words, 'to be avoided'.[25] But Damien had other ideas, which for the moment he kept to himself.

Years later he recalled that when he arrived the people had no medicines other than those concocted by their own healers:

> It was a common sight to see people going around with fearful ulcers, which for the want of a few rags, or a piece of lint and a little salve, were left exposed to dirt, flies and vermin. Not only their sores were neglected, but anyone getting a fever, diarrhoea or any other of the numerous ailments that lepers are so often heir to, was carried off for want of simple medicine.[26]

For a disease that was notorious for *not* killing off its sufferers, there was an astonishingly high mortality rate on Molokai. This was due quite as much to the harsh conditions as to the lack of medicines; despite the lush tropical vegetation, Kalawao in particular was frequently battered by northeast trade winds and squalls of chilly rain; and because of the towering cliffs to the south it lost the sun very early in the afternoon. Kalaupapa was further to the west and enjoyed a better climate, but it was not part of the original leprosy settlement and was subsumed by it only when the numbers became too great to be contained at Kalawao.

Damien's farming background fitted him to tackle the abundant practical problems he encountered at the settlement. But he was first and foremost a priest, and the spiritual challenge of entering a community whose motto was 'in this place there is no law' – impressed upon all newcomers on arrival – was even more daunting.

> In consequence of this impious theory [Damien later wrote], the people, mostly all unmarried, or separated on account of the disease, were living promiscuously without distinction of sex, and many an unfortunate

> woman had to become a prostitute to obtain friends who would take care of her, and the children, when well and strong, were used as servants. When once the disease prostrated them, such women and children were cast out, and had to find some other shelter; sometimes they were laid behind a stone wall and left there to die, and at other times a hired hand would carry them to the hospital. The so-much-praised 'aloha' of the natives was entirely lacking here, at least in this respect.[27]

Damien regarded the anarchy reigning at Kalawao as the product of despair, 'both of soul and body', which drove the leprosy sufferers to extremes of vice, fuelled by the 'horrible liquid' they distilled illicitly, and he sought to counter it by 'kindness to all, charity to the needy, a sympathizing hand to the sufferers and the dying, in conjunction with a solid religious instruction to my listeners'.[28] Should these fail, he was not above taking more direct action and breaking up hula dances by belabouring the intoxicated participants with a big stick until they made themselves scarce. Damien had many human faults; he could be impatient, wrongheaded, stubborn, but he was physically as well as morally courageous. From very early on he understood that if he were to have any influence in his chosen community he had to avoid all squeamishness in his dealings with the afflicted. First he had to conquer fear of the disease in himself. Touch was essential, even if it exposed him to the danger of contracting leprosy – as he knew it must if the disease was indeed 'highly contagious'. Other people might be cowed when threatened by the embrace of leprosy victims prepared to use their stumps and open sores as weapons, but Damien stood his ground; he made himself immune to such threats. When he preached to his congregation, using the words 'We lepers', it wasn't an affectation, as it might have been from the lips of another; it was a simple statement of identification: Damien embraced leprosy long before leprosy embraced him. Thus he earned the respect even of his enemies, though they continued to defy him and the civil authorities by brewing their noxious liquor, holding hula dances and invoking their pagan deities.[29]

In truth, the only authority that could prevail in such a lawless place was moral authority. Threaten offenders with police or prison (Kalawao did have its own gaol, where the insane as well as the criminal were immured) and they would laugh in your face: what was the whole settlement if not a prison? Each and every one of them was already under a life sentence. The 'true governor of Kalawao', as Damien's most penetrating biographer remarks, 'was death'.[30] Death was the one certainty on Molokai, and in the early days it was likely to come sooner rather than later. Damien's trump card, of course, was his unshakeable conviction that death, far from being the end of life (unless you take *end* to mean *purpose*), was the means to a richer life. What he offered was an alternative, not just to indulgence but to the despair that lay behind it.

On a practical level, too, he exemplified energy and purpose. Ambrose Hutchinson, a part-Hawaiian leprosy patient who became resident superintendent of the settlement, characterised him as 'a vigorous, forceful, impellent man with a generous heart in the prime of life and a jack of all trades, carpenter, mason, baker, farmer, Medico and nurse, no lazy bone in the make up of his manhood, busy from morning till nightfall'.[31] Damien proudly wrote to his brother Pamphile, 'I am a grave-digger and a carpenter.'[32] Carpentry had a particular appeal to this follower of Christ; it was hallowed work. But as Hutchinson said, he would turn his hand to anything – even if, as a later colleague observed, he started off many more things than he could ever finish.[33]

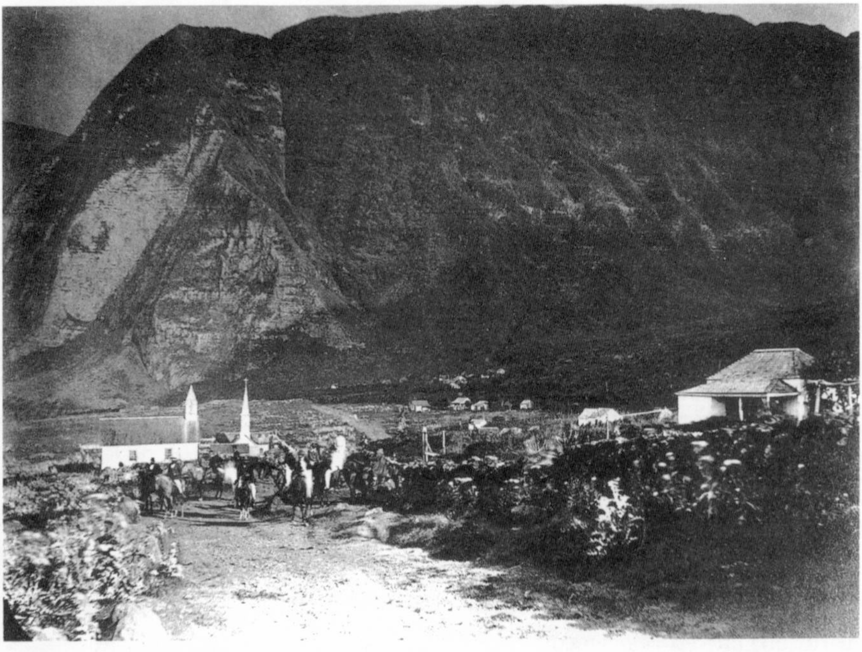

(Hawaii State Archives, unidentified photographer)

Kalawao settlement, c. 1884

His first priority was to lay on a decent water supply so that people would no longer have to carry it in cans on their shoulders over a considerable distance if they wanted to wash themselves or their clothes. He and his helpers found a natural reservoir in a high valley backing on to the precipice, from which they piped fresh water to Kalawao. Secondly, he put pressure on the authorities to provide materials for building proper wooden huts that could be raised off the damp ground and furnish some protection from the elements, and he himself helped to erect these buildings. Thirdly, he campaigned tirelessly to get better food and clothing; the want of both was deeply felt by the patients, and the advocacy of Damien and others led to a change of policy: instead of providing a minimum of clothing, the Board of Health paid an annual clothing allowance of $6 per person and individuals could buy what they needed from a store which opened at Kalawao in 1873; disputes over the quantity and quality of rations continued for years, the patients complaining that they were always hungry, and the Board that they were never satisfied no matter what they got. Last, but far from least, of the practical considerations to which Damien drew attention was the question of medical care. He and the English nurse Williamson did what they could with the limited knowledge and medicines at their disposal but the real need was for a resident doctor. Even if there was no cure for leprosy, much could be done to alleviate the condition.

The Board of Health regarded Damien with some alarm. He might be on the side of the angels, but the authorities found him 'obstinate, headstrong, brusque and officious' in his attempts to cajole them into improving the lot of 'his lepers'. Brother Joseph – as Ira Dutton, an American Civil War veteran who made a bad marriage and took to drink before undergoing a conversion and finding his way to Molokai in 1886 to do what turned out to be a forty-four-year 'penance', came to be known – described Father Damien as he knew him in his last years as:

> vehement and excitable in regard to matters that did not seem to him right, and [he] sometimes said and did things which he afterwards regretted. I am safe in saying that, in all the differences [with the Board of Health], he had a true desire to do right, to bring about what he thought was best. No doubt he erred sometimes in his judgment, as all of us do. These things make his relations with the Government officials more readily understood . . .[34]

The Board might regard Damien as a gadfly, but it could not do without him (nor he without it). For instance, when one of the resident superintendents, a well-connected and flamboyant half-Hawaiian lawyer and leprosy sufferer who liked to be known as 'Governor' Ragsdale, died and Damien refused to serve under Father André Burgerman, who'd got himself nominated as superintendent, the Board had to climb down and offer the post to Damien himself. Damien accepted only in order to keep out his hated rival; he refused payment altogether and as soon as he could sloughed off this unwanted temporal authority, pleading that he needed more time for his spiritual duties. He valued his independence (which frequently strained his relations with his spiritual superiors, too); he wanted to be free to criticise and nag the *Papa Ole* (Board of Health) and not to be in any way identified with what the leprosy patients, in their angrier moments, referred to as *Papa Make*, the Board of Death.

In 1878, during the brief period – a matter of months rather than years – when Damien reluctantly held this administrative position, a Special Sanitary Committee, under the chairmanship of Walter Murray Gibson, visited Molokai in order to report on the state of the settlement at Kalawao. Gibson had brought with him a gift of $100 from the Queen Dowager that was placed in Damien's hands to be distributed among the needy as the priest saw fit. (Damien would attract many more gifts over the years, particularly after it became known that he had contracted leprosy.) Gibson's committee listened to the usual complaints about food and its unfair distribution, and concluded that a 'large-minded, philanthropic, energetic, professional superintendent or governor is the great want and necessity of the unfortunate community at Kalawao'. They ruled out the 'devoted and heroic priest' Damien because he was inevitably absorbed in his spiritual duties and could hardly be expected to devote time and energy to the practical running of the settlement; yet they still maintained that what was needed at Kalawao was 'a priest, a chief and a physician all in one man'.[35] Such a paragon never materialised, though Damien's *bête noire* Father André, who'd had some medical training, regarded himself as perfectly qualified for the role.

Kalawao did acquire a physician, or rather a succession of them since, as the Board of Health report for 1882 stated, 'It is difficult to secure the services of a good one who will reside at the settlement'. The patients were far from grateful, however; they grumbled about these doctors and even said they would 'prefer to be without a regular physician'. This was because the doctors interfered with their freedom of movement, trying to restrict their already tenuous contact with the outside world still further, and refused to touch, or, in some cases, even to approach, their patients, keeping them at arm's length and pushing their medicine towards them with a stick or leaving it on top of fence posts for them to collect. The Board decided that nurses were required: 'It is hardly right to take the lepers away from the care of their friends and leave them alone to care for themselves.'[36] Since *kokuas* were no longer allowed to accompany their loved ones to Molokai, the problem of nursing the helpless had become more acute. Damien argued strongly that 'faithful husbands and wives of lepers should be allowed to accompany their partners to their exile at Kalawao' as *kokuas*:

> Not only is the contented mind of the leper secured by the company of his wife, but [so is] the enjoyment of good nursing and assistance, much needed in this protracted and loathsome disease, and which no other person could be expected to impart.[37]

But he disapproved of unmarried *kokuas* since they were liable to be 'a source of immorality and a temptation to lead the lepers into bad habits' – in other words, they were as destabilising an influence as married *kokuas* were a stabilising one.

The Kalihi Hospital outside Honolulu had closed in 1876, the Board having decided that isolation was impossible in such a location and that 'all parties afflicted with leprosy should at once be sent to Molokai'.[38] Walter Murray Gibson, who became King David Kalakaua's prime minister in 1882 and was disparagingly known by his political opponents as 'Minister of Everything', took a particular interest in leprosy for personal and/or political reasons.[39] While ostensibly supporting the policy of segregation, he empathised with the Hawaiians and understood their antipathy to isolation. As President of the Board of Health he approved the construction of the Kakaako Branch Hospital outside Honolulu in 1881. Like its predecessor, the Kalihi Hospital, it was supposed to function as a staging post for Molokai, but before long it took on a life of its own and Gibson's critics accused the 'Minister of Everything' of setting up a dangerous alternative to Kalawao in which isolation was as impossible to secure as it had been in Kalihi. Worse still, from the point of view of the *haole* Protestant establishment which provided such formidable opposition to Gibson and the king's party, the one-time Mormon missionary seemed to be in league with the Catholics in an initiative to recruit Sisters of Charity to staff Kakaako. The Protestant missionaries and business moguls of Honolulu looked askance at the twin possibilities of contamination by Catholicism and by leprosy. It was bad enough that a Catholic like Damien should have come to epitomise Christian charity in Hawaii without importing a bevy of nuns to partake of his glory.

Recruiting these nuns was no easy matter. The Catholic emissary Father Léonor Fouesnel petitioned more than fifty religious houses in America and Europe and received just one response – from the Sisters of St Francis at Syracuse in upstate New York. But one was enough. Mother Marianne Cope (born Barbara Kopf, her family had emigrated from Germany to the United States in the 1830s when she was still an infant) and six other Sisters arrived in Honolulu in November 1883 and were immediately assigned to the prison-like Kakaako branch hospital, where conditions were scarcely better than they had been on Molokai itself in the early days.[40] Some 200 patients were housed hugger-mugger, regardless of age, sex, or state of health, in a grim collection of neglected and dirty wooden buildings constructed on a salt marsh, surrounded by fences and threatened with inundation at high tide; they were subjected to arbitrary and brutal treatment by attendants who behaved with the petty vindictiveness of prison warders and thought nothing of consigning the more recalcitrant among them to solitary confinement in punishment cells.

The Sisters, undaunted, set about cleaning up and reforming the place, facing down the bullies to such good effect that after a few months, Father Léonor was writing to Damien: '. . . there are 207 lepers at Kakaako; but at present, when they have the Sisters to take care of them *it is* and it will become still more difficult to make them leave for Molokai . . . never will so few people do so much work'. In another, later letter he referred to them as 'our saintly Franciscan Sisters'.[41] Father Damien wanted them to come to Molokai, but the old roué Walter Murray Gibson had become obsessed with Mother Marianne in a religiose way and preferred to keep her close to Honolulu, where he could continue to lavish on her his attention and (unwanted) gifts.

The medical superintendent at Kakaako, Dr George L. Fitch, was popular with the Hawaiians and close to the king and queen. He held unorthodox views about leprosy, insisting that it was nothing more than the 'fourth stage of syphilis'; that 'by the constant use of medicine it may be considerably, but not permanently relieved; and that it is not quickly contagious'.[42] Most doctors agreed with him that the disease was not very contagious and that it was susceptible to temporary relief; but the better informed among them vehemently denied that it had any connection with syphilis. Dr Nathaniel B. Emerson, for instance, who had been medical superintendent at Kalawao in 1880, dismissed this out of hand, saying:

> there are plenty of cases of uncomplicated leprosy among the Hawaiians, who had been and are free of syphilis. It will not do to assume that every ache and rheumatoid pain, every indurated lymphatic gland, every necrosed bone, every cracked and fissured tongue comes of syphilis. Such loose diagnosis as this deserves no refutation . . .[43]

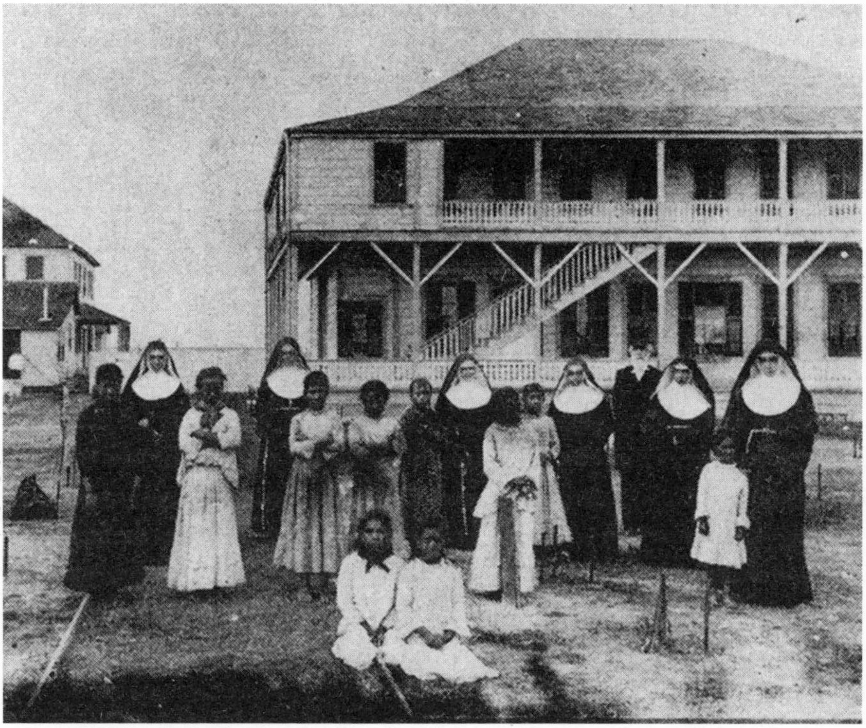

(Hawaii State Archives, unidentified photographer)

The Sisters of St Francis at the Kakaako Branch Hospital, 1886

What worried Emerson and others was that Fitch's pernicious views might lead to 'a sanitary policy that is full of peril, and likely to prove destructive to the Hawaiian people' – i.e., encourage the spread of the disease by relaxing the rules on segregation.

Dr Fitch hit back in his 1882 report, remarking on the reluctance 'of the native to apply to Government physicians for advice and treatment'.

> His great fear that he would be pronounced a leper and hurried off to Kalawao has been partly the cause, and unfortunately in many instances the physicians employed by the Board have been gentlemen too much engrossed in raising sugar or gentlemen of elegant leisure to such an extent that if a native applied for treatment without a liberal fee in his hand, his wants were very poorly attended to.[44]

In contrast, by the simple expedient of offering a treatment involving the use of herbal baths and medicines, developed by Dr Masanao Goto of Tokyo, whom King Kalakaua had invited to come to Honolulu, Kakaako was attracting hundreds of leprosy sufferers who had previously been in hiding.

> That 508 cases should apply for treatment in a single quarter [Fitch argued] shows that the endeavor to enforce the law of segregation as it has been carried on here for years, has been a most complete failure, and considering the kindly, loving nature of the native race, and the heartless manner in which sufferers have been treated, the only wonder is that as many cases have been sent to Kalawao as are there now.[45]

This was heresy, and the *haole* medical profession closed ranks and denounced Fitch as 'a charlatan, quack and a knave' in the press.[46] Fitch sued for libel and the ensuing trial in 1883 was a two-day wonder in which the accuser rapidly found himself in the position of the accused, called upon to defend his record both as an administrator (at Kakaako and on the Board of Health) and as a leprologist. His theory of the relationship between syphilis and leprosy, his denial of the contagiousness of the latter and his conviction that it was, in some cases, curable, all came under scrutiny. The verdict went against Fitch by a ten-to-two majority and the exonerated publication, the *Saturday Press*, opined:

> In reality, the suit was an effort to crush or at least silence the Press for its plain, direct, unsparing and convincing exposure of the criminal mismanagement of leprosy in these islands by the Hawaiian Board of Health, of which body Mr Gibson and Mr Fitch were the officials chiefly responsible.[47]

Fitch was unrepentant. The following year, he was still portraying Kakaako as a model in comparison with 'that hideous brothel' Kalawao:

> For nearly eighteen years that place has been the chosen spot for casting out to a lingering death many hundreds of the most unfortunate of earth's suffering mortals. In addition to the incredible suffering which is the constant feature of leprosy, no care has ever been exercised to make the condition of lepers even tolerable.[48]

No wonder that Fitch, in Dr Mouritz's words, 'gained the inner confidence of the Hawaiian people more than any other foreign physician that I know of'. Mouritz was in a position to know, since he succeeded Fitch as physician to the leprosy settlement, 'and even to the end of my period of service, the lepers were always calling for Kauka Pika's (Hawaiian for Dr Fitch) medicines'.[49]

In gaining his patients' confidence while losing that of his peers, Fitch was like that earlier proponent of the theory that leprosy was simply 'inveterate syphilis', Dr La Billois of New Brunswick. He resembled him in another respect too, in that, far from attracting obloquy from his patients for further stigmatising their disease, he was idolised by them for holding out hope of a cure, however illusory. Furthermore, as Mouritz noted disapprovingly, 'Dr Fitch was one of the most reckless and careless physicians in his contact with leprosy, he seemed to take a delight in putting to proof his non-contagious view of the disease' – in other words, he was not afraid to touch his patients as so many other, more worthy medical practitioners were.[50] That may have been why even Father Damien approved of him.

Fitch poured scorn on the *haole* authorities responsible for creating the settlement on Molokai, and on how they set about it:

> from the very first, numerous *kokuas* have been permitted to live there. And yet this has been called segregation; and there is a political party here

> who established the place, and whose war cry is: 'We will never give up until every leper in the Kingdom is sent to Kalawao, and thus the land become clean.'

'Verily', he went on, with heavy irony, 'sending hundreds to a leper manufactory to establish cleanliness in the land is practising segregation and encouraging virtue, with a vengeance.' After such a rhetorical flourish, it comes as a bit of a shock to discover that Fitch actually approved of segregation – provided it was done in the right way (or by the right party).

Like many other doctors caught up in the debate over whether or not leprosy was truly contagious, Fitch wanted it put to the test and, as early as 1882, he suggested how this might be done: 'Condemned criminals should be given the choice of inoculation with the blood and matter from leprous patients or execution as preferred by them.'[51] Three years later this would happen, but at the behest of a very different sort of doctor to Fitch, one who dismissed Fitch's fourth stage of syphilis hypothesis as 'so extraordinary and self-condemning' as to be unworthy of notice except insofar as it 'has led, and may further lead, the public to consider leprosy as an outcome of licentiousness . . . and to look upon the unfortunate lepers as the victims of their own or their parents' transgressions'.[52]

Dr Eduard Christian Arning hailed from Germany, where he had been a student of Hansen's rival in the discovery of *M. leprae*, the bacteriologist Albert Neisser. Arning arrived in Hawaii in November 1883 at the invitation of Walter Murray Gibson. He was a far more intelligent and better-informed doctor than Fitch, though he, too, seems to have been ambivalent on the question of segregation. In his 1884 report to Gibson, he wrote on the one hand:

> I consider it altogether unwarrantable to call leprosy incurable, and simply to remove the afflicted out of sight. This is a remnant of medieval barbarism which every professional man ought to oppose, more especially so in our relation to a race which has had our civilization forced upon it, and which is accustomed to look up to us for help and support. Is it not fostering their innate sense of indifference to hygienic principles, instead of setting them a fair example, when we gather together very nearly a thousand suffering people in a lonely spot, and let them have only a flying visit of a doctor once a month . . .?[53]

On the other hand, though he refused to be drawn into arguing the respective 'merits and drawbacks' of Molokai and Kakaako except to say that he thought they detracted from each other's value and that 'this condition will last as long as Kakaako is kept up as an overcrowded leper settlement', he concluded, a trifle mystifyingly: 'It will be seen from the foregoing, that I advocate segregation.'[54]

Unlike Fitch, Arning – as a proponent of the germ theory of the disease – did believe in the contagiousness of leprosy. In Hawaii he sought to take forward the work of Hansen and Neisser by experiments in the *in vitro* cultivation of *M. leprae* and through inoculation of a monkey he had acquired. In 1884, however, a crime of passion in which a woman's Hawaiian lover bludgeoned her Japanese husband to death and was condemned to be hanged provided Arning with just such an opportunity as Fitch had earlier sought. The name of this human guinea pig who, naturally enough, preferred to take a chance of contracting leprosy to the inevitability of the hangman's noose was Keanu. Arthur Mouritz took a special interest in this experiment, since he spent much of his time at Kalawao attempting to inoculate willing *kokuas* (of whom there seemed to be an inexhaustible supply) with leprosy; and he recorded that on 30 September 1884:

> Dr Arning excised a leproma [or nodule], about the size of a small hen's egg, from the cheek of a young leper girl, and transplanted and embedded this leprous flesh into an incision which laid bare the belly of the supinator radii longus muscle of Keanu's right forearm, suturing it in position.[55]

Arning ascertained there was no leprosy in Keanu's family, and Keanu, whose death sentence was commuted to life imprisonment, seemed the ideal candidate for Arning's much-publicised experiment. For nearly two years the doctor kept a careful record of developments and by the time he left Hawaii in the summer of 1886 there was nothing to show that he'd had any more success than Mouritz or countless other doctors in different parts of the world who had tried in this way to prove (or disprove) the contagiousness of leprosy. Yet by October that year, according to Mouritz, 'Keanu showed the maculation of nodular leprosy all over his body, and the nerves and lymphatic glands near the seat of the wound also showed implication'.[56] A year later, when it was confirmed that

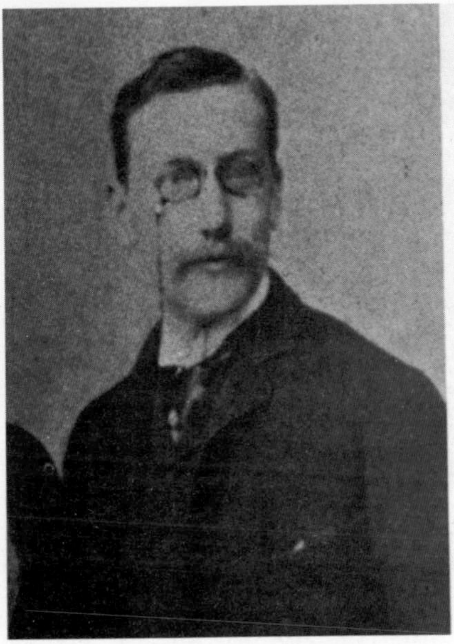

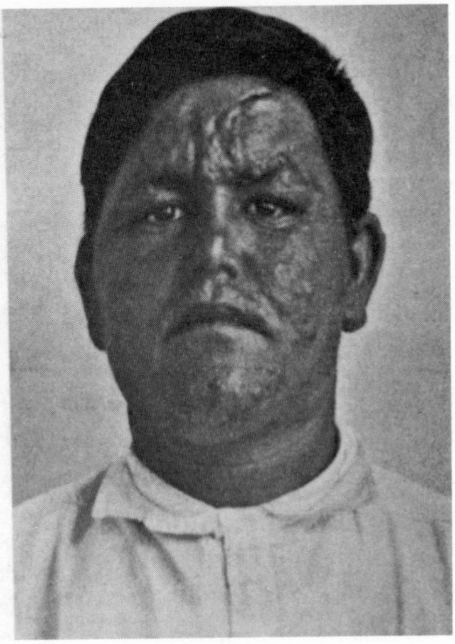

(International Journal of Leprosy)

Dr Eduard C. Arning and the condemned murder, Keanu

Keanu did indeed have leprosy, this was seen as a scientific breakthrough that – along with the fact that Father Damien was now known to have contracted the disease during his long residence on Molokai – established its contagiousness beyond all possible doubt.

But that was not the end of the story. The rapid progress of Keanu's leprosy meant that he had to be removed from Oahu gaol and sent to Molokai, where he arrived in February 1889. The resident physician at the leprosy settlement then was Dr Sidney B. Swift, who found Keanu 'a good-natured, industrious, honest man'. His leprosy was far advanced, but he had a good appetite, looked well and might, the doctor anticipated, 'live long enough to die of old age' (unlike his other famous patient, Father Damien, who was then dying). On Keanu's arrival, Dr Swift placed him in the hospital for observation and noted that he was particularly attentive to a very ill and practically helpless young man of twenty in the bed next to him. It transpired that this young man was Keanu's nephew, his sister's son. This alerted Swift to the possibility that there might be more leprosy in Keanu's family and he started to investigate.[57]

He soon discovered that no less than three other close relatives of Keanu – his son, his brother-in-law and a first cousin on his mother's side

– who'd all lived in the same house with him when he was still a free man were either at Kalawao or had died there. So much for there being no leprosy in Keanu's family. Dr Swift also learned that during the first three months of Keanu's imprisonment in Honolulu he had been in the charge of a gaoler who had subsequently been sent to Molokai and admitted to having had leprosy for as long as twenty years. Once again, the contagiousness of leprosy – at least by inoculation – had been thrown into doubt. Keanu might easily have contracted the disease long before he became the subject of Dr Arning's experiment. It was Dr Swift's opinion that if the inoculation was responsible, the ravages it caused in a very short time were 'such as to make it unparalleled in the history of this settlement'.[58] Far from living long enough to die of old age, Keanu died at Kalawao on 18 November 1892 at the age of fifty-six – just 'eight years and fifty days after his so-called inoculation with leprous tissue', as Dr Mouritz recorded.[59]

Dr Arning and Dr Fitch both left Hawaii for good in the summer of 1886, when their sponsor Walter Murray Gibson's relationship with the *haole* powerbrokers was approaching its nadir. By that time it was widely known that Father Damien had leprosy; Arning himself had diagnosed it. But Fitch's theory on the connection between leprosy and syphilis had gained such currency, and Damien's easygoing intimacy with his Hawaiian congregation was so well known, that his Catholic superiors in the order of the Sacred Hearts subjected him to a humiliating medical examination, not for leprosy but for syphilis – despite his reiterated insistence on his chastity. In his case at least it was firmly established that syphilis was *not* a predisposing factor with regard to leprosy.[60] But while the Catholic hierarchy might regard him with embarrassment, even suspicion, to the world at large Damien had become a hero. The fact that he had contracted leprosy merely set the seal on his living martyrdom among the outcasts of Molokai.

The news of his medical predicament was shortly followed by the publication of a book which, though it appeared in Damien's lifetime, set the pattern for a whole series of posthumous hagiographies. *The Lepers of Molokai* was written by Charles Warren Stoddard, an American professor of English literature from Notre Dame, Indiana, who'd visited Kalawao in 1884. Stoddard's picture of Kalawao is cunningly presented: the beauty of the place with its 'neat whitewashed cottages . . . little gardens of bright flowers, and clusters of graceful and decorative tropical trees', the cheerful greetings of the people who 'seemed to us the merriest and most contented community in the world', and the carefully tended churchyard, where the gate 'was swung open for us by a troop of laughing urchins', all convey the impression of an ideal village. But take a closer look:

> Now, for the first time, I noticed that they were all disfigured: that their faces were seared and scarred; their hands and feet maimed and sometimes bleeding; their eyes like the eyes of some half-tamed animal; their mouths shapeless, and their whole aspect in many cases repulsive.
>
> These were lepers . . . as their number increased, it seemed as if each newcomer was more horrible than the last, until corruption could go no farther, and flesh suffer no deeper dishonor this side of the grave.[61]

Out of the church steps a young priest, making his entrance into this idyllic landscape peopled with gothic monsters.

> His cassock was worn and faded; his hair tumbled like a schoolboy's, his hands stained and hardened by toil; but the glow of health was in his face, the buoyancy of youth in his manner; while his ringing laugh, his ready sympathy, and his inspiring magnetism told of one who in any sphere might do a noble work, and who in that which he has chosen is doing the noblest of all works.

This of course was Father Damien, 'the self-exiled priest, the one clean man in the midst of his flock of lepers'. And just in case we haven't got the message, Stoddard goes on:

> Having with a few words dispersed the group of lepers – it was constantly increasing in numbers and horrors – he brought from his cottage into the churchyard a handful of corn, and, scattering a little of it upon the ground, he gave a peculiar cry. In a moment his fowls flocked from all quarters; they seemed to descend out of the air in clouds; they lit upon his arms, and fed out of his hands; they fought for footing upon his shoulders and even upon his head; they covered him with caresses and with feathers. He stood knee-deep among as fine a flock of fowls as any fancier would care to see; they were his pride, his plaything; and yet a brace of them he sacrificed upon the altar of friendship [as a contribution to the visitors' dinner], and bade us go in peace.
>
> Such was Father Damien of Kalawao.[62]

It is a pretty picture and the stuff of legend – Damien as St Francis of Assisi (who may also have had leprosy[63]). But note how it is achieved, the way the leprosy sufferers are collectively demonised – *the group . . . was constantly increasing in numbers and horrors* – in order that 'the one clean man' in their midst should stand out in the full glory of his sanctity. And the irony – which Stoddard exploits to the full – is that the germs of leprosy are already undermining the robust constitution of the priest (the 'martyr priest' as Stoddard now calls him), though he does not yet know, or at least admit to it. Stoddard quotes Damien's letter to his superior of 25 August 1886, in which the priest acknowledges that the bishop has informed the public of the fact of his leprosy and goes on, in a self-consciously mythmaking manner worthy of Stoddard himself:

> . . . be not surprised or too much pained to know that one of your spiritual children is decorated not only with the Royal Cross of King Kalakaua, but also with the cross more heavy, and considered less honorable, of leprosy, with which Our Divine Saviour has permitted me to be stigmatised.[64]

Dr Mouritz, who had entertained Stoddard during his visit to Kalawao in 1884, regarded *The Lepers of Molokai* as 'pre-eminent' among the many books and pamphlets written about Father Damien, 'a classic of distinction, beautiful, pathetic, soul stirring'.[65] Yet the doctor remained critical of Damien for allowing himself (as Mouritz saw it) to become infected. Mouritz points out that Damien's successor, Father Wendelin, spent almost as long at Kalaupapa as Damien had spent at Kalawao but remained free of the disease:

> Fr. Wendelin took only the ordinary precautions that any prudent man would to avoid leprous infection. On the other hand, Fr. Damien took no precautions whatever; he was kind-hearted, he never forbade lepers entering his house, they had access to it at any time, night or day. I named his house 'Kalawao Family Hotel and Lepers' Rest,' free beds, free board for the needy; this designation I believe could not be improved on; it exactly fitted the daily prevailing conditions.[66]

Mouritz was torn between professional disapproval of Damien for needlessly exposing himself to infection and admiration for his fearless commitment to the people it was his fate to live among. Damien's own view, according to Mouritz, was: 'If Providence sees to afflict me with the leprosy whilst I am working amongst the lepers, I will gain a Crown of Thorns, whether I am worthy or not.'[67]

In the spring of 1886, Mouritz wrote to the bishop on Damien's behalf recommending that he go to Kakaako for Dr Goto's treatment. The bishop gave his consent and Damien took the steamer to Honolulu, where his arrival was eagerly awaited by the Franciscan Sisters who had long since cleansed the Augean stables that Kakaako had been before they came. They whitewashed a room, decorated it for him with a crucifix and holy pictures and made up a bed with sheets (to which he was entirely unaccustomed). Damien was grateful for their loving care, but such attention made him uneasy; he was homesick for Molokai and constantly fretted over what might be going on there in his absence. He studied Dr Masanao Goto's remedy earnestly and convinced himself that the regimen of hot baths (in which medicinal herbs were dissolved) twice a day and pills after every meal, followed an hour later by tea prepared from the bark of a Japanese tree, was doing him good.[68] But it was not in his nature to take things easily and he returned to Molokai within a fortnight.

If one of his less reliable biographers – John Farrow (father of the actress Mia) – is to be believed, Mother Marianne accompanied him to the steamer and he took the opportunity to impress upon her how urgently the Sisters were needed at Kalawao and how concerned he was about the future of the boys and girls who were housed in separate orphanages there and looked after by *kokua* families under his supervision – which Dr Mouritz thought 'was one of the finest works that this priest undertook and carried out'.[69] According to Farrow, Damien's parting words to Mother Marianne were, 'Hurry, there is not much time, you know' – which would show an awareness of the severity of his condition.[70]

The Sisters were already looking after fourteen healthy orphan girls from Molokai who had been shipped to Honolulu at the instigation of Dr Arning and housed in the Kapiolani Home (named after the queen), which was opened in November 1885. Arning was one of the earliest doctors to recognise that children exposed to *M. leprae* were particularly vulnerable, and so he pioneered a kind of reverse segregation in which these leprosy-free children were removed from Kalawao to prevent them developing the disease (as well as to forward their education and protect them from the sexual abuse which was such a common feature at Kalawao despite Damien's best efforts to curtail it). Only one of these fourteen girls later developed leprosy and had to return to Molokai, and the experiment was so successful that from 1894 all children born on Molokai to leprosy-affected parents were separated from them at birth and removed, first to a house at Kalaupapa where they could be kept in isolation, and then to Honolulu, where they were brought up by the Sisters at the Kapiolani Home or farmed out to relatives who might have some claim on them.[71]

Initially, this prophylactic measure had been bitterly opposed on Molokai. The orphan girls were a meal ticket for *kokua* families, who stole their rations and treated them as servants, making them do all the household drudgery; and the motives of the Board of Health in removing them from the island were seen as suspect. Threats were made; and as the girls embarked on the steamer at Kalaupapa there was a scuffle on shore and two policemen were stabbed to death. The two foster fathers who caused the trouble were sentenced to ten years in prison, and the Minister of Everything, Walter Murray Gibson, denounced everyone involved – doctor, priest, and resident superintendent included.[72]

But Gibson was soon fighting for his political life. He managed to win a closely contested and dirty election at the beginning of 1886, the Nationalists holding eighteen seats to the opposition's ten. But the treasury was bankrupt and accusations of extravagance, corruption and a return to 'the [bad] old Hawaiian ways' were being levelled at King Kalakaua and his premier in the *haole*-controlled press with ever-increasing force and bitterness. The opposition organised itself into a new Hawaiian League, or Reform Party, with its own militia, called the Honolulu Rifles, which it invited the unsuspecting king to inspect, while behind his back there were moves to end his reign and bring about American annexation.[73]

Gibson faced problems in his private life as well. While on the one hand he pursued an intense, elevated and spiritual relationship with Mother Marianne that he recorded assiduously in his diary, on the other, as a grey-bearded, but tall, handsome and above all eligible widower he was drawn into an earthier, distinctly physical liaison with an attractive young Californian widow who rejoiced in the name of Flora Howard St Clair. For once his instinct for sliding unscathed out of compromising situations failed and, just when his public life was being subjected to the most intense scrutiny, he found himself facing a legal suit for breach of promise.[74]

The political tragi-comedy ended in farce. The so-called 'Committee of Thirteen' opposition leaders latched on to a scandal over bribes relating to

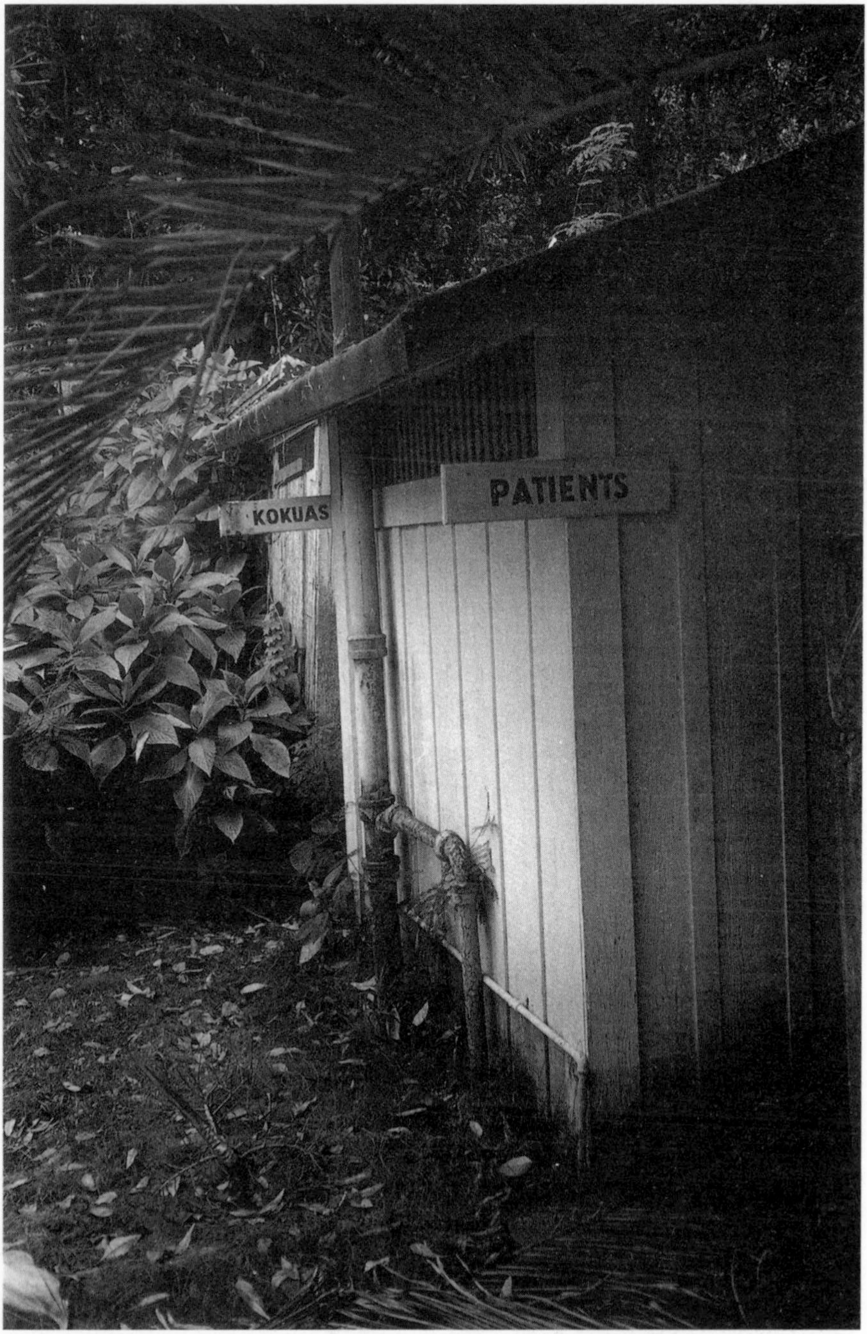

(Wayne Levin Photography)

Separate restrooms for patients and non-patients at Siloama Church in Kalawao, photographed in 1984 by Wayne Levin

the sale of import licences for opium to two competing Chinese bidders, and used the occasion to force the king to dismiss his cabinet, Gibson included. Then the mob, in the form of the militia, took over, arresting Gibson and his son-in-law, who happened to be with him at the time, and marching them off to a waterfront warehouse where the preparations that had already been made to hang one of them had to be speedily amended to accommodate the pair. The lynching was just getting under way when Gibson's daughter Talula, alerted to the likely fate of her father and her husband, made a dramatic entry and loudly demanded their release. But her intervention, however fiery, was less effective than that of Her Britannic Majesty's portly consul, James Wodehouse, who stunned the assembled crowd by announcing that Walter Murray Gibson (who had been born in England and had once boasted to Wodehouse of his British lineage) was a British subject and that if they proceeded with the hanging, they – Hawaii and its American accomplices – would be answerable to the British government. This gave the militia pause. A little local bloodletting was one thing, an international incident quite another. Reluctantly, they removed the nooses from both Gibson's and his son-in-law's necks and marched them back the way they had come.[75] Or so the story goes. There remains some doubt over whether the hanging was ever seriously intended; it may simply have been staged as a piece of street theatre – just as this 'bayonet revolution' (so-called because the spendthrift King Kalakaua was forced at bayonet point to sign a new constitution stripping him of most of his powers) was actually bloodless.

After that, the Committee of Thirteen resorted to legal methods and put Gibson under house arrest on a charge of embezzlement. But they were unable to come up with any evidence against him. So they fell back on trickery and threats; they summoned Gibson to the court and, without telling him there was no case for him to answer, coldly offered him the choice between banishment and prosecution. By now the fight had gone out of him and on 12 July 1887, after saying his fond farewells to 'the dear Mother' and Sisters, as well as to his daughter, son-in-law and their children, Gibson sailed out of Honolulu for San Francisco. Within six months he had died of tuberculosis, but not before news reached him that the court in Honolulu had awarded Flora Howard St Clair $10,000 of damages (though the aggrieved widow was happy to settle for $8,000 when Gibson's lawyer threatened to appeal).[76]

Poor old Gibson. Even the things he prided himself on promoting,

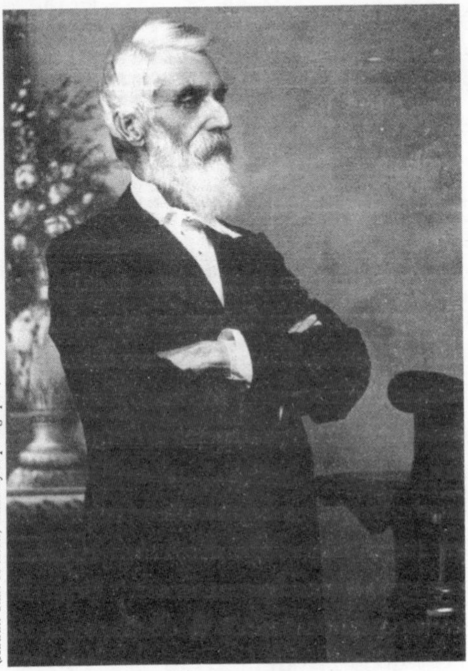
(Hawaii State Archives, unidentified photographer)

The 'Minister of Everything', Walter Murray Gibson

such as an enlightened and charitable approach to the problem of leprosy (after all, wasn't he the man who had brought Dr Arning to Hawaii and done all he could to support the Franciscan Sisters at Kakaako?), had backfired during his final months at the helm – and all because of Father Damien's sudden fame abroad. The vicar of St Luke's Church at Camberwell in London, the Rev. Hugh Chapman, was so moved by Damien's story that, though he was a Protestant, he energetically set about fundraising for the Catholic priest's leprosy settlement on Molokai. He enlisted the help of *The Times* and by the end of 1886 was able to send Damien a cheque for £975. Over the next three years he sent further donations, amounting to £2,625 in all. Gibson took umbrage at the sanctification of Damien and the personalised charity this attracted from overseas, seeing Damien's claim that the money was needed to buy clothes as 'a serious charge of neglect against the Board of Health'.[77] Damien's Catholic superiors were equally unenthusiastic about money coming from such a source, fearing it would undermine the fragile understanding they had with their only ally in power. Damien was fast becoming a law unto himself and they resented this, while he, for his part, was constantly bemoaning his lack of a regular confessor (a problem exacerbated by the fact that he and his superiors could never agree on who would be a suitable priest to partake of his exile).

But Gibson's fall was not so disastrous for the Catholics as they had feared. Damien, in particular, was delighted when Dr Nathaniel B. Emerson succeeded him as President of the Board of Health, since Emerson had been on Molokai and knew the situation there, and was regarded by Damien as a friend. He might be a Protestant, but he was the son of a missionary and an honourable man. He criticised Gibson's 'laxity' over enforcing the segregation law and courted unpopularity in tightening up the regulations, but he conscientiously believed that this was the only way to defeat leprosy. The situation at Kakaako was less happy from a Catholic point of view, since patients were being removed from there and shipped off to Molokai without any consultation with Mother Marianne and the Sisters. But this was all part and parcel of what Emerson called 'the unpleasant duty of segregation'.[78]

One casualty of the change of government was the Japanese Dr Masanao Goto, who resigned from his post when he saw the way things were going at Kakaako. Goto's departure created a problem for Father Damien, who wanted to continue the Goto treatment and to introduce it to other sufferers on Molokai: he found he could no longer get hold of the medicines. Dr Mouritz regarded this as a good thing (despite his earlier recommendation that Damien undergo this treatment) for he disapproved of the results when Damien finally did manage to get 'the much-talked-of Goto bathing and medicines established at Kalawao':

> After a few weeks of vigorous use of this Goto treatment, it had the effect of giving Fr. Damien a semi-asphyxiated appearance, symptoms of aphonia [loss of voice] and dyspnoea [laboured breathing] showed up; he tottered in his walk, his clothes appeared like bags hung on his figure, the lobes of both ears became enormously enlarged, almost reaching to his collar. Bronchial catarrh, oedema of the feet completed the train of grave symptoms. Yet, in the face of this evidence of the unsuitability of the Goto treatment for his case he claimed it was doing him good, and he felt better than he had been for the past two years. He lost at least thirty-five pounds in bodily weight at this time. About the month of June, 1887, many of the lepers began to drop off the Goto treatment. This also influenced Fr. Damien, and he dropped the hot bath part of the treatment to one bath every other day, but the mischief had been done, and his system refused to respond and he grew weaker.[79]

In the absence of an effective treatment for leprosy, there was no shortage of panaceas on offer. One of Damien's many English admirers, the well-connected painter Edward Clifford, who visited Molokai in December 1888, urged on Damien the virtues of gurjun oil, which he had learned about on a visit to India. He even brought a case of it with him; it was not dissimilar to chaulmoogra oil and was extracted from trees only to be found in the Andaman Islands, off the coast of Burma. Damien promised to try it, but by now his leprosy was far advanced and perhaps his experience of the Goto treatment had made him wary of all such nostrums. However, he did have a request to make of Clifford: that he would do a painting of St Francis to be hung in the convent of the Franciscan Sisters, three of whom had arrived on Molokai a month earlier. (He hung in his own room a water-colour of *The Vision of St Francis* by Edward Burne Jones, which Clifford had presented to him at the express desire of the Pre-Raphaelite painter, another member of Father Damien's English fan club.)[80]

The Sisters' influence was soon felt at the settlement; in less than six months people were deferring to Mother Marianne as the only person in authority who really knew what was going on, now that Damien was dying. And in a sense it was as well that Damien was dying; otherwise two such strong personalities would inevitably have clashed. As others had found, Damien was not an easy man to work with.

Damien died in the early morning on 15 April 1889, the Monday before Easter, just as he'd wished – since he fondly hoped to greet his Master on Easter Day. Though illness had reduced him to the condition of a frail old man, he was only in his fiftieth year. Brother Joseph Dutton's kinsman, Charles Dutton, writes of him:

> The life that had started on an obscure little farm in Belgium had ended in an isolated colony of outcasts. Humble in the beginning, at its close the eyes of the world were turned upon it. He had been an unknown and ill-educated priest; he died a hero and a saint.

Furthermore, his demise opened a new chapter in the history of leprosy:

> It may almost be said that the death of Father Damien did more for his lepers than ever his life had done. If the blood of the martyrs be the seed of the Church, this martyrdom sowed the seeds of prosperity for the Molokai settlement . . . money and help that was soon to make of the colony one of the most efficient medical centers in the world, and was to improve also the condition of lepers elsewhere.[81]

In the words of a more recent commentator, Damien 'brought order, peace, and spiritual comfort first, and then helped the kingdom address the temporal problems of adequate housing, better food, water, and

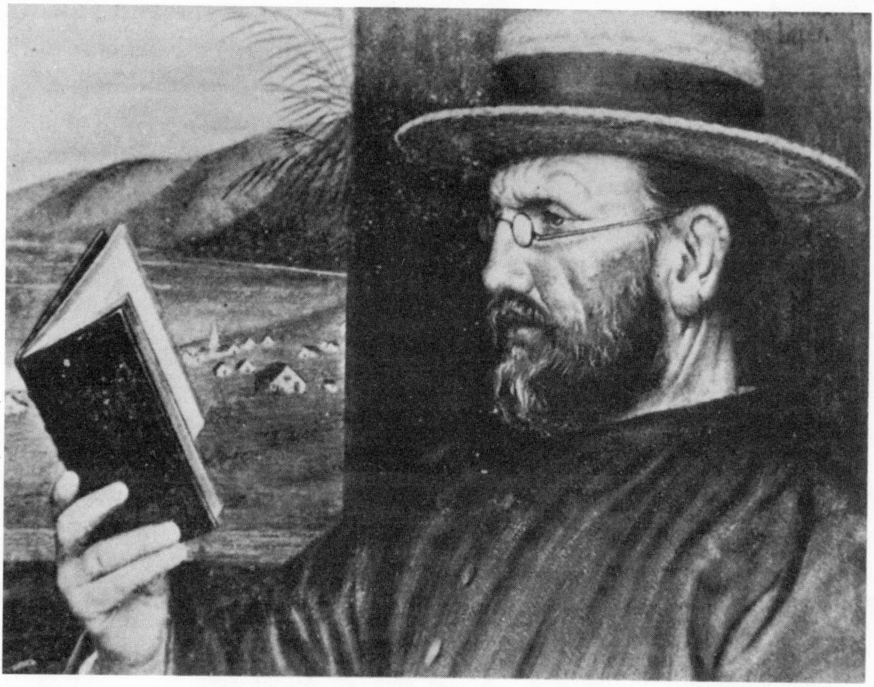
(The Sacred Hearts Damien Collection, Louvain)

Edward Clifford's painting of Damien in December 1888

medicine. In return he endured endless labour and untold physical suffering, but gained inner peace and tranquility'. Because of him, 'What might have turned into a squalid, forgotten village of outcasts became instead a model leprosy colony with the aid of the government and charitable funds and through individual tenacity'.[82] Others had come, kept their distance and gone away again; Damien remained. He identified with his chosen flock, knew that he must become 'one with them', and if that meant eventually becoming 'one of them', so be it. He was not the only one to make a significant contribution to improving conditions on Molokai: Fitch, Arning, Emerson and many others, including Gibson, all made a difference during his lifetime; and his successor Father Wendelin, Brother Joseph Dutton, Mother Marianne and the other Sisters of Charity would continue his work after his death. But he remains unique in his total commitment and fearless zeal in the promotion of the welfare of the outcasts he served. Even Brother Dutton, who did his 'penance' on Molokai for close on half a century without once leaving the island, is but a pale shadow in comparison.

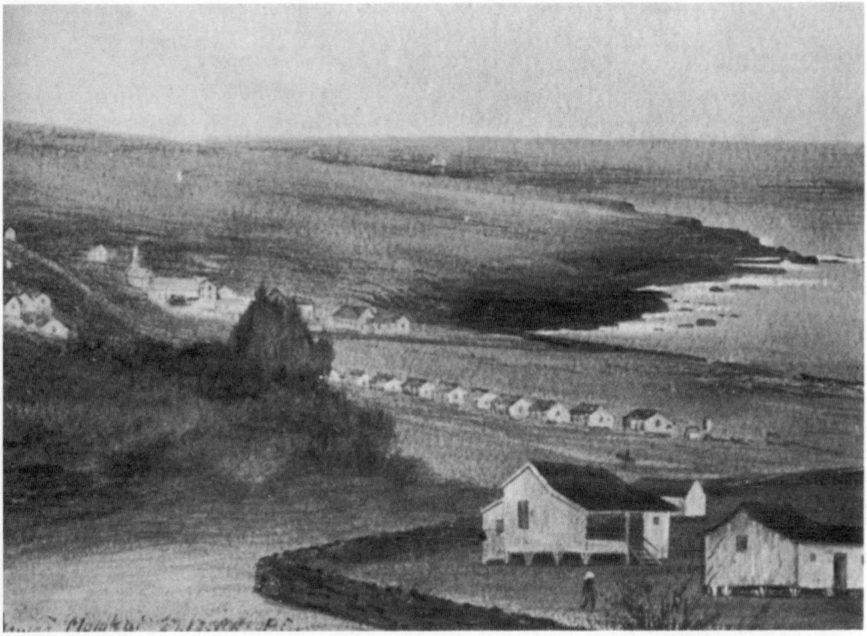
(The Sacred Hearts Damien Collection, Louvain)

Molokai in 1888, painted by Edward Clifford

Chapter 4

MR STEVENSON AND DR HYDE

It may be a matter of regret that the last foreign visitor to see Father Damien before his death should have been the painter Edward Clifford and the first to come after it was Clifford's friend, the writer Robert Louis Stevenson, himself mortally ill with tuberculosis of the lungs and travelling in the Pacific in search of a kinder climate in which to live out his days. What if it had been the other way round? What sort of a portrait might Stevenson have provided had he actually met Damien? As it was, RLS busied himself excavating the truth about the priest as if he knew that one day he would be called upon to defend his memory.

Stevenson sailed to Molokai on 21 May 1889, little over a month after Damien's death. With him on board were two Sisters of St Francis from Syracuse, New York, on their way to join Mother Marianne and the other Sisters already on the island. He befriended the nuns and took comfort from their presence, telling his wife Fanny, 'My horror of the horrible is about my weakest point; but the moral loveliness at my elbow blotted all else out.'

His first sight of his destination was unpromising:

> Presently we came up with the leper promontory, low-land, quite bare and bleak and harsh, a little town of wooden houses, two churches, a landing-stair, all unsightly, sour, northerly, lying athwart the sunrise, with the great wall of the *pali* cutting the world out on the south.

As for the people, 'there was a great crowd, hundreds of (God save us) pantomime masks in poor human flesh, waiting to receive the sisters and the new patients.' Once on land, however, he felt better: 'All horror was quite gone from me; to see these dread creatures smile and look happy was beautiful.' On his way through Kalaupapa he exchanged cheerful *alohas* with everyone he met:

> One woman was pretty, and spoke good English, and was infinitely engaging and (in the old phrase) towardly; she thought I was the new white patient; and when she found I was only a visitor, a curious change came into her face and voice – the only sad thing, morally sad, I mean – that I met that morning.[1]

Stevenson worried that he was there 'for no good'. He wanted to be of use and he soon found a way. In Honolulu he had heard of the Bishop Home for orphan girls, now run by the Sisters, and he had sent a croquet set as a present (after this visit he would send another, more expensive gift, a Wetemayer piano). Now he discovered there was no one to teach the girls how to play the game. So he volunteered his services and, despite Mother Marianne's protests that he was unnecessarily exposing himself to infection, set to with a will. Sister Leopoldina recorded (in her shaky syntax and sparse punctuation):

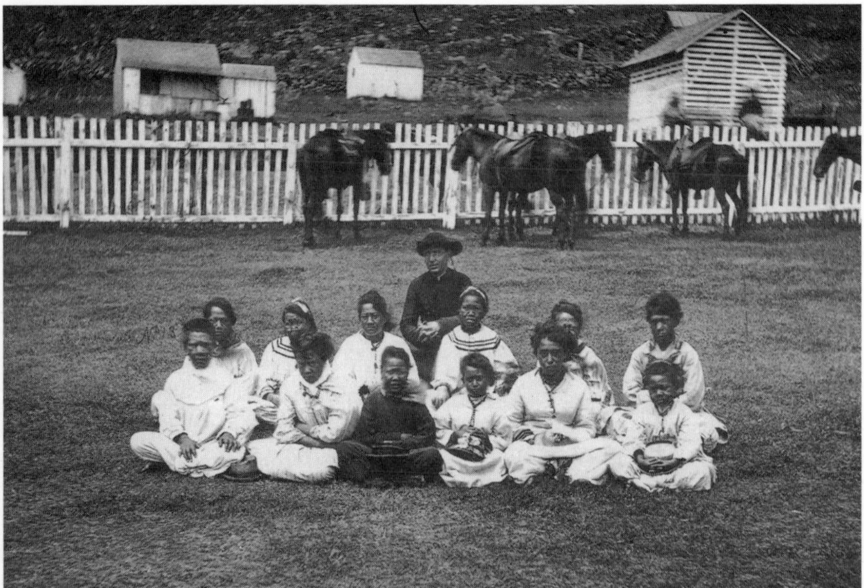

(Hawaii State Archives, unidentified photographer)

Father Damien, c. 1880, with girls of the settlement whom Robert Louis Stevenson taught to play croquet soon after Damien's death

> Poor dear children could hardly believe that a fine well white man would not be afraid, and why he did not shrink from them and shun them as all other white men do. The next morning quite early he came, the girls were ready but they kept away thinking it could not be possible but when he called to them come girls I only have a few days to teach you, and you must know your game well so that you can beat me or I shall not be happy leaving you . . .[2]

The girls responded enthusiastically and one eighteen-year-old, Waika-hi, soon proved a formidable opponent. Stevenson would pretend to be upset when he was beaten, but the girls knew better.

> In the evening [Sister Leopoldina recalled] it was funny to hear the little girls talking about him. *Sister he only one howlie (white man) not scart of us all the other white man too much fraid he our good friend we like he stay with us he not fraid us leper.*[3]

Stevenson himself wrote to a friend:

> I am fresh just now from the leper settlement of Molokai, playing croquet with seven leper girls, sitting and yarning with old, blind, leper beachcombers in the hospital, sickened with the spectacle of abhorrent suffering and deformation amongst the patients, touched to the heart by the sight of lovely and effective virtues in their helpers, no stranger time have I ever had, nor any so moving.[4]

To the 'Reverend Sister Maryanne [*sic*], Matron of the Bishop Home, Kalaupapa' he would dedicate a poem:

> To see the infinite pity of this place,
> The mangled limb, the devastated face,
> The innocent sufferers smiling at the rod,
> A fool were tempted to deny his God.
>
> He sees, and shrinks. But if he look again,
> Lo, beauty springing from the breast of pain! –
> He marks the sisters on the painful shores,
> And even a fool is silent and adores.[5]

To another friend, Sidney Colvin, he tempered his enthusiasm for 'Catholic virtues' somewhat:

> The passbook kept with heaven stirs me to anger and laughter. One of the sisters calls the place 'the ticket office to heaven'. Well, what is the odds? They do their darg [day's work], and do it with kindness and efficiency incredible; and we must take folk's virtues as we find them, and love the better part.

All this by way of preamble to a thumbnail sketch of the man who put Molokai on the map and acted like a magnet to visitors such as RLS himself:

> Of old Damien, whose weaknesses and worse perhaps I heard fully, I think only the more. It was a European peasant: dirty, bigoted, untruthful, unwise, tricky, but superb with generosity, residual candour and fundamental good-humour: convince him he had done wrong (it might take hours of insult) and he would undo what he had done and like his corrector better. A man, with all the grime and paltriness of mankind, but a saint and hero all the more for that.[6]

That might have been it as far as Stevenson was concerned – eight days and seven nights in a place he had been drawn to but dreaded visiting, over which a 'horror of moral beauty broods' (a phrase he partially disowned as 'bad Victor Hugo'),[7] and which in the end he was glad to leave – had it not been for a certain Dr Hyde.

Rev. Dr Charles McEwen Hyde was the very model of a New England Protestant missionary, a pillar of the new Hawaiian establishment, the ruling *haole* Reform Movement. Mouritz describes him as 'scholarly, polished, and refined; belong[ing] to the best class of Americans . . . He rather reminded me of a college proctor or don, such as we have in European universities, or even the rector of the same institution'.[8] When asked his opinion of the celebrated Father Damien by the Rev. H.B. Gage, a fellow cleric in San Francisco, Hyde wrote in a private letter that the recipient promptly published:

> The simple truth is, he was a coarse, dirty man, headstrong and bigoted. He was not sent to Molokai, but went there without orders . . . He had no

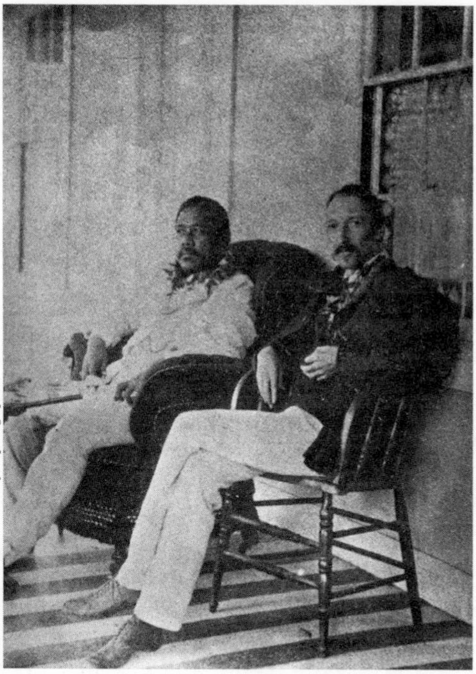
(Hawaii State Archives, unidentified photographer)

Robert Louis Stevenson with King Kalakaua

> hand in the reforms and improvements, which were the work of our Board of Health . . . He was not a pure man in his relations with women, and the leprosy of which he died should be attributed to his vices and carelessness . . .[9]

The quixotic Stevenson, who was by then in Australia, read these words in the Sydney *Presbyterian* and fired off a rebuttal in the form of an open letter to the Rev. Dr Hyde (whom he'd met in Honolulu), which was published and republished until it became part of the Damien myth.

Given that he himself had heard similar things on Molokai, Stevenson accepts many of the epithets Hyde used to describe Damien but turns them against the fastidious Hyde. He does not so much defend Damien (some devout readers have been as offended by his apologia as by the letter that occasioned it) as attack Hyde. He depicts the plump missionary sitting in the comfort of his Beretania Street house – which the cab driver who'd taken Stevenson there had envied for its size and luxuriousness – and affecting a cultural and religious superiority to a better man than he:

> . . . when we sit and grow bulky in our charming mansions, and a plain, uncouth peasant steps into the battle, under the eyes of God, and succours the afflicted, and consoles the dying, and is himself afflicted in his turn, and dies upon the field of honour – the battle can not be retrieved as your unhappy irritation has suggested. It is a lost battle, and lost forever.

He chides Dr Hyde for never having set foot on Molokai: 'If you had, and had recalled it, and looked about your pleasant rooms, even your pen perhaps would have stayed.' He makes much of his own brief experience on the island by way of contrast, saying of Hyde:

> I imagine you to be one of those persons who talk with cheerfulness of that place which oxen and wainropes could not drag you to behold. You, who do not even know its situation on the map, probably denounce sensational descriptions, stretching your limbs the while in your pleasant parlour on Beretania Street . . .[10]

There is much more in the same vein. The gist of Stevenson's accusation is that Hyde is really ashamed of the fact that it was an upstart Catholic, not one of God's own New England Protestants, who set an example of Christian charity, and therefore seeks to belittle the man he secretly envies. It is a powerful, but flawed, polemic. If you argue *ad hominem* you must make sure you get your facts right, and RLS was wrong about Hyde. Hyde had been to the leprosy settlement on Molokai in 1885 and would go again; he had met Damien and admired what he was doing to the extent of using his influence with wealthy parishioners in Honolulu to raise money to build new orphanages for the boys and girls at Kalawao. Illogically, since he believed his friend Dr Fitch that leprosy resulted from licentiousness and he himself led an exemplary personal life, Hyde had a deep personal fear of contracting the disease. Indeed, a year before he visited Molokai he was in an agony of apprehension when he developed a rash after donning clothes that had been washed in a Chinese laundry.[11] It turned out not to be leprosy, of course, but in the circumstances it took some courage for him to go to Kalawao. So whatever else he might have been, Hyde was scarcely the armchair critic of his betters that Stevenson had portrayed.

Hyde was devastated by Stevenson's attack – 'I have received the worst blow of my life,' he said after reading it.[12] But in public, at least, he adopted an attitude of *sang-froid*, dismissing the author as 'a Bohemian crank, a negligible person, whose opinion is of no value to anyone'. Although he complained to friends that his own letter had been published without his permission, he never retracted anything he had written about Damien but repeated his accusations, maintaining that Stevenson had merely confirmed them. Charles Dutton comments wryly:

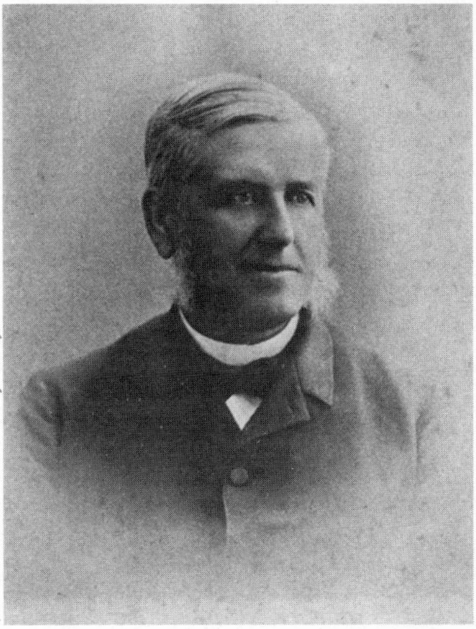
(Hawaiian Children's Mission Society Library)

Rev. Dr Charles McEwen Hyde

> If – that is – Damien washed none too often, that proves that he was immoral. If he came from the peasant class, that proved that his leprosy was the result of syphilis. If he was bigoted, then of course he deserved no credit for having reformed conditions on Molokai. There is a certain charm in such a line of reasoning.[13]

The question is, why did Hyde turn against Damien between September 1885, when he referred to him in print as 'that noble-hearted Catholic priest . . . whose work has been so successful'[14] and August 1889, when he dismissed him so contemptuously in his letter to the Rev. H.B. Gage? Three reasons suggest themselves: one, that Damien's apotheosis in the world's press, by eclipsing the work done by other sects at the settlement, had kindled his resentment; two, that he was influenced by the persistent rumours suggesting Damien's personal habits were in marked contrast to his public image; and three, that if leprosy was, as Hyde so firmly believed, the product of a licentious lifestyle linked to syphilis, then Damien's developing it surely confirmed those nagging rumours. According to one of Damien's biographers, Gavan Daws:

> it was leprosy that made for Hyde's ultimate difficulty with Damien. To Hyde, who could never permit himself to link sanctity with dirt, the self-surrender of Damien, who made himself a 'leper', was not only repellent

> but somehow morally perverse. Hyde could never have made a sacrifice that matched Damien's.[15]

Hyde finally overplayed his hand, making a specific allegation that could be checked. He claimed that Damien had contracted leprosy before he went to Molokai in his parish on the island of Hawaii, where he 'left behind him an unsavory reputation'. It turned out that it wasn't Damien but his successor on Hawaii who had been accused of immorality and was taken to court in 1880. When he learned of his mistake, Hyde made no effort to withdraw his false accusation but simply kept quiet and the facts were not published till well after his death in 1899. In his last years he became an isolated, self-pitying figure, a 'leper' himself as he saw it, even a martyr:

> No one in this world can know with what stress of pain I have taken the stand I have maintained as a witness for the truth, assailed on the one hand by the arrogant pretentiousness of the Roman hierarchy, and betrayed on the other by the fanciful falsities of sentimental humanitarianism.

Yet if his initial letter had never been published, or had not come to Stevenson's attention and aroused his withering scorn, Hyde might have lived out his life in decent semi-obscurity, continuing to perform modest good works. As it was, when there was an outbreak of cholera in Honolulu in 1895, he volunteered his services as an inspector and patrolled the streets in an affected area.[16] He was not a bad man, merely one whose imaginative sympathies did not extend far enough to encompass a saint who didn't conform to his idea of sanctity or to appeal to an exceptional writer who was also exceptionally popular.

Stevenson was not the only famous writer drawn to Molokai by the Damien legend; Jack London was another. London visited Kalaupapa in 1906 and wrote several short stories featuring leprosy, which dramatise western fear and loathing of the disease and, by extension, its victims. But there is one story – 'Koolau the Leper' – which, though it too lays on the horror with a trowel, is told from the point of view of a leprosy sufferer on the island of Kauai who holes up in the hills with a motley crew of other sufferers and shoots anyone who attempts to capture him, rather than submit to segregation on Molokai. The eponymous hero actually existed and, though the story is considerably embellished, it is based on a real incident recorded by Arthur Mouritz, among others.

Mouritz prefaces his account of 'The Leper War on Kauai' with the remark that armed resistance to deportation was rare: perhaps a dozen cases over a period of thirty years, the 'most serious and successful' of which was this one. It took place in the remote mountain valley of Kalalau in the northwest corner of Kauai during the first week of July 1893. A month earlier, Mouritz recalls, he had been enjoying a yarn with his friend Marshal Edward G. Hitchcock in the Merchant Street police station in Honolulu when a slightly built man in his late thirties was ushered into the office. Hitchcock, whose short way of dealing with offenders had earned him the nickname of 'The Holy Terror', introduced the visitor as Deputy Sheriff Louis H. Stolz of Kauai and told him (in Mouritz's presence):

> Stolz, you had better wait a little until I can spare you some of my foreign police officers, you cannot trust your Hawaiian officers, just as things are at present [with the Americans consolidating their hold on Hawaii by deposing the last Hawaiian monarch, Queen Liliuokalani]. You are foolish to think of going alone to Kalalau, because I hear the people and lepers in that valley are practising target shooting. Let this leper business go over for the present, we are not yet out of the woods in Honolulu.[17]

The marshal urged Stolz to wait a month or two, and then he would join him. But Stolz objected that the stretch of coast at Kalalau became surf-bound at the end of September, making access almost impossible. Whatever the reason, Stolz's impatience got the better of him once he returned to Kauai; he ignored Hitchcock's advice, armed himself with a Winchester rifle and announced that he was going after Koolau, who had a reputation as a marksman. Using local guides, he approached a hideout where Koolau was waiting for him. Koolau challenged the deputy sheriff, 'Stolz, you have a gun, are you after me?' Stolz admitted that he was. Koolau took aim and shot him in the stomach, severely wounding him, then called out to the Hawaiians near Stolz to ask if he were dead; when they said no, he fired again. This time he made no mistake; the deputy sheriff was killed instantly. 'This story', Mouritz insists, 'came to me from the lips of eye witnesses, some of whom were with Koolau. They were lepers, and I met them at Kalaupapa three months after the shooting.' Mouritz was convinced that the local guides had deliberately led Stolz into an ambush.[18]

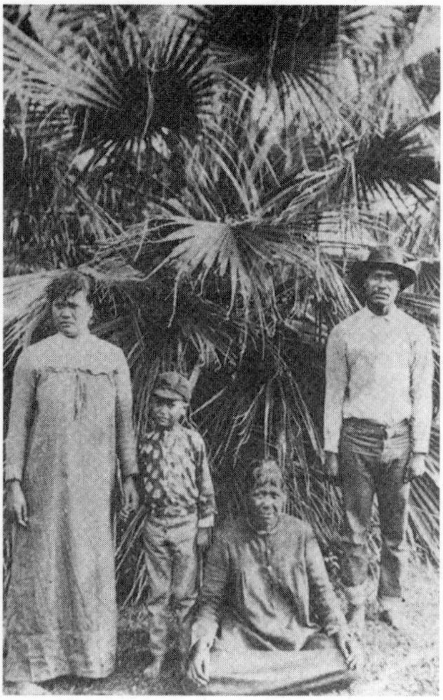

(*Hawaii State Archives, unidentified photographer*)

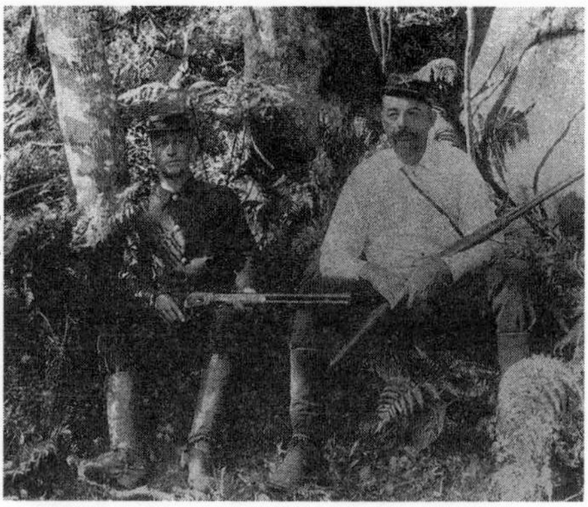

(*Hawaii State Archives, unidentified photographer*)

(*Left*) The outlawed marksman Koolau with his family in 1893. (*Above*) Troops sent to apprehend Koolau

Koolau was now doubly an outlaw, wanted for murder as well as for leprosy. The *haole* government despatched a platoon of soldiers with a field gun to capture him. He was encamped with his wife Piilani and son (the son also had leprosy), on a narrow ledge high up one side of the valley – an impregnable position well camouflaged by the dense tropical vegetation. In such a terrain a field gun was virtually useless and the soldiers attempting to scale the ridge provided a sitting target for such a skilled marksman as Koolau. He picked off one on the first day of the assault and another the next day (a third soldier was shot through the brain from under the chin, but the angle of entry of the bullet suggests that this was an accident). After that the government gave up, recalled the soldiers and left Koolau and his family to their own devices.[19] They remained hidden in the valley for a couple of years, during which first the son died and then Koolau himself. Piilani then returned home and was eventually persuaded by a sympathetic *haole* to tell him her story. Its publication in 1906 inspired Jack London to write his version and more recently the poet W.S. Merwin has made of it an epic novel in verse.

Piilani's story is essentially that of a family that wanted to stay together. Koolau would have accepted his fate and gone to Molokai if he could have taken his wife as well as his son. But that had been denied him; at that time, when the law of segregation was being rigorously enforced, there was no place for *kokuas* at Kalaupapa (and no Damien either to make the case for married *kokuas*); leprosy had indeed become the 'separating sickness'. In his story, London transforms Koolau into a kind of Ned Kelly, an outlaw rebel with a cause, urging his tattered band of grotesques to make a stand against the 'men who preached the word of God and the word of Rum [and] brought the [Chinese] sickness with the coolie slaves who work the stolen land'. His Koolau is a rabble-rousing demagogue preaching the gospel of 'Hawaii for the Hawaiians'. But he is also a loner; there is no mention of a wife or child. He kills not in self-defence but in anger at the injustice of it all, as an avenging angel. And his own people ultimately betray him, one of them cursing him as they troop off to Molokai, defeated.[20]

W.S. Merwin's *The Folding Cliffs* sticks much closer to the original.[21] For a start, its central figure is not Koolau but the storyteller, Piilani. It is no less political, or anti-colonial, than London's story, but the tone is elegiac: a lament for a lost way of life. It might almost be described as a work of anthropology in verse, with its sensitive evocation of a dying culture – except for the brooding inwardness that provides its poetic power, the feeling that, yes, this is how it must have been. There is no ranting of the kind that mars 'Koolau the Leper', in which the protagonist seems more like a displaced westerner than a native Hawaiian.

During Jack London's 1906 visit to Molokai he met Brother Joseph Dutton. Dutton was unimpressed by the writer. He grumbled in a letter: 'The less said about London's visit, the better. After all, these people see the colony only for a few hours or days and know little about it.' In another letter, he wrote:

> There is much public misapprehension regarding Molokai. It is no longer a pest-hole, no longer a place of suffering . . . Writers picture horrors, mostly in their own minds. Perhaps the world likes to hear of horrors more than of cheer. But it's not what it was in Damien's day, or when I first came. Up to 1902 or 1903 things [were] not good here; after that a great change [took place], until today the place [is] as orderly, as happy, as any spot in the world . . .[22]

In other words, once Uncle Sam took it over it became the best of all possible worlds – it was now called 'Molokai the Blest', the patriotic

Dutton proudly told the Governor of Hawaii in 1908. That was the year in which the federal government began a building project at Kalawao that would take nearly two years to complete and cost the then huge sum of $300,000. This complex, consisting of hospital wards, research laboratories and handsome houses for doctors, technicians and their families, as well as dwellings for a number of Chinese servants, stables for horses and sheds for cows, was called the United States Leprosy Investigation Station, or USLIS for short – an unfortunate and, as it turned out, all-too-accurate acronym. Patients and staff at Kalaupapa stood outside the two high barbed-wire fences surrounding these gleaming structures and gawped in amazement when the electricity was turned on for the first time, flooding them with light (Kalaupapa itself would not acquire electric lights until 1931[23]). But neither patients nor staff were invited to attend the official opening on Christmas Eve 1909.[24]

The message could hardly have been plainer: this palace of science was dedicated to research, not to the welfare or cure of leprosy patients. Tragically, nobody took the trouble to explain to the patients that you couldn't have one without the other. So by the time the doctors and technicians were ready to lower the barricades and invite the people it was designed to benefit into their sanitised environment, the patients boycotted it; scarcely anyone volunteered to act as a guinea pig and the few that did were so alienated by the clinical surroundings, chemical smells, face masks and rubber gloves, the lack of companions, the sheer boredom of life in a bare hospital ward, that they escaped as fast as they could.[25]

This is how a visitor in 1916 saw it:

> At Kalawao we alighted to inspect the federal leprosarium. Not a room, not an alcove, not a workshop of the great congeries of buildings escaped us. 'But nothing in the sounding halls he saw.' The leprosarium has been finished for seven or eight years, and for only some six weeks of that time has it harboured patients. Four or five caretakers keep the frame of it from utter ruin; but, except for the vast laboratory where the federal physician (absent on leave in the States at the time of our visit) struggles heroically with what to a scientist must be very like despair, the place is disused . . . Even the uninformed visitor must feel bitterness to see the dynamo purring as vainly as a cat by the fire, when, a few miles away, the Settlement itself, the homes, the nursery, the very hospital must do with lamps and candles because the Territorial government cannot afford a dynamo. The truth is

> that the leprosarium was 'queered' in the early days of its being, and since then the federal appropriation has been greatly cut down – not unnaturally, since no apparent results came from the larger sum . . . Not without relief did we turn from this grave of humanitarian hopes . . .[26]

Though the research station had closed in 1911, this white elephant remained standing for a further eighteen years, a monument to the mutual misunderstanding and mistrust between *haole* and *kanaka*, coloniser and colonised, that characterises the history of leprosy – and much else besides – in nineteenth- and early twentieth-century Hawaii.

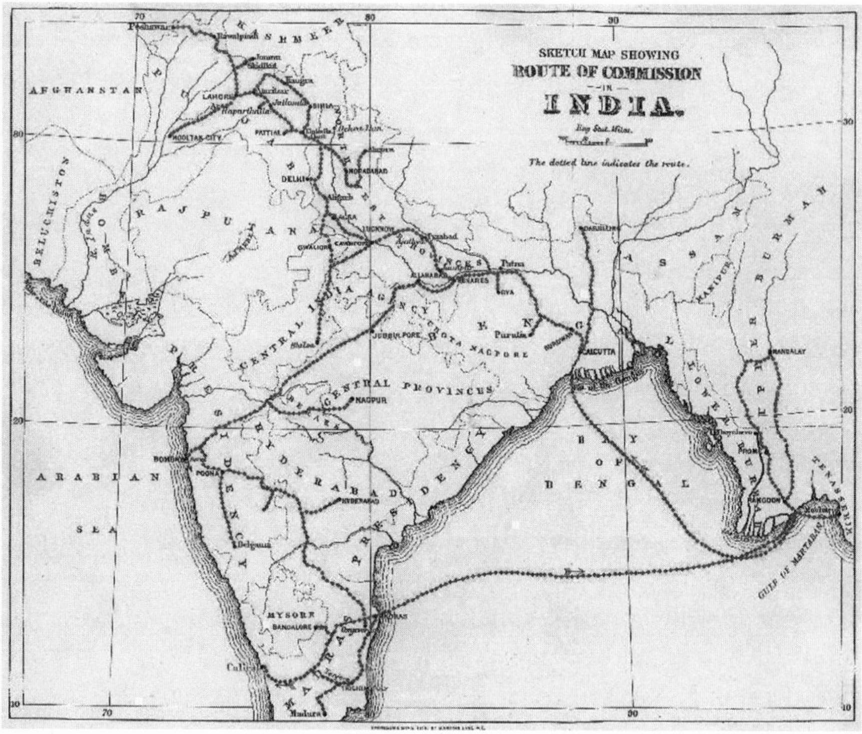

(from 'Leprosy in India: Report of the Leprosy Commission in India, 1890–91)

Map of India, giving the route followed by
the Indian Leprosy Commission in 1890

Chapter 5

AN IMPERIAL DANGER

Nowhere outside Molokai did the death of Father Damien in 1889 have such a strong impact as in England. A 'Father Damien' Memorial Fund was immediately set up with a committee of the great and good, headed by no less a personage than the Prince of Wales. Its aims were threefold: to commemorate the martyr saint with a monument placed over his earthly remains on Molokai (though these were later removed to his native Belgium); to encourage the study of leprosy by opening a 'leper ward' in London, to be attached to a hospital or school of medicine there, and by endowing one or more travelling scholarships; and to instigate a 'full and complete inquiry into the question of leprosy in India'.[1] This last objective, in particular, chimed in with the public mood of apprehension – to put it no stronger – over the 'imperial danger' associated with the disease. These were the words Archdeacon Henry Press Wright, rector of Greatham in Hampshire, used in the title of a book he compiled, *Leprosy: An Imperial Danger*, which was published (appropriately enough) in the year of Damien's death. Wright wrote in the introduction:

> I believe that leprosy is by far the most trying malady that has ever afflicted man, and that, in these days of general travel and easy intercommunication of nations, there is a possibility, nay a great probability (unless due care be taken) of its again assailing Europe and the British Isles.[2]

This was the nub of the matter. If leprosy was indeed a contagious disease – no matter that, in the words of a *British Medical Journal* editorial of 15 June 1889, it might well be 'the least frequently contagious of all known contagious diseases'[3] – then in these days of wholesale migrations of peoples brought about by colonial activities it would surely not be long before those European countries that thought they had rid themselves of this scourge centuries before had to face up to it again. Hadn't the Prince of Wales himself, in his speech proposing the Damien memorial scheme, alluded to 'a leper with his hands distinctly affected by the disease, engaged in his business in one of the large London meat markets' (identified, in a subsequent number of the *BMJ* as Edward Yoxall, a butcher)?[4]

Nor was this the first apparently home-grown case to be noted in London during Victoria's reign. In 1868 Johanna Crawley, an Irishwoman of fifty-four, who had lived for thirty years in Stepney beside the Limehouse basin, just half a mile from both the West India and the East India docks, featured in *Guy's Hospital Reports* as a case of leprosy. Her body and limbs were covered in large brown patches; she had lost part of the little finger on her right hand and had no feeling in her arms up to the elbows. Her face was described as puffy, her lips and ears as swollen. Dr W. Munro, who wrote a series of articles on leprosy in the *Edinburgh Medical Journal* a decade later, enquired after Johanna in Stepney and learned from her daughter that she had died in 1874, after losing 'a part of *all* her fingers and toes':

> Although undoubtedly indigenous, I cannot look upon this case as necessarily an autochthonous one, although, from the information given me by Mrs Suckling [the daughter], I could not trace any actual source of infection, as her mother never, as she remembers, kept lodgers, and her father had never been abroad, – but Johanna was a sailmaker, working in a factory with many others, and living in a district crowded with people *in constant communication* with the East and West Indies and in which there are many coloured people . . .[5]

The Rev. Henry Wright urged that every case of leprosy in England should be reported to the authorities and registered, so that a careful check might be kept on the progress of the disease: 'If it return not to its old haunts, well; but if there be any sign of such return, then active precautions should be speedily taken that the plague may be stayed.'[6]

But the medical profession was resistant to the idea of making leprosy a notifiable disease in Britain (and would remain so for another sixty years). As the *BMJ* editorial cited above put it:

> It is well to bear in mind that lepers have freely moved about in this country, have been received into general hospitals and have mixed freely

with other patients, and that neither in London nor Paris does it appear that a single case of contagion has occurred.

True, there had been a strange case in Ireland where a man who had only ever left the country once (to visit England) had developed the disease; but the circumstances had been most unusual in that he had for a year and a half shared a bed and clothes with his brother, who'd contracted leprosy after living for many years in the West Indies. Those were hardly grounds for the introduction of 'panic-stricken legislation'. But it was different in a country like India, where leprosy was rife: 'the practice of partial segregation, in itself surely a good thing, could be and should be at once extended.'[7]

In India itself, opinions were mixed. Surgeon-Major Henry Vandyke Carter, the doctor who'd gone on a fact-finding tour of Norway in the early 1870s, was now a convinced segregationist. He foresaw that objections would be made to the construction of asylums in India:

It may be said that the natives themselves have not asked for the intervention of Government: that the majority of executive and other officials have not expressed the necessity of intervention: that the design of leper-asylums for the whole country is novel, costly, ill-suited to the character of the people, and after all not certain of success: and that for carrying it out special agency might be required; perhaps fresh laws needed.

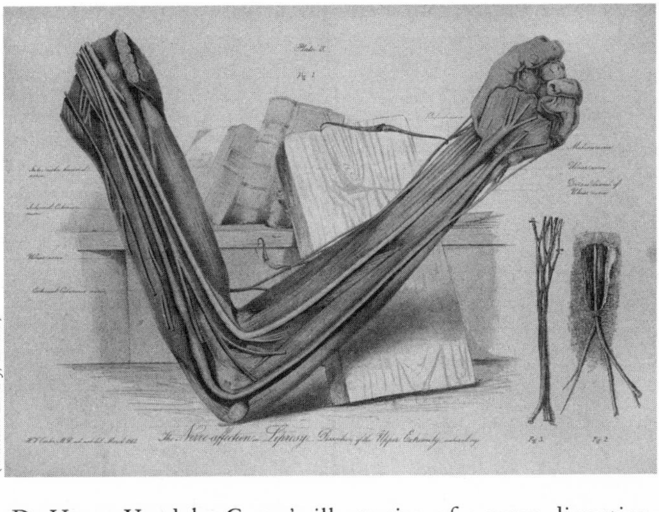

(Wellcome Library, London)

Dr Henry Vandyke Carter's illustration of a nerve dissection he carried out on a leprosy-affected upper limb

But he dismissed all these objections, asserting 'that the malady under notice is an altogether peculiar one in severity and extent, and claims special consideration'.[8]

Carter was particularly concerned about the susceptibility to leprosy of European residents in India. At present, there might be relatively few cases (he had recently seen three 'well-marked instances . . . a boy at school, a young woman, and an adult military man'), 'but present immunity (or comparative immunity) may not continue under circumstances so much changing as those we live in, in these days of increasing social contact with the native-born'. Indeed, if so many medical authorities were warning of the danger to England presented by the importation of an infinitesimal number of leprosy sufferers, then how much more 'would prudence dictate that Europeans permanently living in India should be careful of their surroundings'.[9]

Soon after his return to India in 1875, Carter enlisted the help of private subscribers to set up an asylum for about 150 'pauper lepers' outside Bombay, to be officially opened by the Prince of Wales. In a vast country where the number of leprosy sufferers was known (through census figures) to be over 100,000 and reckoned to be more like 250,000 all told, this initiative would barely scratch the surface of the problem; as the viceroy Lord Dufferin told Edward Clifford (when the latter was in India en route to Hawaii to visit Father Damien), 'one might as readily undertake to rid India of its snakes as of its leprosy'.[10] But as Carter saw it, it was a gesture in the right direction. Unfortunately, it remained a gesture, since the government of Bombay preferred to mark the prince's visit by erecting a statue of him mounted on a black horse (which has long since been removed from its original site and relocated in the Mumbai zoological gardens).[11]

What was perhaps the first leprosy asylum in British India was opened back in the 1840s at Almora in the Himalayan state of Kumaon. The credit for setting this up and supporting it should go to General Sir Henry Ramsay, Commissioner of the North West Provinces, who was then a lowly lieutenant. In 1877 this asylum was visited by two doctors, T.R. Lewis and D.D. Cunningham, billed as 'Special Assistants to the Sanitary Commissioner with the Government of India' – whose report therefore carried considerable weight. They noted 'a very interesting experiment is now in progress at Almora': this was an orphanage for a dozen children, one or both of whose parents had leprosy. The children

> have been removed from the surroundings under which the disease manifested itself in their parents, have been well fed and carefully attended to, and their subsequent history cannot but throw light on the extent to which the influence of heredity can exert itself, or may be modified and kept in abeyance by ameliorated conditions of life.[12]

(It is not clear whether or not these children were separated from their parents *at birth*, but this experiment predates Dr Arning's Hawaiian initiative by at least a decade.)

Unlike Carter, Lewis and Cunningham found 'no satisfactory evidence of contagion and none of a rapid *increase* of cases due to hereditary influences' (italic in the original). Certainly, the prevalence of the disease remained high enough to justify efforts to reduce it. But the 'means for effecting this can hardly be looked for in attempts at forcible repression of the disease, such as the compulsory imprisonment of lepers in Asylums'. Not only did this reek of 'tyranny'; it was also impractical in that it 'would not be sufficient merely to confine those suffering from developed disease'. Lewis and Cunningham believed in heredity, and posed the question: 'had all those predisposed to be secured, how and by whom could the existence of predisposition be determined?' Yet that 'Asylums, properly so called, are very useful and desirable institutions in districts where chronic diseases like leprosy prevail, is just as true as that prisons ought not to be substituted for them'.[13]

In opposing compulsory isolation, Lewis and Cunningham endorsed the conclusions of the Royal College of Physicians' 1867 report on leprosy. But in the wake of Hansen's discovery of *M. leprae* many doctors were coming to regard this weighty tome as *un*authoritative and thoroughly pernicious. In an article of 1889 entitled 'The Dreadful Revival of Leprosy', Sir Morell Mackenzie went so far as to say that by giving official support to the view that leprosy was not contagious it had 'probably done more to propagate the disease than any other single agency since the Crusades'. For Mackenzie, an ear, nose and throat specialist whose mishandling of the German crown prince's throat cancer was to bring him some notoriety, there was no mystery over leprosy's mode of transmission: 'The evidence in favour of contagion is to my mind quite overwhelming. The contagiousness of the disease was never doubted till it had nearly died out; men ceased to believe in contagion when they no longer saw daily instances of it.'[14]

He rehearsed what he called the 'miserable story' of the involvement of the Royal College of Physicians; how in 1862 as a result of an expression of alarm at the spread of leprosy in Barbados the Colonial Office had sought the advice of the RCP, and the RCP had drawn up a questionnaire to be circulated to medical officers and other officials throughout the British empire and dependent territories, the resulting evidence from which would be sifted by a committee appointed by it. The trouble was, there were only two physicians on this committee with even the slightest practical acquaintance with the disease: 'One of them, the late Dr Owen Rees, had met with one remarkable case [that of Johanna Crawley, outlined above], and another, Dr Gavin Milroy, paid a hurried visit to Demerara, where he was egregiously hoaxed even by dull-witted lepers.'[15]

Milroy was the most influential figure on the committee and its spokesman; he was also a member of the anti-contagionist 'sanitarian' lobby that was so active in Victorian Britain. Sanitarians believed that poor diet and unhygienic conditions – not contagion – were responsible for many diseases, including cholera; quarantine was therefore unnecessary, if not completely useless. So when he visited the penal settlement at Demerara in British Guiana and heard from a leprosy sufferer that his disease was the result of the salt diet the prisoners were given, he believed him and ignored the fact that the man's wife and child both had leprosy, too.[16] Unsurprisingly then, with only a quarter of the number of replies that would eventually be received to the RCP questionnaire on leprosy in, Milroy and his committee were already advising the government that they contained 'no evidence which in their opinion justifies any measures for the compulsory segregation of lepers'.[17] This incensed Sir Morell Mackenzie: that 'incompetent' judges, taking the word of 'untrustworthy' witnesses, many of whom 'knew little and cared less about the disease', should arrive at unjustifiable conclusions 'that led at once to practical consequences of the most far-reaching importance':

> The measures devised by humane and enlightened statesmen for the mitigation of the scourge were abandoned; the leper-houses throughout Her Majesty's dominions were thrown open, each discharging its measure of pollution into the stream of healthy life near it; and a general relaxation of sanitary discipline with regard to leprosy supervened [one in the eye for the sanitarians there!]. It may without much exaggeration be said that if leprosy slew its thousands before, it has slain its tens of thousands within the confines of the British Empire since 1867.[18]

In fact, in India during the decade 1881–91 there was a reduction in the number of leprosy sufferers recorded in the census from 120,000 to 110,000. Though both these figures may be underestimates and leprosy may well not have decreased, it was certainly not increasing in the manner Mackenzie – 'without much exaggeration' – was suggesting.

When Dr N.C. Macnamara, of the Bengal Medical Service, subjected the hundred or more Indian replies to the RCP questionnaire to independent analysis, he reached a very different conclusion from Milroy and his committee. He found plenty of support for the view that the disease was contagious and inoculable, and that 'neither climate, kinds of food, nor filthy habits are capable of generating leprosy'.[19] But as Mackenzie said of the RCP committee:

> . . . like their prototypes in *Tristram Shandy*, 'they concerned themselves not with facts – they reasoned.' . . . Sterne must have foreseen these learned Thebans when he described the disputations of the Strasburg doctors: ' "It happens otherwise," replied the opponents. "It ought not," said they.'[20]

In the nineteenth century the British established their hegemony in India piecemeal; the transformation of the swashbuckling trader-soldiers of the East India Company into the 'heaven-born' civil administrators of the British Raj was a gradual process involving an ever-increasing assumption of moral authority along with political power, the turning point being the suppression of the sepoy rebellion known as the Indian Mutiny in 1857 and the subsequent takeover of the country by the crown. Traditional Hindu or Muslim practices that had been tolerated as 'native customs' in the days of the 'John Company' came under critical scrutiny once the British began to regard it as their destiny to rule India. The self-immolation of widows on their husbands' funeral pyres, known as *sati* (or 'suttee' in Anglo-Indian parlance), was an example of a Hindu custom that the British found so repugnant that they outlawed it as early as 1829. The 'assisted' suicide of advanced leprosy sufferers was another traditional practice that caused concern.

In 1812 the early Baptist missionary William Carey happened upon the 'burning of a leper' at Katwa, in Bengal. He described the process: first, a fire was lighted at the bottom of a deep pit; then the man rolled himself into it but the moment he felt the flames he began to struggle and beg to be helped out; his pleas were resisted by his mother and sister, however, who, far from rescuing him, thrust him back into the flames. Though Carey was appalled at the cruelty of doing away with a man 'who to all appearances might have survived several years', he explained that this

> poor wretch died, with the notion that by thus purifying his body in the fire, he should receive a happy transmigration into a healthful body; whereas, if he had died by the disease, he would after four births, have appeared on earth again as a leper.[21]

Another pioneer Baptist missionary in Bengal, William Ward, witnessed the drowning of a man who'd lost his fingers and toes to leprosy but otherwise appeared to be in good health, also in 1812. From the boat on which he was travelling Ward couldn't tell whether the man had gone into the water of his own accord or had been pushed. All he knew for certain was that, despite the man's struggles, the current carried him far out into the river and eventually he sank. Once again, the victim seems to have been a party to his own fate, since he was seen 'eating very heartily in the presence of his friends' before he drowned.[22]

By the 1840s, when the British annexed the Punjab following the Sikh Wars, the new breed of high-minded and mostly very young administrators groomed by the Lawrence brothers, Henry and John, were no longer content to observe and record native customs; they had such confidence in their own sense of rectitude that if they didn't like what they saw they intervened. A typical example was Robert Needham Cust, who wrote of himself:

> I was appointed District Officer of one of the newly annexed Provinces of the Jalandhar Doab, Hoshyarpur, at the age of twenty-five, with a salary of £1,200 per annum. I took charge on April 6, 1846, and met for the first time my great Master, John Lawrence, with whom I was officially connected till the day of my leaving India, December 1867 . . . I built myself a small house in a beautiful garden. I issued the famous Three Commandments:
>
> 'Thou shalt not burn thy widows;
> 'Thou shalt not kill thy daughters;
> 'Thou shalt not bury alive thy lepers.'[23]

These 'commandments' are often attributed to John Lawrence himself, and they certainly bear the stamp of his overweening personality. But if the evangelical rulers of the Punjab, who became a role model for British Indian civil servants in general, were against the burying alive of leprosy sufferers in a literal sense, they – or their successors – were quite happy to bury them alive metaphorically, in asylums, whether or not they believed in the contagiousness of leprosy. Assisted suicides of advanced cases of leprosy may have struck them as barbarous, but the proliferation of these unsightly sufferers in public places offended their sense of decorum and constituted 'a public nuisance', requiring legal action.

On 6 April 1889, for instance, the *Bombay Gazette* carried a report of a meeting of the Bombay Municipal Corporation in which an educational inspector, T.B. Kirkham, described how 'a colony of lepers had taken up their abode on the flagstones surrounding the large Nacoda Tank', a body of water separating two educational establishments for which he was responsible, the Elphinstone High School and St Xavier's College, and were 'dressing their terrible sores with stones lying about them, and then flinging away those stones, to be picked up or trodden upon by anyone'. The police had no powers to arrest them; they might move them on, but a couple of days later they would be back again. Kirkham called this 'the artificial propagation of leprosy' and questioned whether such people should be allowed to do as they pleased in such close proximity to 2,000 young men and boys.

Dr Arnott of the Health Department admitted that they were 'utterly powerless to interfere in the matter' and, citing Dr Vandyke Carter as an authority on leprosy 'who deserved respectful attention', said how Carter 'had over and over again urged the pressing necessity of providing suitable asylums for lepers, and taking measures to prevent their being a danger to the community', but to little avail. The coroner, Dr Blaney, told the meeting that every year he had to give orders for the disposal of a dozen or so bodies of leprosy victims who had either died on the roadside or drowned themselves in wells:

> He said he did not think there was a single well on the Esplanade in which a leper was not drowned. All over Bombay, in dark corners, in gullies, where rats and bandicoots had taken their abode, these lepers were hiding themselves, thrown out by their families, to pine away neglected and forlorn. Lepers were to be seen in all parts of the city, and not at the Elphinstone School and the St. Xavier's College alone.[24]

Local pressure to introduce anti-leprosy legislation was resisted by central government on the grounds of cost. The initiative the Father Damien Memorial Fund (renamed the National Leprosy Fund) took in creating the Indian Leprosy Commission in 1890 was seen as a heaven-sent opportunity to postpone any action 'for the present'. (See chapter frontispiece for map of the route.) In the course of its deliberations, the government noted how divided public opinion in India was, with Indians questioning the need for segregation and concerned about the possibility of misdiagnosis and its consequences, while Europeans and Eurasians clamoured for more stringent measures than it was prepared to consider.[25]

The composition of the Indian Leprosy Commission suggested that the Royal College of Physicians was up to its old tricks again. There were three doctors appointed in London and two in India. Four out of the five had no previous experience of leprosy, and the one who did, Dr Beavan Rake of the Trinidad leprosy asylum, an RCP nominee, was a known sceptic in the matter of the contagiousness of leprosy (and he it was who became chairman of the commission). He had been a leader of the diehards who'd challenged the unanimous finding of the thirteen experts who made up the 1875 British Guiana Commission that leprosy was indeed contagious. Rake even questioned whether Damien's leprosy arose out of contagion, arguing that the priest might have 'absorbed the specific virus . . . in many other ways, e.g., in food, water, air, etc'.[26] (Though the words *contagion* and *infection* have become virtually interchangeable, in the nineteenth century contagion meant transmission through direct contact, or touch, while infection involved a medium such as air or water. Similarly, *heredity* covered a multitude of meanings from some structural bodily defect or abnormality to a morbid tendency towards a disease that would manifest itself only later in life, characterised as a 'hereditary predisposition', and including atavism, which was the term used when a disease was thought to 'skip a generation'.[27])

The commissioners produced a curiously contradictory report, which they concluded by saying that '*no legislation is called for on the lines either of segregation, or of interdiction of marriages with lepers*' – a kind of a-plague-on-both-your-houses to contagionists and anti-contagionists alike. They saw no occasion for an Imperial Act directed against leprosy sufferers, 'for these are far less dangerous to a community than insane or syphilitic people'. Yet in the same breath they suggested that 'municipal authorities be empowered to pass by-laws preventing vagrants suffering from loathsome diseases from begging in or frequenting places of public resort, or using public conveyances', and recommended 'the adoption of a voluntary isolation as extensive as local circumstances allow'.[28]

If the commissioners are to be congratulated for not allowing themselves to be panicked into criminalizing leprosy, they are open to criticism on the grounds of inconsistency. As no less an authority than Hansen pointed out in a generally temperate critique:

> The position of the Commissioners as regards leprosy is that of those who will not admit the propagation of tuberculosis to be dependent on contagion, or, let me say, bacillary infection; they will not concede isolation to be a necessity, but, unable to deny its use, they are willing to go half-way.[29]

For better or worse, though, the legislative recommendations made by the commissioners would form the basis of the government of India's Lepers Act, 1898.

This provided 'for the segregation and medical treatment of pauper lepers and the control of lepers following certain callings'. A 'pauper leper' was defined as one '(a) who publicly solicits alms or exposes or exhibits any sores, wounds, bodily ailment or deformity with the object of exciting charity or of obtaining alms, or (b) who is at large without any ostensible means of subsistence'. The police were licensed to arrest any such person without a warrant, and local governments were empowered to prevent leprosy sufferers from trading in food, drink, drugs or

Extract from the Abstract of the Proceedings of the Council of the Governor General of India, assembled for the purpose of making Laws and Regulations under the provisions of the Indian Councils Acts, 1861 and 1892 (24 & 25 Vict., cap. 67, and 55 & 56 Vict., cap. 14).

The Council met at the Viceregal Lodge, Simla, on Thursday, the 30th July, 1896.

* * * * * * *

LEPERS BILL.

The Hon'ble MR. WOODBURN moved for leave to introduce a Bill to provide for the segregation of pauper lepers and the control of lepers following certain callings. He said:—"In 1890-91 a Leprosy Commission visited India, and a couple of years later submitted a Report to the Government of India pressing upon it very earnestly two questions—the segregation of lepers and the restraint of lepers in certain callings in which they were brought into immediate contact with the food or the clothing of their neighbours. The Government of Bombay had already taken action in that direction with the help of a very munificent donation from Sir Dinshaw Petit. They constructed in 1890 a leper asylum in Bombay. That asylum, I believe, contains accommodation for about 300 lepers, and the result has been to free the City of Bombay from the beggars who extorted alms by the exhibition of their sores. The unfortunate creatures subjected to this dreadful malady have now been removed to a hospital in which that comfort and attention are given to them to which their pitiable condition gives them a just claim. The Government of Bengal followed that example last year and passed through their local Council a Bill for the two purposes I have mentioned—the segregation of lepers and their prohibition from certain callings; but the Act in its application was very carefully restricted. In the first place, the Act could not be introduced at all except into an area in which a leper asylum had been previously constructed; in the second place, as far as the segregation of lepers is concerned, it was confined to pauper lepers, that is, lepers who were beggars and had no ostensible means of subsistence; in the third place, no leper could be removed to an asylum except on the certificate of a medical authority, and the leper was provided with means for making an appeal from the order for his removal to an asylum; and last of all a very careful definition was made in regard to the callings from which the lepers in that area were expressly precluded, such as the sale of food and the washing of clothes. The Bill as is usual was circulated to a very large number of officials and non-officials in the Province and to Associations interested in the matter, and it was eventually passed through the Bengal Council, where it met with general approval and support. The Chief Commissioner of Burma has since applied to have the provisions of that Bill extended to Burma, and it is understood that several other Local Governments are also desirous of having the provisions of the Bengal Act applied to their Provinces. It has been considered more desirable, however, that, instead of having a separate Bill for each Province, a general measure should be framed upon the lines of the Bengal Act which each Government in turn may apply or not as the circumstances render expedient. That is the Bill which I have now the honour to ask leave to introduce."

The motion was put and agreed to.

The Hon'ble MR. WOODBURN introduced the Bill.

The Hon'ble MR. WOODBURN moved that the Bill and Statement of Objects and Reasons be published in the Gazette of India in English, and in the local official Gazettes in English and in such other languages as the Local Governments think fit.

The motion was put and agreed to.

(from 'Abstract of the Proceedings of the Governor General of India, 1892')

Facsimile of the government of India's Lepers Bill, 1896

clothing, from bathing, washing clothes or taking water from a well or tank from which they had been debarred, and from driving, conducting or riding in any public conveyance other than a railway carriage.[30] A missionary doctor working in India forty years later commented:

> the Leper Act was not framed or passed by the Government of India with the idea that it was of any value from the public health standpoint, for the Government did not believe leprosy to be contagious to any appreciable extent. The Act appears therefore to have been framed merely with the idea of mitigating a public nuisance, or possibly in deference to public opinion which in India has always believed that leprosy is contagious.[31]

Though it remained on the statute book for many years, this act was seldom invoked. It had one significant consequence, however. Since leprosy did not impinge on any of its vital interests, the government was intent on spending as little money as possible on controlling the disease; so rather than build institutions of its own it went for the cheaper option of providing grants-in-aid to existing leprosy asylums, most of which had been set up and were run by missionaries. This meant reappraising government policy on missionary activities.

Even the most Christian of British Indian officials had an ambivalent attitude towards missionaries. Robert Needham Cust, for instance – he of the 'Three Commandments' – wrote in his memoirs:

> After the Mutinies there were signs of a fanatical spirit, and a desire to introduce the Bible into the State-Schools, to push Christians forward in Government-offices, to let Missionaries interfere, to preach to the Prisoners in Gaols. To all this I was totally opposed, and successfully; it would have been followed by appropriation of Hindu and Mahometan places of Public Worship, State-grants to Missions, disabilities to non-Christians, and all those features which disgraced the conversion of Europe in the Middle Ages . . .[32]

Cust wrote an article on 'Leprosy and Lepers' for the *Churchman* in 1890. In it he envisaged a chain of state-controlled secluded rural 'retreats' for leprosy sufferers, who would be lured there by the promise of free food, gentle treatment and medical care, all at the expense of urban taxpayers (who would presumably be willing to pay up to get rid of a public nuisance). But, he wrote:

> the missionaries must be excluded, as, under the unwritten law of British India, the State is prohibited from any act of direct or indirect proselytism, and the very *raison d'être* of the missionary is to proselytize . . . the great Central Government cannot afford to move one inch from the grand position, which it has always occupied, as the impartial protector of each one of its meanest subjects in the observance of such religious duties and feelings as he or she may please to practise or adopt, being of sufficient age to be a judge of the matter. This is the very mainspring of our power in India, and any attempt to depart from it on the solicitation of short sighted missionaries and ignorant philanthropists must be sternly resisted.[33]

That might have been the government position when Cust was in India, but things had changed by the end of the century. Fear of forcible conversion to Christianity of the entire population – Hindu and Muslim – had been one of the causes of the sepoy rebellion of 1857, and the suppression of the uprising had done nothing to remove that fear. On the contrary, missionary activity increased, particularly in the decades following the 1870s, and if the government now looked upon it more favourably than before that was because missionaries had – in the words of a historian of Christian missions who was also a bishop – 'to some extent yielded to the colonial complex':

> Only Western man was wise and good, and members of other races, in so far as they became westernised, might share in this wisdom and goodness. But Western man was the leader, and would remain so for a very long time, perhaps for ever . . .[34]

From this perspective the early life of the founder of a 'special mission to lepers' whose growing 'extent and usefulness' Cust applauded in his essay – despite his firm views on the separation of church and state in India – is revealing.[35] Born in Queen's County, Ireland, in 1846, Wellesley C. Bailey went as a very young man to New Zealand and New Caledonia in search of adventure, trying his hand at gold digging and stock riding, before making his way to India. He was intending to become an officer in the North-West Police when a chance encounter with an American missionary in the Punjab changed the direction of his life. The missionary, Dr J.H. Morrison, took him to visit the small leprosy asylum at

Ambala on a crisp, clear morning in December 1869. Bailey later recalled how shocked he'd been at the 'woebegone expression' on the faces of the inmates, their 'look of utter helplessness'. Some were in the early stages of the disease, others in the advanced stages 'terrible to look upon'. He wrote:

> I almost shuddered, yet I was at the [same] time fascinated, and I felt, if ever there was a Christ-like work in this world it was to go among these poor sufferers and bring to them the consolation of the Gospel.[36]

He had found the cause to which he would dedicate his life. But if he hadn't met Morrison, he might easily have gone on to become an imperial police officer and served Mammon just as devotedly as he would serve God. His granddaughter's assessment of him bears this out:

> He was not a saint, nor even a clever man. But I do not ever remember hearing from him an ungenerous remark, or seeing him angry apart from minor irritations. His great gift was single-mindedness, and a simplicity that perhaps could not see the difficulties which a more sophisticated mind might see.[37]

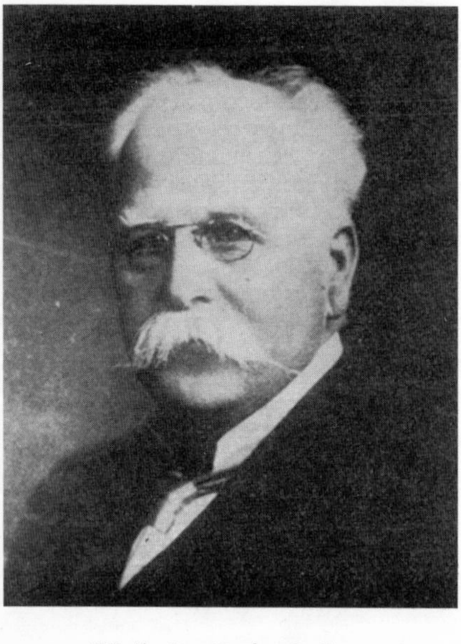

Wellesley Cosby Bailey,
founder of the Leprosy Mission

Bailey married an Irish girl from Dublin, Alice Grahame, who joined him in India in 1871. By the end of 1873 they were obliged to return home because of her poor health, and it was in the following year, at an informal meeting in Dublin, that Alice's friends, the three Misses Pim, volunteered to raise money for leprosy sufferers in India. Charlotte Pim asked Wellesley Bailey to write a pamphlet they could circulate, and he composed *Lepers in India* (which became known as 'the original beggar'); in return, the sisters undertook to come up with not less than £30 a year.[38] In the event, they did much better than that, raising nearly twenty times that amount in the first year alone. (The Leprosy Mission's centenary year, 1974, saw its income top a million pounds for the first time – a far cry from its modest beginnings.)[39]

The money was more than Bailey needed for the Ambala asylum, so he gave grants in an *ad hoc* way to other missionaries engaged in leprosy work. This was the real beginning of The Mission to Lepers, as it became known once it was properly established. Strictly speaking, it was not a missionary society; it did not send missionaries out into the field; it did not even call itself a mission to begin with – its original title was 'Friends to Indian Lepers'. It acted more as a kind of ecumenical agency, supporting a range of international and (non-Catholic) interdenominational missionary initiatives devoted to leprosy sufferers. At first Wellesley Bailey himself was not employed by the mission but by the Church of Scotland, which in 1875 sent him to the tiny Native State of Chamba, north of the Punjab. Education rather than leprosy work was his brief, so when he set up a small leprosy asylum there he turned to the British Resident for help, not to the missionary society that had sent him out. In 1879 he was transferred to Wazirabad, but by 1882 his wife's health had again broken down and he and his family (there were now young children as well) had to return to Britain, where they settled in Edinburgh. It was not until 1886 that he became full-time Secretary (later, Superintendent) of The Mission to Lepers, making periodic trips to India and, as the mission expanded, to other parts of the world as well.[40]

From the start the mission had a dual purpose: Bailey recognised that in addition to providing the consolation of the Gospel, 'a good deal more was needed, e.g. good living rooms, good food, clothing, medical attendance, sanitary regulations etc'. Though he spoke of 'medical attendance' rather than 'treatment', Bailey always hoped that leprosy would prove as treatable as other diseases; for instance in 1875, when he heard about gurjun oil, he immediately wrote off to the Andaman Islands and ordered a fifty-four gallon cask of it. He supported the pioneering efforts of Dr Arthur Neve to relieve nerve pain by surgical intervention. Neve was ahead of his time in another respect as well: he admitted leprosy patients to the general wards of his Church Missionary Society hospital at Srinager in Kashmir instead of isolating them – though this was probably out of necessity rather than choice; in acknowledging a grant from The Mission to Lepers he wrote, 'The roof is now being put on a special place for them, which will, I trust, by your help, be the germ of a leper asylum . . . From the data I have collected I am inclined to believe in the contagiousness of the disease . . .'[41]

Purulia, in what is now West Bengal, became the mission's largest leprosy asylum and hospital in India and, in the early days of the twentieth century, a centre for government-sponsored drug trials, where chaulmoogra and a number of shorter-lived 'cures' were tested.[42] Collaboration with government was not achieved without some tough negotiation, but the mission had got itself into a strong position and could to some extent dictate its own terms. It already accepted the principle that 'no person [should be] compelled to receive religious instruction or deprived of any privileges for declining to do so'; but it was not prepared to give any more ground: 'the Mission to Lepers cannot assent to any restriction being placed upon missionaries who have dedicated their lives to work among the heathen.'[43]

The Lepers Act of 1898 introduced an element of compulsion into the segregation of leprosy sufferers, which the Mission to Lepers initially opposed. Bailey informed the government of Bengal that the mission would take responsibility for leprosy beggars forcibly removed from the streets of Purulia by the police in accordance with the act only if 'the free exercise of missionary work in the Government Retreat' to be attached to the asylum were permitted. The Bengal government had no alternative but to agree. This was the price the mission exacted for doing the government's dirty work, so to speak. It did not wish to incur the hostility of those whom the authorities paid it to care for, or to place missionaries in 'a difficult and *in the eyes of the natives invidious position*'.[44] But despite this risk, it recognised that it stood to gain far more by co-operating with government agencies than if it held itself aloof. This was too good an opportunity to miss, and could be justified as a case of rendering unto Caesar . . .

Purulia's attraction for leprosy sufferers predated missionary involvement with it. It was a Hindu place of pilgrimage and they gathered there to beg for alms. A kind of shanty town had grown up to the north of Purulia proper, but in 1883 the district officer, who regarded it as an eyesore and its inhabitants as a public nuisance, had ordered it to be razed to the ground and its inmates loaded on to bullock carts and despatched to the villages whence they had come. Since their reason for coming to Purulia in the first place had been to escape from these villages which had made them outcasts, the upshot was predictable: no

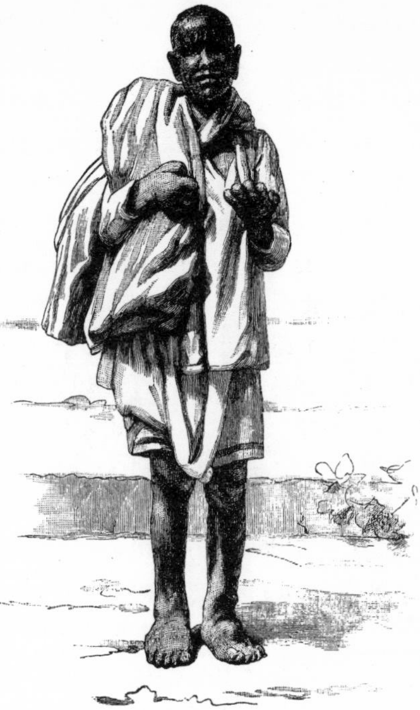

(from 'My Leper Friends' by Mrs M.H. Hayes, London 1891)

A 'pauper leper'

welcome awaited them on their enforced return and 'being left "without the camp" they dragged their way back to Purulia to beg again in the streets and encamp under the trees, where their old huts had been'.[45] Here they caught the attention of the Lutheran missionary Heinrich Uffmann, who had returned to India from his first home leave in Germany in the mid-1880s. Uffmann had been obliged to come back without one of his seven children, a daughter called Maria, who had contracted leprosy and would die in a Berlin hospital at the age of thirteen. He vowed he would never turn away a leprosy sufferer who came to him for help, and was as good as his word, founding and running the leprosy asylum at Purulia.[46]

When Wellesley Bailey visited Purulia in December 1890, Uffmann drew his attention to the 'brightest and happiest looking' of all the inmates, a woman whose history Bailey recounted in a letter to his wife:

> She lived in a village about 9 miles from Purulia, & when her husband & friends saw that she had become a leper, they sent her away to lie on her face before an idol until she should be healed . . . for about 3 weeks [she]

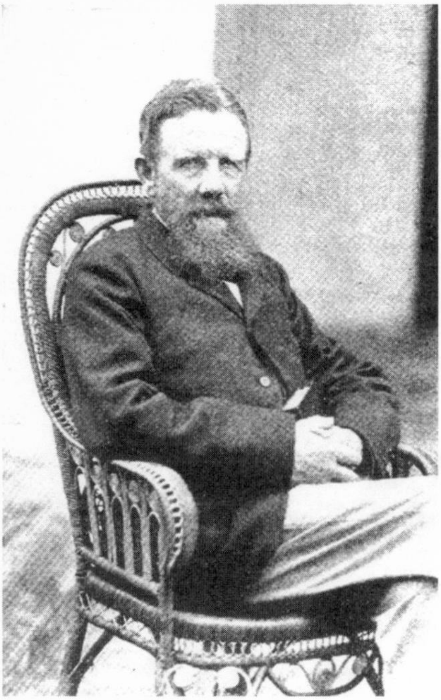
(©TLM)
Rev. Heinrich Uffmann

lay on her face before the idol, sleeping only as little as possible, & taking only a little dry grain in the evenings, just to sustain life. At the end of that time she returned, & the unnatural husband & friends said to her: – 'Well, the god has not healed you, so you had better be off to Purulia'! Accordingly she left, with a breaking heart. Mr & Mrs Uffmann met her outside their compound & were horrified at the awful appearance she presented. She was the picture of a consuming despair. She implored admittance & was taken in at once. She improved rapidly under kind care & good treatment. She drank in the gospel message, & in about two months God gave her a new heart & she is the brightest woman in the whole Asylum now.[47]

This 'good looking young woman', whose name was Dayamony – 'a pearl of grace, or mercy' – became a favourite of all the Europeans who visited Purulia. Like many of the inmates of the various asylums who embraced Christianity she was 'adopted' by a subscriber to the mission in Britain, to whom reports were made of her progress. Dayamony herself wrote letters to her 'new mother in Scotland', a Miss Gurney. In one dated 27 October 1897, she described how all the leprosy survivors, 500 or more of them, had moved from their old asylum to a newly built one on the edge of the forest, 'a very fine place'. There were trees and space and fresh air, but its chief virtue in her eyes was that 'none is able now to persecute us as people did in the other place'. She praised the Lord, who 'has opened the hearts of the Europeans, the dear friends for us, to provide for us bodily and spiritually, and especially the last the Bread of Life':

> In this year we have had an awful famine here, but by the blessings of God we did not feel very much about it. By this famine my sister and her two children came also; there are now ten of us here from one family, one child died. I have also one son but he is with his father. I went once to see him, my child, but could not do so because my husband and his relatives got very angry with me and said 'Do not come back again, and if so we will give you a good thrashing through the scavenger [i.e., person of the lowest caste, the sweeper], and will kill [you] and have your remains thrown away by the pariahs.' My relatives are so cruel to me that they do not allow me to see even my child. That is very hard, but my heavenly relatives will not drive me away, not when I see Christ; how they love me!
>
> I do not much think on my former condition, but my husband, my child and those belonging to my family are as yet heathen; that will break my heart. For my own sake I begin to understand, I am happy to say, that the Christian religion is the only true one . . .
>
> Many of our relatives come to the Asylum to see us in a happy and contented life, and do not persecute us now; and many of them have become Christians. I hope the rest will also come . . .[48]

It is impossible to say to what extent Dayamony, writing out of gratitude, was influenced by what she knew her 'mother in Scotland' would like to hear; most likely, though, every word she wrote was heartfelt. As one missionary in India put it:

> To be welcomed, instead of being told to 'clear out'; to be fed, instead of being semi-starved most of the time; to be clothed, instead of being in rags and tatters; to be told that there is hope of salvation through a Saviour, instead of having it dinned into them that the gods have cursed them; what a heaven it is to the leper![49]

The contrast in how they were commonly treated by their own families and by these European strangers was indeed so marked that it was no surprise that, in the words of another missionary, the 'heathen patients are often puzzled, and sometimes "imagine vain things," and assign the most mistaken of motives' to their benefactors.[50] A missionary such as Uffmann, who almost single-handedly transformed Purulia into a model asylum, suffering more than one breakdown of health in the process and hastening his own end through physical and mental exhaustion, deserves the kind of praise that has been heaped on Father Damien. But missionaries did have mixed motives: succouring the sick and needy was part of a larger agenda. It was the thin end of the wedge in the grand plan to convert the 'heathen' and evangelise the world. As Dayamony reported, the Bengal famine of 1897 had brought several of her relatives (if not the ones she cared for most) into the fold. 'It is these Christian lepers,' Uffmann's friend and admirer, the Rev. F. Hahn, wrote, 'who work as a light and are . . . frequently the means of bringing new comers to the feet of Jesus.'[51]

There was some resistance even among those leprosy sufferers on whom the missionaries lavished their love and attention. An American missionary called Mary Reed had contracted leprosy in Calcutta and, like Father Damien in Molokai, devoted the remainder of her – long – life to the inmates of the Chandag Heights asylum in the Himalayan foothills, becoming something of a legend and having books written about her (one of them by the missionary John Jackson, mentioned by her below). Her letters are full of pious sentiments and money matters and as such are mostly unrevealing; only when she writes about her charges do we get any insight into life in the asylum.

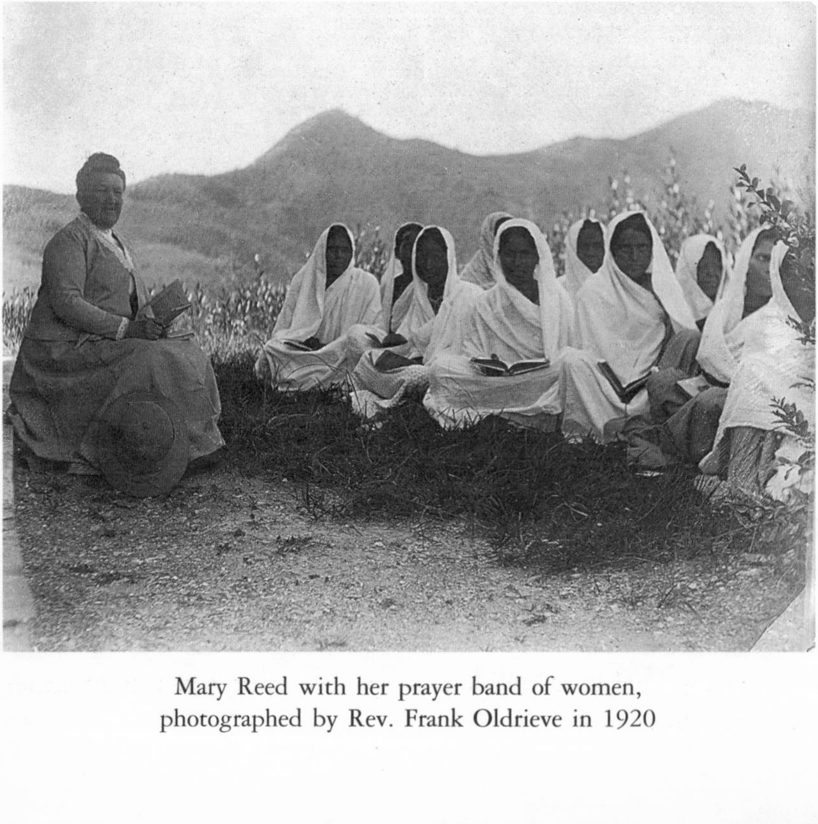

(©TLM)

Mary Reed with her prayer band of women, photographed by Rev. Frank Oldrieve in 1920

From the beginning a major problem in leprosy asylums was segregation of the sexes, particularly in the case of married – and sometimes not-married – couples. At Purulia, for instance, men and women lived on opposite sides of a building with a wall down the middle; even the asylum shop opened on one side to men, and on the other to women.[52] At Chandag, men and boys were removed to another building which was built in 1895 at nearby Panahgah. For three years after that there were no 'runaways' from Chandag, but in 1898 Mary Reed was distressed to have to report to Wellesley Bailey an 'exodus' of two couples:

> You will be shocked and grieved to hear that *one* of the four who chose the downward way and set out therein a few days ago, is, or *was* formerly my little girl Minnie! She had grown much in stature during the past three years since Mr. & Mrs. Jackson adopted her, but disease having made much progress I was obliged to remove her to the women's barracks, and unfortunately instead of choosing [good women] as her most intimate companions, she had as I noted with sorrow for some time past, taken up with those who had not yet 'chosen the good part'. And with her went Manwa, the little Nepalese boy in whom Mr. Jackson was also interested, as he was supported by a Young People's Society at Sidcup. I say 'little' Minnie and 'the boy Manwa' for I can think of them as *children* only, though Manwa is nearly or quite 18 and very small of stature, and Minnie only about *13*!! but not a child [any] longer in innocency and goodness! These two were led astray by a wicked woman who had fallen some years ago and after months of a wicked wandering life she professed and seemed earnestly and truly repentant and was again admitted to the Asylum – but it turns out now that her repentance was not 'true repentance' . . .[53]

For a girl like Minnie, growing up petted and adored and with no experience of life outside the asylum, the desire for love, sexual fulfilment and a normal life must have been very strong to have enabled her to resist the considerable moral pressure exerted upon her by Miss Reed and her Christian votaries. The price of remaining in the asylum was to accept its monastic values and renounce worldly love in favour of spiritual love. Minnie voted with her feet. Another girl in the same asylum, Chandra, 'who is supported by Miss Hogg', was in a more difficult situation, as Reed recorded:

> She, with her old and decidedly queer mother who lives with her here at Chandag, and her old and very obstinate father who is an inmate of Pana[h]gah, are all three here. Chandra knows I believe what experimental religion is; but to awaken, develop, and enlighten the mind, to create hunger and thirst for spiritual life in the hearts of this old couple I have made a complete failure so far, after all these years of effort. From childhood heathenism their hearts became darkened and they are still in bonds of sin and of great darkness and are yet tainted with falsehood and deception and heathen ideas; for instance, the old woman had shaking spells hideous to behold now and again, and says an evil spirit has taken possession of her (!); and only two or three weeks ago she had what I call a tantrum, a great shaking and trembling. But oh, how she uses her tongue in abusing any who may happen to try to displease her or chide her! She endeavoured the other day to smite – by blowing mightily with her breath – one of the most earnest and exemplary sweet Christian women here, saying 'May this evil spirit go into you!' She looks worse than an insane person when she goes off into one of her spells. The old father is one of the most obstreperous characters, 'set' in his crooked ways; and sometimes Chandra is influenced by her parents, and becomes entangled and hindered in her heart and gets hardened and cold; but she repents of her backsliding after a time and comes back to the Saviour of sinners, our blessed Jesus, and then I have the joy of seeing her make some progress in the heavenly race for a time. At present she has not fully recovered from a stumble she made not long since because of her mother's doings and influence. She will I trust be saved finally, but her progress and growth are greatly hindered by this untoward influence.[54]

Caught between the wicked old world of her parents and the brave new world of the missionaries, no wonder Chandra vacillated in her loyalty and was occasionally guilty of 'backsliding'. Her predicament illustrates more clearly than any argument how the Mission to Lepers' stated policy of 'on the one hand an absolute equality of welcome and treatment for all, of whatever faith and without pressure to hear the Christian message; and on the other freedom for Christian teaching to be made available to those voluntarily desiring it'[55] (which still applies today) was at odds with the practice of missionaries for whom proselytism was, as Robert Needham Cust pointed out, their 'very *raison d'être*'.

On balance, however, leprosy sufferers in India and, later, in the Far

East and elsewhere had reason to be grateful to Wellesley Bailey and the Mission to Lepers. By 1904, when it had been in existence a mere thirty years, the mission already had forty-two asylums of its own and helped to support another sixteen. It also had twenty homes for the 'untainted children of leper parents'. It worked 'in happy co-operation with 24 Protestant churches or missionary societies, representing America and the continent of Europe, as well as Great Britain and Canada'. Provincial governments all over India recognised its pre-eminence in the field of leprosy and were glad to hand over to its care several of their own asylums; much of its income now came from the government.[56] Though the twentieth century would see a gradual secularisation of leprosy work as scientific medicine wrestled with the problems of the disease, missionaries would remain at the forefront of the struggle throughout the period. The urge to proselytise remained just as strong, of course, but increasingly these missionaries were themselves doctors and their contribution to the scientific understanding and treatment of leprosy was as great as their dedication and commitment to improving the lives of their patients.

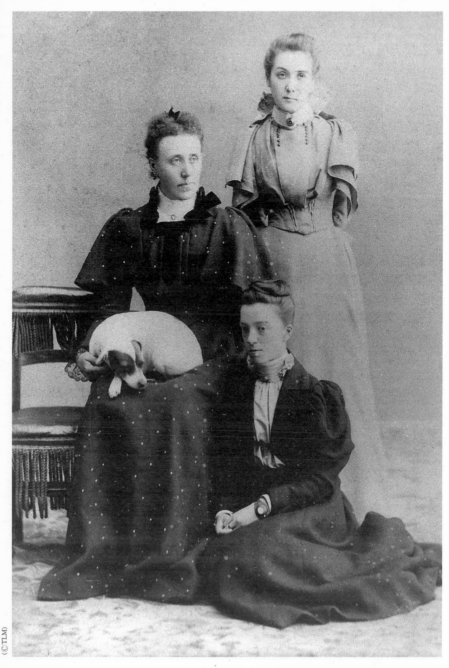

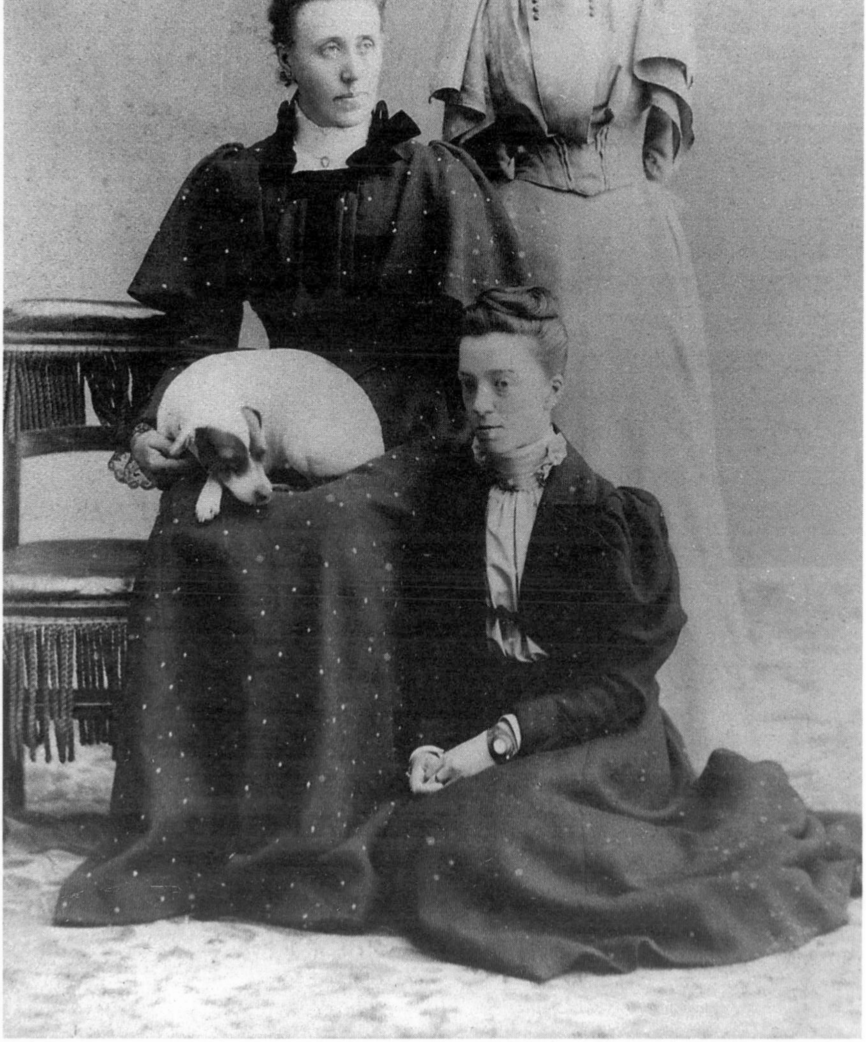

(©TLM)

Hannah Riddell (*left*) and her niece,
companion and secretary Ada Hannah Wright

Chapter 6

TWO WOMEN WITH A MISSION

The minutes of the Mission to Lepers' committee meeting for Thursday 9 March 1893 record that the Secretary read out 'a deeply interesting letter from Miss Riddell of the CMS [Church Missionary Society]' from southern Japan pleading for help 'to establish a Home for outcast lepers'. It was 'unanimously resolved to make a grant of £200'. Two years later, a further grant of £50 was made to Miss Riddell, 'leaving the continuance of the grant for future consideration'.[1] Who was Miss Riddell, and what was she doing, setting up a leprosy asylum in Japan?

Hannah Riddell was one of the pioneering women missionaries sent abroad by the Church Missionary Society. She was the oldest of a group of five young women who sailed from Southampton to Japan on 14 November 1890. While some of the others were barely out of their teens, Hannah was already in her mid-thirties and accustomed to earning her living. In this respect she differed from most of the other Victorian middle-class spinsters recruited by the CMS in those early years for work overseas; her biographer tells us that of 'the thirty-one ladies sent abroad by the CMS between 1888 and 1889, nearly half were honorary missionaries who could contribute to their own support and who had probably never before worked for a living'. As her subsequent life would demonstrate, Hannah was not the malleable sort of young lady the CMS might have preferred her to be.[2]

She began her missionary work as a teacher in the city of Kumamoto on the island of Kyushu, but in her first annual report to the CMS, dated 1 December 1891, she was already revealing an interest in the plight of leprosy victims and volunteering her services to ameliorate the condition of those who had wasted all their money on doctors before seeking refuge at the Honmyoji temple:

> Destitute, homeless, in unutterable misery, sleeping under bridges or by the road-side, they drag out the remainder of their wretched lives. They want a Father Damien. Is there not one among the CMS recruits? I have no medical experience, but I could see that advice was carried out and take a little comfort to them.[3]

Hannah had found her calling, the reason she believed God had guided her steps to Japan, but the CMS responded cautiously. Leprosy work might have a place in the missionary scheme of things, but the main function was to make converts to Christianity. While the CMS prevaricated, failing to see, in the words of Riddell's biographer, 'that Hannah, with her genuine longing to do something for a wretched group of human beings, was preaching the most powerful Christian message of all', Riddell went ahead with her plan for a leprosy asylum, involving influential Japanese figures such as the most senior garrison doctor stationed at Kumamoto, as well as a missionary friend, Grace Nott, who had sailed out to Japan with her. She 'liked to identify a problem and then deal with it, and if misguided people chose to place obstacles in her way, she was adept, some might say even Machiavellian, in circumnavigating them'. If the CMS would not support her project, then she would apply to the Mission to Lepers, which was already supporting leprosy work in China, and persuade it to contribute towards the cost of building the asylum. The sanatorium was opened on 12 November 1895 and named Kaishun, meaning 'resurrection of hope' and conveying a message of renewal to the afflicted.[4]

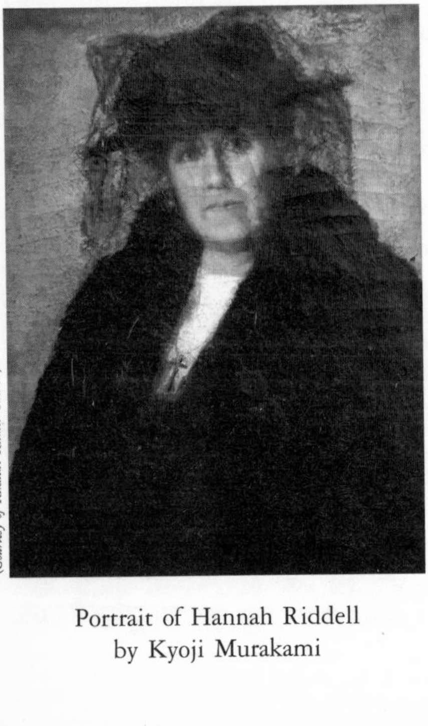

(Courtesy of Kikuchi Reimei Church)

Portrait of Hannah Riddell
by Kyoji Murakami

This was not the first asylum to be opened in Japan during the Meiji era (1868–1912), in which the country was exposed to western influences after a long period of isolation from the outside world. On 9 January 1892, the *British Medical Journal* reported:

> Another missionary who devoted himself to the succour of lepers has completed his sacrifice by giving his life in their service. Father Testevuide, who may be called the Damien of Japan, established the first leper house in that country in 1886. At that time no provision whatever was made either by the Government or the public for the care of lepers, and it was only by the most persevering efforts that the energetic priest was able to collect sufficient funds to build a leper house on Mount Fusi. This institution he personally managed until his death. His example has been fruitful, and now there are three asylums for the victims of leprosy in Japan, all apparently owing their existence to private charity.[5]

Private charity was all very well and in Japan, where government intervention would be even more draconian than elsewhere, had much to recommend it. But for the recipient there was a price to pay in individual freedom, as this comment from the CMS's *Church Missionary Gleaner* of 2 July 1902 makes plain:

> If a nurse becomes a missionary her one object must be the winning of souls. Her work is not only nursing; she must be able to explain the Gospel of Christ to her patients in their own language, and she needs to be as skilled in dealing with sin-stricken souls as she is in relieving bodily pain.[6]

Among the foreigners in Japan at this time, there was at least one, the writer Lafcadio Hearn, who did not welcome the missionary invasion. 'For myself,' he wrote in a letter:

> I could sympathize with the individual but never with the missionary-cause. Unconsciously, every honest being in the mission-army is a destroyer – and a destroyer only; for nothing can replace what they break down. Unconsciously, too, the missionaries everywhere represent the edge . . . of Occidental aggression. We are face to face here with the spectacle of a powerful and selfish civilization demoralizing and crushing a weaker and, in many ways, a nobler one . . . and the spectacle is not pretty.[7]

Hannah Riddell would not have understood such cultural sensitivity. She may have been too determinedly outspoken and energetic to fit comfortably into the disciplined and self-negating world of the missionary, but she shared the religious outlook and values of her Christian brothers and sisters and was just as keen on the winning of souls as they were. Even in the early days of the Kaishun refuge, ten out of its twenty-four patients were Christian. But the success of her initiative did not mean that the CMS was prepared to let her have things her own way. Back in England in 1900, Riddell was told that she would no longer be stationed in Kumamoto when she returned to Japan. She made it clear that she intended to go back there willy-nilly, and pre-emptively resigned from the CMS.[8]

This was a brave decision. For two years after her return to Kumamoto, Hannah struggled to keep the Kaishun sanatorium going financially. Her sheer determination, combined with the support she had gathered in England and her ability to make friends in high places in Japan, carried her through this difficult time. She was taken up and promoted by two influential Japanese in particular, the educationalist and politician Shigenobu Okuma and the financier Eiichi Shibusawa. In November 1905 they invited her to address a select gathering of politicians, businessmen and journalists at the Bankers' Club in Tokyo on the subject of 'What Should We Do for the Lepers in Japan?' This was the first public airing of a social problem to which Japanese officialdom had previously responded by turning a blind eye, and it not only pushed the government into introducing a leprosy prevention bill, educating the public about the disease and providing funds for medical research; it also raised Riddell's status from that of a humble missionary pleading for funds for her little-known provincial institution to that of an expert, advising the government and, in return, receiving financial support for the asylum she had created.[9]

In her own eyes, too, she had become something of an expert. Like many other self-appointed authorities, she now had very definite opinions about leprosy: in defiance of informed, up-to-date medical opinion on the contagiousness of the disease, she remained convinced that it was hereditary and that the only way to prevent its spread was to segregate the sexes. As late as 1914, she was writing to her friend and patron Okuma, now prime minister of Japan for the second time, about the children of parents affected by leprosy:

> They should of course be allowed every possible chance in life . . . but I think they should not be allowed to marry for two generations, and

> although that seems a very stringent thing, I believe their patriotism could be appealed to, and boys and girls would grow up with the idea that marriage was not for them, though every other joy and comfort in life might be theirs.[10]

How convenient it was for her, if not for her charges, that the medical view to which she subscribed should make the eradication of the disease dependent on celibacy, since that was not just the ideal of the gospel she was always urging upon them but her own personal choice as well. As her biographer remarks, 'she could not abolish original sin. However, she could justify banishing sex from the Kaishun Hospital and from her hypothetical leper communities on the spurious grounds that total abstinence was the only way to halt the spread of the disease.' Couples in love or those whose concupiscence could not be concealed were expelled from the asylum. But the martinet in Hannah was tempered by kindness and she did not abandon even those who, in her terms, had fallen by the wayside; she would write to them and send them presents long after they had left her domain. This was part and parcel of the maternal relationship this tall and commanding Englishwoman sought to establish with the patients. She liked to be thought of as their 'Mother' and would in turn address them as 'My dear Child' in letters she wrote, regardless of their actual age. The younger ones, in particular, or those who had entered the asylum at an early age, were happy to comply with her wishes, since she was the only mother figure many of them had ever known.[11]

Riddell clashed with Japan's leading leprosy doctor, Kensuke Mitsuda, over the need for sexual segregation. Mitsuda was the architect, along with Hannah's second wealthy friend and patron Shibusawa, of the 1907 leprosy law.[12] According to the first-ever leprosy patient survey conducted in 1900, there were 30,359 victims of the disease in Japan – a prevalence rate of 6.43 per 10,000 population. Law No. 11, enacted in 1907, was Janus-faced: it was ostensibly philanthropic and charitable, in the manner Hannah advocated, providing refuges for stigmatised outcasts; but these refuges were at the same time places of confinement for undesirables, run by former police officers. Japan, victorious in both the Sino–Japanese and Russo–Japanese Wars, aimed to create a modern nation-state free from embarrassing sights such as the clusters of leprosy-affected vagrants who had first caught Hannah's attention.[13]

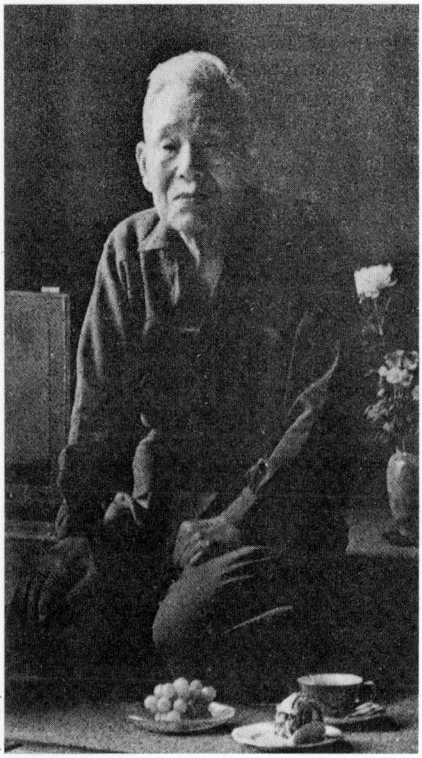
(The Star)

Dr Kensuke Mitsuda, Japan's most influential leprosy specialist

The law provided for the construction of five leprosaria in different parts of Japan. Kumamoto was the site of one of them, the Keifu-en, which opened in 1909; and once the state leprosarium had come into being Hannah Riddell could afford to be more selective about whom she admitted to the Kaishun asylum. Vagrants had become a state responsibility, so she offered a refuge to those who had led more respectable lives or were better educated. Her charges included 'university professors, maids, farmers, policemen, Shinto priests, screen makers, and artists', who would certainly have appreciated the gentler treatment they received at her hands than in the state institution, even though some of them might find her determination to convert them irksome. Riddell's biographer learned of a patient who died in 1993 at the age of ninety-two and had kept a diary at the beginning of the 1930s 'in which he described how irritated he had been at the attempts to move him into a room with a Christian leper who, Hannah hoped, would influence his beliefs'.[14]

But that sort of pressure was nothing compared to what awaited the poor vagrants housed in state leprosaria once the gloss of providing a refuge for the sick and destitute had worn off. Dr Kensuke Mitsuda might have taken a more liberal line on sexual segregation than Hannah Riddell, but the Zensho Hospital, the state leprosarium of which he was director, became notorious for the harshness of its discipline. In 1915, Mitsuda himself proposed a revision to the law, enabling prison facilities to be built within the leprosarium 'in order to contain the incorrigible patients'. The head of a leprosarium acquired the right to impose all sorts of disciplinary restraints, ranging from reprimands and reduction of rations for up to seven days to confinement for up to thirty days in this prison within a prison. But the real villain of the piece at Zensho-en was not Mitsuda but Hiroshi Kegai, a man who'd been hired as a clerk in 1914 and became so influential that people would say there were 'two directors in the Zensho Hospital'. Deserters were taken to a cell and flogged on his orders; they were given as many as 100 or even 200 lashes, and their screams could be heard all over the leprosarium. But Kegai was far from unique; there were plenty of other sadists among the staff. The history of the Tama Zenshoen patients' association relates:

> Some of the clerks never caught a patient but then there were those who lived to catch a patient in the act of gambling or to get their hands on a patient who had tried unsuccessfully to escape. There was no shortage of successors to Kegai.[15]

Kegai and his successors regarded all leprosy vagrants as potential or proven criminals and instituted a reign of terror in state leprosaria, a

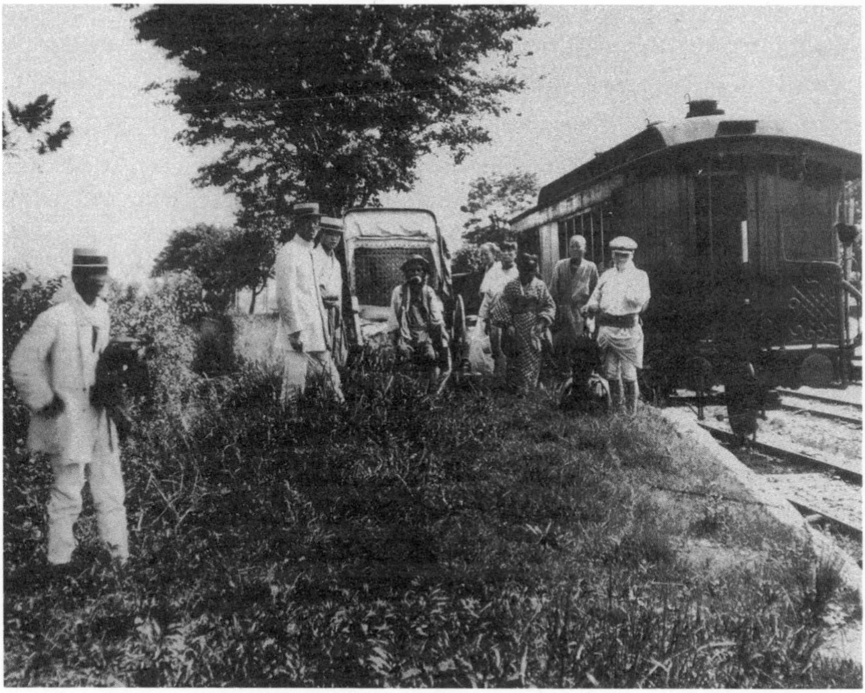

(HIH Prince Takamatsu Memorial Hansen's Disease Museum)

Higashi Murayama Station, where patients sent to the Tama Zenshoen state sanatorium near Tokyo were 'unloaded' on a separate platform

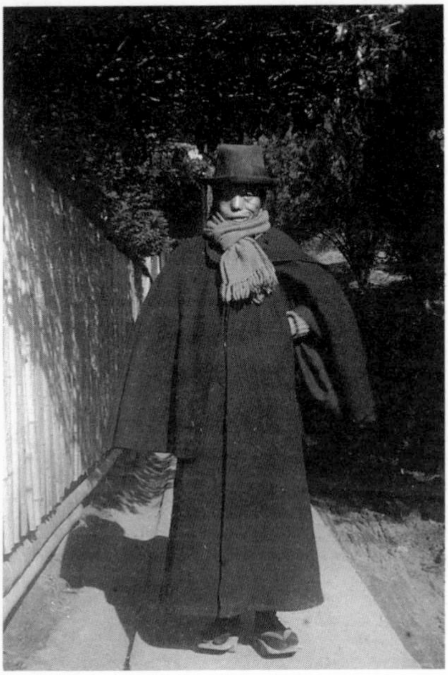
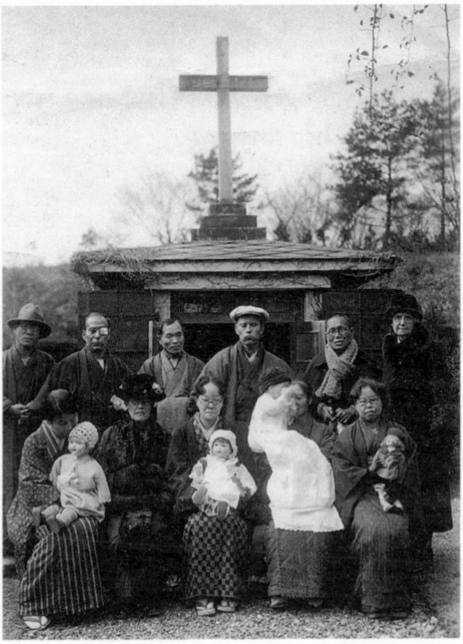

(©TLM)

Patients at the Kaishun Sanatorium

strategy that received official sanction as Japan became increasingly militarised and leprophobic. There might be a militaristic element in Hannah Riddell's British boarding school-type regime, but by comparison it was entirely benign. Patients at the Kaishun hospital had happy memories of recreational activities, music and sport and gardening. There were occasional treats, too, as when patients were sick and Hannah brought them ice cream.[16] The disadvantage of a Christian asylum might be its ceaseless efforts to make converts, but its advantage – and it was a huge one – was that it cared for, and about, its patients. They were not branded as a class of criminals, but seen as individual souls worthy of salvation.

Fortunately for Hannah Riddell, she did not live long enough to see the destruction of her life's work. She died on 3 February 1932, nine years to the day before the Kaishun sanatorium was forced to close by the unrelenting hostility of the Japanese authorities.[17]

In her later life she'd acquired a taste – and a reputation – for an extravagant lifestyle. This did not trouble her unduly. As her perceptive biographer expresses it:

> She was convinced that living the life of a grand lady was the only way she would be accepted as an equal by those who had the means to keep the hospital going. In this assertion she was almost certainly right, and it did at least give her the moral justification to follow her natural inclinations.[18]

To her credit, she recognised the importance of medical research and set up a laboratory at Kaishun hospital. But then she proceeded to make life difficult for researchers by her vehement opposition to the use of animals in medical experimentation, as well as by her refusal to acknowledge any findings that clashed with her own preconceptions. She was opinionated, bossy and none too scrupulous in gaining her objectives, but she had a kind heart and gave her all to her patients and her project. In fact, she was not entirely unlike the Catholic priest she had set out to emulate.

Father Damien's example also served as an inspiration for Kate Marsden. A near contemporary of Hannah Riddell (she was born just four years later, in 1859, and died a year earlier, in 1931), Kate had a similar Victorian middle-class background. Her father was a prosperous solicitor, practising in London's Cheapside, and the family home was in the leafy village of Edmonton, north of the city. 'Kitty' was the youngest of eight children, four boys and four girls, and quite unlike her brothers and sisters; she was the 'harum-scarum tomboy of the family', according to a biography that she herself seems to have had a hand in writing.[19]

In that book she is presented as 'a child of nature', who fought against the constraints of 'the severest domestic discipline' – her mother is rather oddly described as 'a woman in whom the gentleness of her sex was strongly developed, combined with strict ideas of family discipline'. The sense Kate had of herself as 'naughty' – a 'bad', even 'a very bad girl' who got her clothes dirty splashing around in puddles and falling into ditches – was merely confirmed when she went away to boarding school. Her 'home record of laziness and good-for-nothingness' was reproduced there, and domestic discipline gave way to the 'oft-repeated punishments of the schoolroom'.

At home, she escaped from the house whenever she could, especially when ill, 'and shut herself up with the animals, believing that she had their sympathy as much as they had hers in their sufferings'. Like St Francis of Assisi (who else?), 'she regarded animals as her friends and kinsfolk, and talked to them in a familiar way, believing that they understood all she said'. She also 'nursed them in babyhood, tended them in sickness, and buried them when dead'. Her dolls, too (a reassuringly feminine touch here), were treated for 'broken arms and sawdust-bleeding legs'.[20] Even members of her family were not immune from the precocious nursing talents of this budding Florence Nightingale when they fell ill.

If there is an element of hindsight about the suggestion that this gauche, tomboyish girl, who was in all other respects such a failure at home and at school, had a vocation for nursing, there can be no question of the need for it in her family. As *The Life* states with unusual terseness, 'Consumption was the mortal enemy in the household.'[21] First, Kate's father died when she was in her teens, reducing the family to genteel poverty (but releasing Kate from her hated boarding school); then her siblings were picked off one by one. By the time Kate was forty, she and one of her brothers were the only family members to have been spared by tuberculosis. Indeed, so many close relatives had died of this dreaded disease – first cousin to leprosy, and just as incurable then – that the younger generation of Marsdens is said to have abjured marriage (though if Kate was the source of this information, it should not necessarily be taken at face value, as the sequel will show).[22]

Her father's unexpected and untimely death left the family without an income; they had to sell the large house in Edmonton and move into a more modest dwelling elsewhere. Kate looked for work, answering adverts for nursing jobs; but first she needed to be trained. She approached the Tottenham hospital (which became The Prince of Wales's General Hospital in 1893) because it was close to her old home, and was accepted for training there. A German Jewish doctor by the name of Michael Laseron, who had settled in England after converting to Christianity, had developed the hospital out of a Ragged School. There was an orphanage of 800 girls attached to it and a deaconess, also from Germany, trained some of the older orphans to work in the slums of Tottenham. The Tottenham Community, we learn, 'was conceived as an Evangelical counterpart to the Roman Catholic Nursing Sisterhoods'.[23]

Guilt-ridden and intense, the young Kate Marsden was a prime candidate for religious enthusiasm. Whether it had a stabilising or destabilising effect on a highly-strung teenager who had just lost her father is another matter. But in 1877 her new-found missionary zeal led her to volunteer, while still a probationer at Tottenham, to join a group of nursing sisters heading for Bulgaria, scene of the so-called Bulgarian Atrocities reported in the press in lurid detail, to nurse sick and wounded Russian troops engaged in a war with Turkey. In view of the fact that this was her first exposure to travel, war and front-line nursing, her contemporary biographer's treatment of this episode is absurdly perfunctory and adds to the suspicion that he was merely a mouthpiece for his subject: 'It is needless to describe Kate Marsden's war experience in detail. Though full of horror, it broadened her sympathies, tested her courage, inured her to hardship, and developed the highest qualities of womanhood . . .'[24]

Nothing could be less revealing than these empty generalisations. Even the information that it was in Bulgaria that Kate first became aware of leprosy and the needs of its victims seems like an afterthought, given that she showed no further interest in the subject for several years to come. Back in England she pursued an orthodox nursing career; after a spell at the Westminster hospital in London, she became Sister-in-Charge of the Woolton convalescent home in Liverpool, where she remained for nearly five years. She resigned through illness, giving rise to fears that she would become the latest victim of the family scourge.[25] It turned out she did not have tuberculosis; but one of her sisters, who had gone to New Zealand in the vain hope of finding a cure there, was now terminally ill and wrote home pleading with her mother and sister to come to her. Kate and her mother left for New Zealand in November 1884. They arrived just in time to witness the death of this invalid sister.[26]

Stranded on the other side of the world with no money and her mother to support, Kate had to find work. Like Hannah Riddell, she already seems to have developed the knack of making friends in high places that would be so important to her later. 'Among the friends who rallied round Miss Marsden,' her biographer records without comment or explanation of how they met, 'were Sir William Jervois (at that time Governor of New Zealand) and Lady Jervois. Sir George Grey also showed her great kindness . . .'[27] She took a job as Lady Superintendent of Wellington hospital and busied herself in various ways, introducing first aid and forming a branch of the St John's Ambulance Brigade.[28]

After this promising start, however, her world suddenly collapsed. Once again, her biography conceals more than it reveals: 'Miss Marsden met with a severe accident in the hospital, and for several months was dangerously ill. She was compelled to resign her post, and, on partial recovery, removed to Nelson.' Some kind of nervous breakdown is indicated, the phrase actually used being 'a most trying mental illness'.[29] Marsden herself spoke of this as 'the period when I took many backward steps and turned away from Christ',[30] leading a later writer to surmise that she was experiencing 'a kind of revulsion against the intense religious training of her youth'. Perhaps, but this writer is on firmer ground when she goes on: 'There is a suggestion of a guilt complex, a desire to atone for something, in the intensity with which on her recovery she decided to devote herself to the cause of the world's lepers . . .'[31]

Certainly this was the moment when her thoughts turned seriously to leprosy. On her return to England, she was caught up in the publicity surrounding the death of Father Damien and sought out the Hawaiian consul to offer her services at the leprosy settlement on Molokai, only to be rebuffed with the remark that the government intended to make its own recruiting arrangements. Then she read Sir Morell Mackenzie's article in *The Nineteenth Century* on 'The Dreadful Revival of Leprosy', and thought about going to India to minister to 'Christ's lepers' there.[32] But before she made a move in that direction, she received an invitation from the Russian Red Cross to go to St Petersburg to be awarded a medal for services rendered in Bulgaria during the Russo–Turkish war of 1877–8.

This was just the sort of opportunity she had been waiting for, and she used it to promote her own private investigation of leprosy in the Near and Middle East as well as in Russia. She arranged to be presented at court in London in March 1890 and persuaded the Princess of Wales to provide her with a letter of introduction to the Empress of Russia. She met the Empress at the beginning of May and gained her support, without which she could not have got far in Russia. She went to France to pick the brains of the scientist, Louis Pasteur, who in the course of a long interview gave it as his opinion that leprosy was incurable. She also sought the advice of Florence Nightingale before setting out on her journey.

In Jerusalem she found 'fresh inspiration' in being 'where the Great Healer Himself had been amongst the lepers'. She visited the Moravian leprosy hospital outside the Jaffa Gate and, on her way back into the city, was appalled at the number of vagrants she encountered seated against the walls begging, their sores covered in flies:

> It was a matter of great surprise that the poor creatures should prefer living thus on casual charity to accepting the comforts of the Hospital, and also that they were permitted by the authorities to frequent public places, and so, probably, spread the disease.[33]

Constantinople, though outwardly beautiful, was 'a place of abomination and uncleanness', its 'Leper Home' in the middle of a burial ground quite literally 'an abode . . . of the dead':

> We drove through this cypress forest, and lost sight of the sea. Into the midst of this vast cemetery some few lepers were admitted by the Government. The sun seldom penetrates their lonely dwelling, whilst the wind howls through the trees, and rushes in at the open door, making the poor creatures huddle together for warmth.
>
> Notwithstanding the remonstrances of my guide, who looked horrified at my intention of going into the house, I entered, and wondered how any nation could subject some of its people to such misery.
>
> Thank God! There was a ray of light in this dark picture. This was the ministrations of good Dr. Zambaco [Pacha], who is devoted to the lepers, and is their one comfort. He has done everything in his power to induce the Sultan to provide properly for them; but in such a country, and with such a people, he is almost powerless.[34]

Kate went from Constantinople to Tiflis, where she heard about a herb that grew in the north of Siberia, which could cure leprosy. Impulsively, she at once determined to go there and discover this plant 'so that the lepers of India and of every other country might be benefited, and delivered from death', as well as pursue her investigations into the plight of leprosy sufferers in that inhospitable region. She crossed the Caucasus Mountains and made her way to Moscow, where she arrived in November 1890.[35] There and in St Petersburg, though she knew hardly a word of Russian, she prepared for her epic journey into the Siberian wilderness. Apart from the patronage of the Empress, she secured the support of the highly orthodox and reactionary Head Procurator of the Holy Synod, Konstantin Pobedonostzeff, and of Countess Alexandrine Tolstoy, a cousin of the great Russian novelist. It has been suggested that her appeal for such luminaries was 'due to the fact, more acceptable in Victorian times than today, that she was a philanthropist and not a

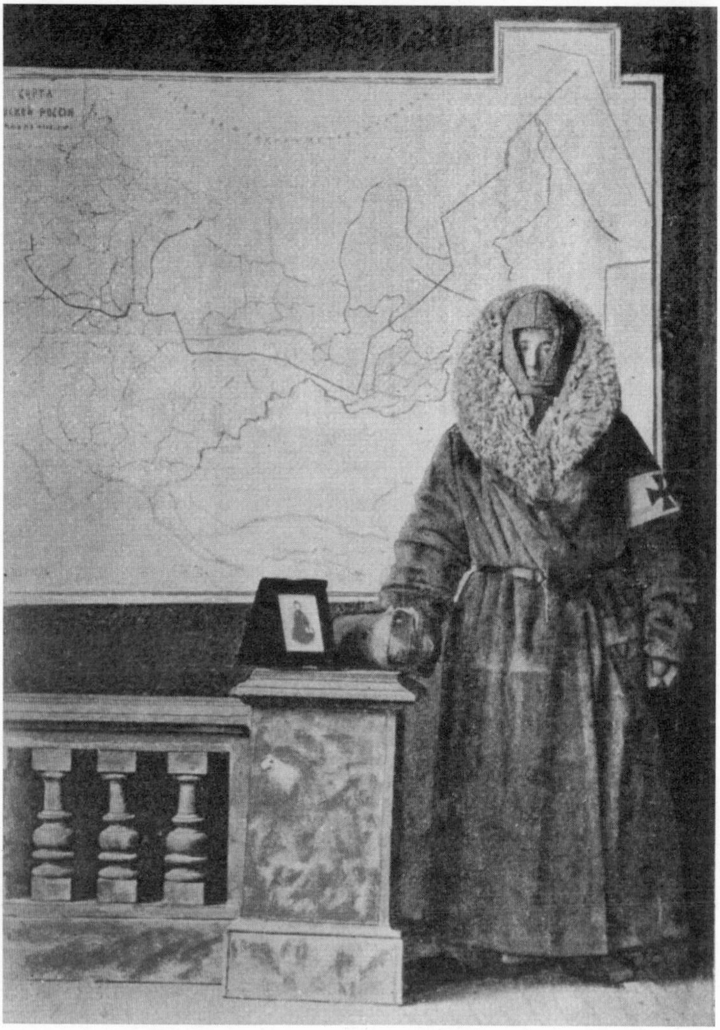

Kate Marsden, dressed for Siberian travel,
in front of a map showing her route across Russia

reformer', that she could 'speak of "a charming leper colony" and "a splendid prison" without a trace of irony'.[36] She had no desire to change the world, only to succour the needy.

She set out to cross a wintry Russia by sledge with a companion and interpreter, Miss Ada Field; their destination was the great forest extending from Yakutsk to Vilyuysk in north-eastern Siberia. The journey as far as Yakutsk was arduous but comparatively straightforward, though it was too much for Ada Field; by the time they reached Omsk, around the halfway mark, she was already so ill she had to turn back. Kate was undaunted; she found a Russian soldier who could speak some English and, though from time to time she came under suspicion of being a British spy, continued on her way. As she wrote later:

> Siberia then was a place principally for prisoners and officials. True Siberians remind me very much of British Colonials – they are frank, honest, truthful and loyal, they give help to every stranger and to every one in need, but why a strange English lady should take it into her head to choose that one spot of all others to ferret out a lot of useless hated Lepers was a problem difficult for Russian officials to understand, and they could not believe that some sinister motive was not behind it.[37]

Once these Siberians had got over their initial mistrust and scepticism, however, they became 'true and valued friends, only too anxious to help at every turn'; and at Irkutsk, near Lake Baikal, Kate organised a supportive committee before proceeding to Yakutsk. She also gathered together a party of Yakuts to act as guides and bodyguards. She must have cut a curious figure there, dressed in a huge hat to protect her from the sun, a mosquito net draped like a veil over her face, a long jacket with wide

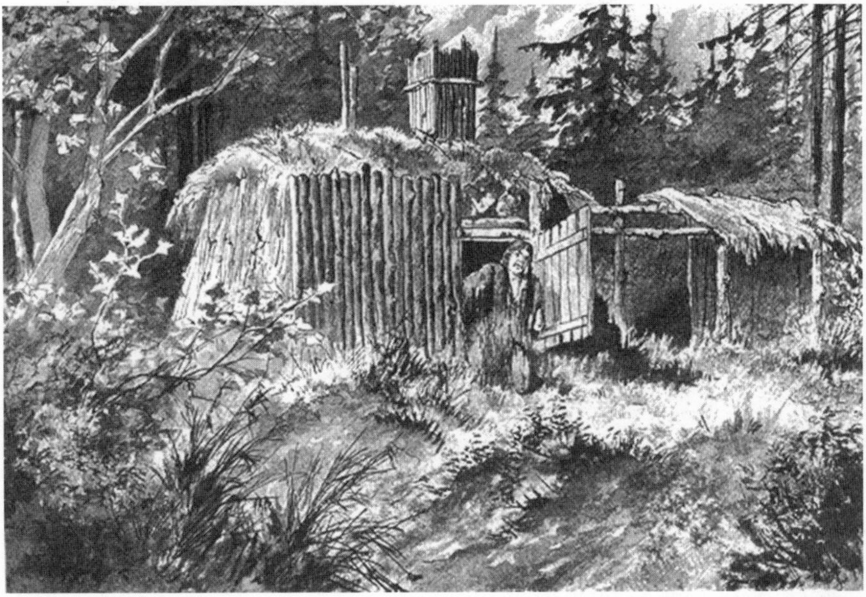

(from 'Review of Reviews', July–Dec 1892–©O. Renard Moscou)

A leprosy sufferer emerges from a primitive *yourta* (hut) in the Siberian forest sleeves and trousers which tucked into her boots at the knee. She carried a revolver and a whip, as well as – a more homely touch – her bag. Riding side-saddle was unknown in those parts, so she had to sit astride her horse like a man. Before the expedition departed the local bishop gave it his blessing, and the cavalcade set out in midsummer 1891, carrying tents and provisions that included an inordinate amount of plum pudding.[38]

'She rode for over two thousand miles through the woods,' an admiring contemporary wrote, 'one of the longest rides that ever a lady knight errant made even in olden times.'[39] The going was hazardous; there were no roads; the horses waded through marshes of uncertain depth and stumbled over tree roots; bears were a constant threat: the horses had only to smell them and they bolted through the dense forest, endangering the lives of their riders; and mosquitoes were an ever-present aggravation, particularly at night. If the Holy Grail in this instance was a herb with magical properties that would cure leprosy, then Kate Marsden's expedition was a signal failure. She found no such thing. But if the purpose of her mission was to draw attention to the plight of leprosy-affected outcasts cowering in the depths of the forest, then it succeeded beyond all expectation.

In her account of it, Marsden wrote:

> for sixty-four years the lepers of Yakutsk pleaded in vain for a permanent place of shelter. It is enough to make one's heart bleed to read that the hospital opened in 1860 for forty lepers had to be closed three years later, 'owing to insufficiency of means' . . . So, after their brief respite from awful loneliness and misery, these poor creatures were turned adrift to seek again, in the untrodden depths of the forest, the only home which their fellow creatures would allot them.

Once a person was discovered to have leprosy, he or she was driven out of the village – 'as if he were some noxious animal' – to some isolated spot on the marshes or in the forest and 'doomed to a living death'.

> The only shelter he can find is some filthy little *yourta* (hut), which may have been tenanted by another leper, who now, perhaps, is buried near the threshold. His first duty is to make a cross, which he is bound to place outside, as a warning to anyone who may happen to pass to shun him. And so he begins his outcast leper life . . .[40]

Some of the leprosy sufferers Kate came upon lived alone except for a dog – and that was not so much for companionship as out of necessity to keep away the bears. Others sought out fellow sufferers and formed small settlements, like the one called Hatignach, which she found 'too horrible to describe fully':

> Twelve men, women, and children, scantily and filthily clothed, were huddled together in two small *yourtas*, covered with vermin. The stench was dreadful; one man was dying, two men had lost their toes and half their feet; they had tied boards from their knees to the ground, so that by this help they could contrive to drag themselves along . . . On my approaching them they all crouched on the ground, as if almost terror-struck at the very idea of anyone coming near to help them . . .[41]

If food was put out for them, it was generally putrid; they had no bread and lived mostly on rotten fish – unless they were lucky enough to own cattle. One old woman would creep back to her village to sift through the refuse in an attempt to assuage her hunger, but when she was discovered the headman ordered that she be stripped and all her clothes removed, so she would not come back again. Soon afterwards her naked body was found; she had frozen to death.[42] Father John, the priest at Vilyuysk – 'one of the quietest places I ever visited' – told Kate that the Yakuts had a superstitious dread of leprosy, which they regarded as diabolic: ' "Small-pox, measles, scarlet fever," they say, "were appointed by God; but leprosy was sent by the devil." '[43]

Marsden managed to rescue one little girl who was herself untouched by the disease but had been expelled from the community along with her leprosy-affected mother. Children were particularly vulnerable to chicanery. The fact that the afflicted lost their property rights meant that unscrupulous individuals could take advantage of those who were unable to defend themselves.

> Information was received at Viluisk, two years before my visit, that a supposed child-leper had been starved to death. After an investigation, the true facts of the case became known. This child's father and mother [had] died and left him a few cows. His uncle took charge of him and his sister and at once began to practise upon him unheard-of cruelties. After

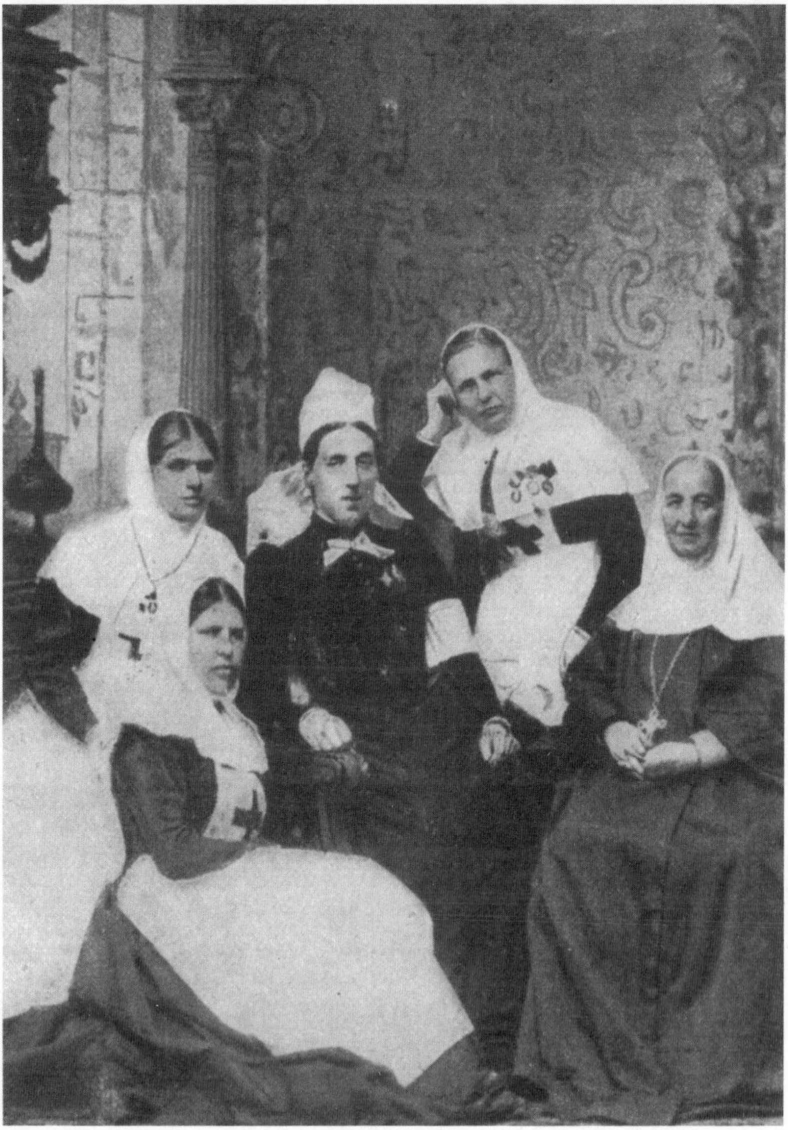

(by kind permission of the St Francis Leprosy Guild)

Kate Marsden (*centre*) with the Russian Princess Shachovsky and three of her nursing sisters

murdering the sister, he conceived the inhuman plan of getting the community to believe that the boy was a leper, in order to secure the cows. His plot succeeded, and he at once drove the lad into the depths of one of the densest forests in the district, where, in truth, the only inhabitants were bears. This occurred in the midst of a Siberian winter.

> The uncle had formed a kind of kennel in which the child was to pass the rest of his days. It was made simply of a few sticks thrust into the ground, lightly covered with cow-dung and snow; and there the child was left to starve, or to be frozen to death . . .[44]

Such stories of peasant avarice were by no means confined to Siberia; they were familiar to leprosy workers in many other parts of the world: for example in India, where only the climate was different. Drs Lewis and Cunningham spoke of the 'great ill-usage' to which leprosy sufferers there were exposed:

> The aversion with which they are regarded, and the disgrace attaching to the occurrence of the disease in a family, are inducements to make outcasts of them, and the temptation to do so is increased by interested motives, as, by turning them adrift, their relatives are enabled to appropriate to their own use the share of the family property belonging to the sick.[45]

Kate Marsden resolved to raise money to found a Siberian settlement that would achieve what the short-lived hospital in Yakutsk had set out to do in 1860 but lacked the funds to carry through. Because she had an entrée into Russian high society, she had no difficulty in galvanising support for her project on her return to Moscow and St Petersburg. She had already raised some money through her committee in Irkutsk, and now a group of five nursing sisters from the Princess Shachovsky Sisterhood in Moscow volunteered to go to Siberia and care for the leprosy sufferers. The princess herself described their departure from Moscow station on 29 May 1892:

> I saw a man of venerable appearance approaching me, who asked me to accept 51 roubles (£5 2s.) for the travelling expenses of the Sisters. Another gave me 100 roubles (£10), a third 200 roubles (£20), half for the Sisters and half for the poor unfortunate lepers. Again a fourth brought 25 roubles (£2 10s.). Very touching prayers were offered by an earnest pastor, a great number of people being present, all surrounding the Sisters, and with tears wishing them a happy journey. It was indeed a solemn hour. Why could not our good angel, our loved Kate Marsden, have been present at this beautiful religious service, which would, indeed, have filled her heart with inexpressible joy?[46]

Kate could not be there because she was being swept along on a tide of triumph. On her return to England, she had an audience with Queen Victoria, who wrote a letter on 27 October, expressing her 'deep interest in the work undertaken by Miss Marsden amongst the lepers'. W.T. Stead's *Review of Reviews* carried an enthusiastic article on her 'Quest for the Holy Grail', describing her work as 'so important, so full of humanitarian charity, that we cannot fail to see in Miss Marsden an instrument chosen by the Lord Himself to alleviate the miserable condition, moral as well as physical, of the poor lepers'.[47] The Royal Geographical Society made her a Fellow – one of the first women to be so honoured. Even the *British Medical Journal* could scarce forbear to cheer, though it pooh-poohed the 'so-called plant remedy' that was 'the chief object of her journey', remarking that it was 'the first time that good work has been done en route in aimless searches for a philosopher's stone'.[48]

But as Marsden prepared her own account of her journey for publication and planned a lecture tour of the United States to raise more money for her project, critical comments began to appear. As early as 3 December 1892, the *BMJ* ran the following note:

> A great deal of money is being subscribed for 'the lepers of Siberia'. Is it ungracious to suggest that a duly audited financial statement and balance sheet should be published up to date, and that a duly constituted committee and financial officer should be appointed for further purposes?[49]

Three weeks later, the *BMJ* struck again, but from a different angle:

> From a report in a newspaper of a lecture given by Miss Kate Marsden on her visit to Siberia it appears that the lady now admits that she had seen not more than 73 lepers, and she stated her belief that there were only between two or three times that number in the whole of the vast Yakutsk district . . . What special claims the comparatively few Siberian lepers have on the charity of the British public it is not easy to see.

According to the *BMJ*, the Russians should 'support their own lepers': British folk should direct their assistance to the colonies and India.[50] The journal continued sniping at Marsden throughout 1893, in January noting the publication of her book and the 'sympathetic notices' of it appearing in the press and questioning the need for charity when 'Dr Smirnoff, the Government Medical Inspector, could find no more than 62 [leprosy sufferers] in the leper district of Viluisk',[51] and making much the same point again in July, quoting a *Daily News* correspondent reporting from Irkutsk:

> 'Not only are the lepers few, but they are well provided for. A Russian Medical Inspector – Dr Smernoff [*sic*] – had visited them all, and made what arrangements were deemed necessary for their comfort before any English lady thought of doing so . . . They eat good Siberian bread, wear good Siberian clothes, live in good Siberian cottages, and even possess good Siberian cattle . . .' We have already given warning in this direction more than once. But the leper mission fund is now being boomed in Chicago, and probably will make a tour of the world.[52]

The Chicago reference is to the World's Fair that was held there in the spring of 1893. Kate Marsden had planned to exhibit in it and was expecting a friendly welcome. But according to *The Life*, 'she found a whole "heaven of storm" raised against her. Her motives and all her actions in connection with the leper work were questioned and traduced, and both she and her work were looked upon as frauds'.[53] Through sheer persistence, she was eventually and grudgingly allocated a tiny space.

In the *BMJ*'s last salvo, dated 20 January 1894, it did not even bother to name the guilty party, merely remarking that 'the lady – whose *début* in the realms of "Philanthropy" was, some few years ago, duly "boomed" *secundum artem* by a sympathetic interviewer of the *Pall Mall Gazette* – is still on the warpath'.[54] Now the Charity Organisation Society was investigating Marsden and her London-based committee's attempt to raise £10,000 to found a leprosy settlement in Siberia. The fact that its findings, though confidential, were sent to a Miss Katherine Willard of Evanston, Illinois, may help to explain Marsden's hostile reception in Chicago.

The COS absolved the committee, largely composed of 'Miss Marsden's personal friends', of any wrong-doing over the money raised: all that had been received was duly transmitted to Russia. But its assessment of Kate herself, based on 'a mass of information as to [her] career from the age of 19 years', was damning. This might not have mattered, except insofar as she proposed 'to live in the colony, and superintend it', which meant that the money would eventually find its way back to her – 'She is admitted by her friends to be utterly unbusiness-like, and she has shown herself to be extremely careless in dealing with money'. Not only that, but the evidence showed that she had 'habitually romanced about her doings and adventures in Russia and New Zealand'; that she had 'fallen out with, or forfeited the confidence of, a large number of persons, many of them of undoubted standing and repute'; and that 'her conduct has in many ways been such as to lead her friends to the conclusion that she has not always been responsible for her actions'. Though widely regarded as 'a person of commanding influence', in the estimation of the COS she was decidedly not 'a suitable person to undertake the administration of Charitable funds'. Nor, in its view, was 'the scheme of a Leper Colony . . . necessary or practicable'.[55]

On 11 March Marsden's erstwhile supporter, the pastor of the British-American Church in St Petersburg, Rev. Alexander Francis, wrote to warn her not to return to Russia 'for at least some months':

> Reports adverse to yourself are so numerous and widely spread, and opinion, here and in Siberia as well as in England and in America, is so divided that you have no prospect of successfully accomplishing, in the meantime at least, any good work for the lepers.

By August he was openly repudiating her in a letter to the Editor of *The Times*, which stated that a committee of investigation, consisting of 'friends of Miss Marsden' in Russia, had looked into 'serious charges preferred against [her] by various people in England, America, and New Zealand' and, as a result, 'Miss Marsden's leper work is necessarily at an end'. He claimed that Marsden had 'at last' acknowledged in writing 'the truth of the gravest charges against her', but gave no indication of what these might be, contenting himself with saying that he had 'the sad satisfaction of knowing that no possible injustice is done to her'. He publicly thanked the Charity Organisation Society and a number of individuals for their help, especially 'Miss Isabel F. Hapgood, of New York, U.S.A., to whom all who have the interests of true philanthropy at heart are deeply indebted for her public-spirited work in connexion with this case'.[56]

Kate retorted by publishing an earlier report by her 'friends' in Russia that fully exonerated her from the charges of falsifying the record of her adventures in Siberia, exaggerating the need for her mission and mishandling the money subscribed to it. In addition, she threatened to take legal action against Francis, whose letter, she wrote, was 'calculated to do me so much harm'.[57] Francis, given the chance to reply in the same edition of *The Times*, explained that the document the paper had reproduced was merely a draft that Marsden had acquired and got committee members to sign by taking it round to them herself while 'abundant and convincing evidence . . . from many quarters' was still coming in. Francis said he had withheld his own signature when he 'was informed where and how complete proof of the charges against Miss Marsden could be procured'. These charges remained unspecified, but Francis was able to use Kate's threat of legal proceedings to make a counter threat of 'a complete *exposé*'.[58] Whether from fear of that or for pecuniary reasons, Kate did not pursue the case against Francis.

In an appendix to *The Life of Kate Marsden*, which was published in the midst of this furore, her *alter ego* or amanuensis gives an account that suggests it was the former rather than the latter:

> Her Committee in London, after much enquiry, found that the rumours concerned her past life (previous to commencing the leper work), during the period in which she suffered a prolonged illness, with seasons of partial recovery, followed by relapses, consequent upon her accident in the hospital in New Zealand. In the course of this most trying mental illness, and at times of convalescence when, physically, she was in fairly good health, she said and did things for which she could not justly be held morally responsible. It therefore appeared to the Committee that to bring up charges, based upon actions which occurred under the influence of mental aberration, for the purpose of destroying Miss Marsden's reputation, was both unfair and cruel . . .
>
> All persons of fair minds and unbiased judgment will not hesitate to exonerate Miss Marsden from culpability with regard to the events referred to. But in her own eyes she was culpable, and, behind her intense sympathy for the lepers, there was a motive, hitherto not mentioned, which to a very large extent prompted her to face hardship and suffering in the depths of Siberia. It was the motive of expiation, or, in her own words, '*living her repentance and sorrow.*' And when she returned from her mission – her health undermined for life – she devoutly hoped that the past was buried. But her hope was not realised, for not long had

> she been in this country when rumours affecting her reputation passed from mouth to mouth. It may be said, without any exaggeration, that her sufferings in Siberia were slight compared with the persecution which she has endured in England from various sources . . .[59]

In 1895, having converted to Catholicism, Marsden was instrumental in founding the St Francis Leprosy Guild. Almost immediately, she felt obliged to resign because of the controversy surrounding her, but the Guild soon reinstated her, noting in the minutes that 'any enemy of hers is unlikely to be a friend of the Guild'.[60] In the wider world, however, the damage was done and, although the sum of 32,000 roubles (£3,200) raised by Kate's efforts went to the founding of a leprosy hospital at Vilyuysk in 1897, she took no further part in that scheme. The number of patients in the hospital never exceeded seventy-six (in 1902) and had fallen to nineteen by 1917, but it performed an invaluable service, providing food, shelter and medication for those Siberian outcasts who might otherwise have been left to starve or freeze to death.[61] Kate might be reviled, then neglected and finally forgotten in her own country, but in those parts she was, and continued to be, revered.

She tried to make a new life for herself in the United States, that land of opportunity. But her reputation had gone before her, as we have seen, and she was *persona non grata* there, too. One of the more bizarre twists in a bizarre story is revealed in correspondence preserved in the US National Archives, involving the Secretary of the Treasury and the Secretary of State in Washington DC, over 'the case of Miss Kate Marsden'. It stemmed from a letter Kate had written to the Marquis of Lansdowne from an address in Bayswater on 25 November 1901, in which she begged for government help 'in a matter which has caused me over three years of intense suffering'. She informed his lordship that she had been living in Philadelphia for the past five years and intended to return there forthwith, but feared she might be prevented from staying because it was said she had leprosy.[62]

Three years before, a Philadelphian doctor had examined her nose and, suspecting she might have the disease, told her she must either submit to segregation by the Board of Health within twenty-four hours or take herself to Hawaii and consult the leprosy specialist Dr L.P. Alverez in Honolulu (though why she should have to go so far when there were perfectly competent leprosy doctors closer to home is a mystery, unless it was hoped that she would be detained there and sent to Molokai – where she had once volunteered to go, only to be rebuffed). She chose to see Dr Alverez, who confirmed that she had the symptoms of leprosy. Through the intervention of the acting British consul she was permitted to return to England. There she underwent further examinations by Harley Street doctors, who could find no sign of the disease and gave her a clean bill of health. But this did not satisfy the Americans. On her return to Philadelphia, she was again told to leave. She consulted other European doctors, who also denied that she had leprosy. But, she wrote, 'I am allowed to remain nowhere in peace, owing to the certificate of the Board of Health, Honolulu'. No English doctor would employ her as a nursing sister; no boarding house would take her in as a guest. She had lost her home in America and spent all her money 'in trying to right myself of this terrible stigma'. And all to no avail.[63]

Her next letter on file was written a month later, on 20 December, from the Hotel Normandie on Broadway, New York City, and was addressed to the British ambassador to the United States, the Rt Hon. Lord Pauncefote. She reported that three leading New York specialists had examined her the day before and were unanimous in their verdict that she did not have leprosy or show the least bacillary evidence of it. She reiterated how much mental distress and pecuniary embarrassment she had suffered as a result of the false diagnosis and thanked the ambassador for a small loan he had made her.[64] At the ambassador's request the Secretary of State took up the matter with the Secretary of the Treasury (the department responsible for the Marine-Hospital Service, forerunner of the US Public Health Service) and asked that she be allowed to resume her residence in Philadelphia, provided an examination by government experts confirmed that she was free from leprosy. The Secretary of the Treasury replied that Philadelphia had its own health laws and regulations and 'if the City Health Officer of Philadelphia believes that Miss Marsden is suffering from leprosy and issues an order debarring her from residence in that city, it is not a question in which the Treasury Department can interfere'.[65] And there the matter seems to have rested: Kate became a victim of bureaucracy, and had no choice but to leave Philadelphia.

Back in England she was lucky enough to find a devoted companion, with whom she lived for the rest of her days in various locations mainly on the south coast, for Miss E. LL. Norris was a painter of seascapes and skies 'full of storm, full of atmospheric environment, full of sunshine, and at all times wonderfully true to nature'.[66] Kate's frequent letters to the Secretary of the Royal Geographical Society, apologising for falling into arrears in payment of her subscription to the RGS journal, bear witness to her poverty. Eventually she hit upon a means of maintaining this vital connection – 'I love the Geographical Society,' she wrote – without having to make further payments. In 1916 she presented the RGS with the jewel that Queen Victoria had given her in 1892 on her return from Siberia: 'It represents the Angel of Victory standing upon the World & I value it beyond words . . . ' The RGS, in return, made her a Free Life Fellow.[67]

This gave her the impetus to make one last attempt to clear her name. In 1921 she published a résumé of her original book under the title, *My Mission in Siberia: A Vindication*, in which she rehearsed all the old arguments. But nobody cared any more. The world had moved on, and Kate retreated into silence, poverty and invalidism. When the chairman of the council of the Professional Classes Aid Council wrote to the RGS for confidential information about Marsden, the secretary replied dismissively, referring to her as 'a rather tiresome old woman' who occasionally bothered him 'about calumnies'.[68] Her friend Miss Norris also got short shrift when she asked 'if it would be any good to try and get up a private subscription for her among some of the Fellows of the RGS'.[69] But that did not prevent this loyal friend from carrying out Kate's wishes and giving the RGS all that was left of her Siberian journey – her watch and a whistle she had taken with her – when Marsden died in 1931.[70]

In August 1994, exactly 100 years after it had contributed to Kate Marsden's ruin by publishing the Rev. Alexander Francis's letters about her, *The Times* made partial amends by running an article by William Millinship that put these letters in context and provided the missing piece of the jigsaw puzzle, without which the story would remain incomprehensible. Millinship discovered in the Russian State Archives a letter Francis had written to the Prefect of St Peterburg in 1894 – a letter, he says, which 'reeks of fear of the Russian authorities, whose goodwill Francis needed to preserve his church'. In it Francis had written, 'It would be terrible for all concerned were it to be known that immorality with women is, according to Miss Marsden's own written confessions, one of her sins.' Not to spare her, but to protect her wealthy

Russian patronesses from guilt by association, he hit upon the plan of publishing 'facts concerning her fraudulent transactions, in order that the public may suppose that that is the greater offence'. His letter to *The Times* would, he was convinced, 'suppress Miss Marsden', as long as she received no further encouragement from Russia. And so it did.[71]

Behind Francis was a more implacable enemy, a woman Marsden had never met who nevertheless conducted a relentless campaign against her. Isabel Hapgood, whom Francis had thanked effusively in his original letter to *The Times*, was an American translator, the first to render the great nineteenth-century Russian novels into English.[72] At this remove it is impossible to say in what way Kate had earned the enduring enmity of this 'public-spirited' woman who pursued her like a fury.

What is certain is that England, or London – at any rate, the press – was enjoying one of its periodic hysterical outbreaks of morality. The year 1895 saw the failure of Oscar Wilde's libel action against the Marquis of Queensberry and his own trial and imprisonment for homosexual acts; and though the recently enacted legislation did not apply to female homosexuality (such a thing apparently being inconceivable to Queen Victoria), Kate's lesbianism would have been equally stigmatised had it been made public, as Francis well knew. Hence Marsden's frustration: since her real offence in the eyes of her accusers could not be made public without damaging her reputation still further, she was unable to defend herself in any but the vaguest, and therefore least convincing, terms.

In the end, the woman who is remembered as a heroine in Vilyuysk for what she did for Siberian leprosy sufferers more than a hundred years ago herself became, in that hideous and tautological phrase, a 'moral leper' in her own country.

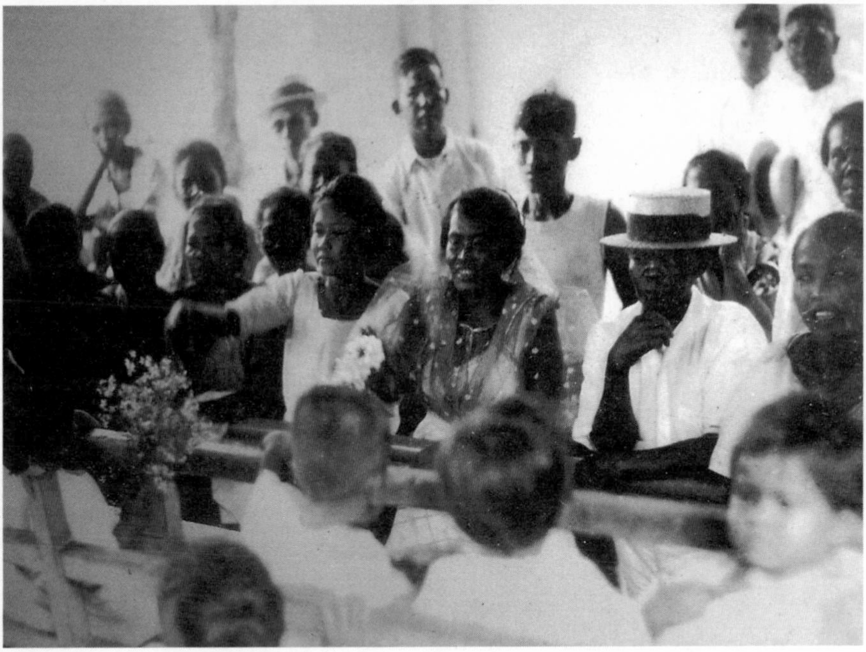

(Culion Museum)

Children at Culion leprosarium,
separated from visiting family by a pane of glass

Chapter 7

VETERANS OF THE SPANISH–AMERICAN WAR, 1: 'NED LANGFORD' AND CULION

Ned Langford was a real person, though this was not his real name. His story, based on what he'd written himself and told in the first person with considerable empathy and skill by Perry Burgess, an influential figure in the world of leprosy, became an instant bestseller when it was published in 1940.[1]

In 1898, while he was still at college, Ned volunteered along with a roommate to serve his country in its newly declared war against Spain over Cuba. By that time the West was well and truly Won and the United States had run out of (continental) land to conquer. The only direction in which an expansionist nation could expand was overseas and the problem there was that it would encounter opposition from other nations. In the words of Gore Vidal:

> Fortunately Cuba wanted to be free of Spain; and so the United States, a Goliath posing as David, struck down Spain, a David hardly able to pose at all, and thus Cuba was freed to become a client state, the Philippines conquered and occupied, and westward the course of empire flowed.[2]

Of course, the young Ned Langford could hardly be expected to take such a cynical view of the adventure on which he embarked to the accompaniment of military bands and the suddenly shy and awe-struck glances of hitherto impudent younger siblings.

The two football-playing roommates enlisted in the 1st Regiment, Colorado Volunteers, but the unit they yearned to join was (Teddy) Roosevelt's Rough Riders, whose glamour was enhanced when its colonel,

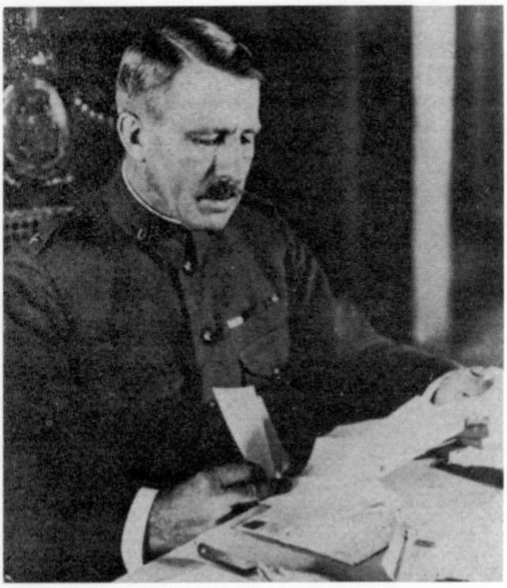
(The Star)

Major-General Leonard Wood

Leonard Wood – 'an army medico who had covered himself with glory fighting Indians, and particularly Geronimo' – stopped by to inspect the new troops. They failed to get a transfer to this already oversubscribed outfit, but the 'tall, straight, bronzed and lean' Wood smiled at Ned when Ned ran into him off parade. Their paths would cross again many years later in circumstances neither could have predicted.

Ned was thrilled to be heading out to the Philippines, along with the other soldiers on board the general's flagship, appropriately named the *China* – since having an advanced trading post with China was one of the (unspoken) objects of the exercise. By the time they arrived and made their way to Manila, he and his friends found the Spanish army cut off inside the city, on one side by Filipino nationalists and on the other by the American navy and troops. The outcome was inevitable. The volunteers, who were disappointed to have come so far and seen and done so little, expected to be on their way home once the city had fallen. Then they heard rumours of an 'insurrection' and learned that the Filipinos 'were demanding immediate independence, which the American leaders were unwilling to grant'.

The people they had been helping to throw off the Spanish colonial yoke had suddenly and mysteriously become their enemy. They would have their fight after all, only it would be against the 'insurgents' rather than the Spanish, who had done a face-saving deal with the Americans whereby they not only avoided the *coup de grâce* in Manila but received compensation into the bargain. 'In this fashion', the novelist and historian James Hamilton-Paterson writes, 'the Philippine Islands and their entire freight of souls changed hands like any piece of real estate for $20 million, made over at the Treaty of Paris in December 1898.'[3]

Mark Twain might object, 'We cannot maintain an empire in the Orient and maintain a republic in America,' but Theodore Roosevelt, who became US President in 1901, was contemptuous of such criticism. Roosevelt's unashamed imperialism was very much of his time, and he saw the conquest of the Philippines as part of a smooth and logical progression from internal to external expansion: 'Every argument that can be made for the Filipinos could be made for the Apaches . . . As peace, order and prosperity followed our expansion over the land of the Indians, so they will follow us in the Philippines.'[4] The career of Roosevelt's henchman and Ned Langford's hero, Leonard Wood, was an embodiment of precisely this sort of progression: from successful Indian-fighter to commanding General in Cuba and, many years later, Governor-General of the Philippines.

Langford's term of enlistment soon came to an end, but he volunteered to remain as a regular. As a foot soldier in war, one of his main preoccupations was simply staying alive. So when he came under fire while taking a message to a neighbouring unit he dived for cover in the gateway of an imposing building he mistook for Command HQ. Shouts from behind him – 'Where do you think you're going, you damned fool?' and 'That's a home for lepers!' – brought him up short.

> I jumped back from that gate as though I'd been hit. My heart missed a beat. A home for lepers? It must be a joke. I had heard about lepers in Sunday School but I didn't dream they still existed . . . As the firing increased I could see the inmates of the house across the way going hell for leather through the fields. Lepers, it seemed, had no more relish for hot lead than anyone else. I couldn't understand it. Why wouldn't they welcome death? I was certain that if I were a leper, a bullet would seem a good out.

Ned spent the remainder of his service in the Philippines on garrison duty in the south, where he was billeted with an upper-class Filipino family. The Nolascos had a beautiful daughter called Carita – Spanish for 'little face' – with whom the youthful Ned fancied he was in love. He daydreamed about marrying her and settling in the islands, but the lure of home was stronger and when his time was up he returned to his family in Missouri. He did write to Carita a couple of times, but put her out of his mind when she failed to reply. Then he got a letter from his old college friend, who'd joined the constabulary and stayed in the Philippines. The friend wrote that he'd visited the Nolasco family and Carita had asked him to explain why she hadn't written: her younger brother Sancho had been diagnosed with leprosy and sent to the San Lazaro

Hospital – the very place where Ned had sought cover during the battle with the insurgents – and she had been too concerned, not just about Sancho, but over the possibility that other members of the family might be infected, to write. Ned was horrified; he grieved for the family and worried about Carita. Insofar as he had thought about leprosy at all he had supposed it was a sexually transmitted disease, but Sancho was too young for that to have been the means by which he contracted it. Only then did it dawn on Ned that he, too, might be at risk; he'd lived in their house, slept on their floor and eaten their food. He had a moment of panic before dismissing the thought.

He joined his father's trucking and warehousing business, and took it over when the old man sickened and died. Nine years after his return from the Philippines Ned fell in love with a music student called Jane. They were engaged within a month, but she would not marry him until her studies were over – to cut them short would have been unfair to her parents, who had made sacrifices for her education. Ned was now set up for life: his family owned two small farms; he was running a business; he was wildly in love and engaged to be married; his younger brother Tom was doing well at college . . .

The first sign of trouble came when a fire broke out in a stable and warehouse building and Ned burned his arm badly as he struggled to free the trapped horses. The doctor was surprised to discover that while the hand was very painful, the arm, which was far more severely damaged, did not hurt at all. In time the burns healed, but the numbness of the arm remained, mystifying the doctor, who put it down to an old and forgotten injury. Jane went away for her last year at college and Ned looked forward to the following June, when they planned to be married. Everything would then fall into place.

In another letter from his friend in the Philippines, he learned that Carita had got married but her husband had died soon after and she'd had a stillborn baby. The letter also informed him that her brother Sancho had been moved from the San Lazaro Hospital to an island called Culion, two hundred miles south of Manila, on the edge of the China Sea, where 'the Americans had established a leper colony'.

In their anxiety to avoid such telltale words as 'colony' (except in the context of leprosy) and 'colonialism', the Americans dreamed up a 'Bureau of Insular Affairs' as a subdivision of the War Department, through which they would rule the Philippines for thirty-six years.[5] The man appointed Director of Health for the Islands in 1905 was Dr Victor Heiser, who published a bestselling memoir in the 1930s and lived to a very grand old age. Confronted with Filipino apathy and fatalism over disease, Heiser used his near-dictatorial powers to good effect. In fifteen years plague was eradicated, fatalities from cholera and smallpox dramatically reduced and the rampant tuberculosis checked.[6]

With leprosy, he wrote, the 'foundation stone on which I built my policy' was the fact that the disease 'does not occur in areas in which there is no leper'. One of his 'most important duties', as he saw it, 'was to isolate the lepers'. The model was Molokai, where he spent a month in 1908, and while he admitted that segregation was cruel, his line was that 'segregation is cruel to relatively few, whereas non-segregation threatens an entire people'.[7]

So in May 1906, 365 inmates of the San Lazaro Hospital were shipped – not without difficulty, since 'as we were about to sail the entire crew deserted' – to the small island of Culion, twenty miles long and at its broadest point twelve miles wide. On arrival, they were met by a Jesuit priest and four sisters of the French order of St Paul de Chartres. This was the beginning of what soon became the largest leprosarium in the world. Heiser did his utmost to publicise the attractions of Culion as a way of encouraging leprosy sufferers to go there voluntarily rather than wait to be apprehended by health officials on 'leper-collecting trips' – or worse, go into hiding:

> There was a young leper girl in Cebu whom the local authorities were never able to produce when we arrived. Finally her brother was stricken and taken to Culion. On our next visit she gave herself up voluntarily. When I asked her how she had eluded us so long, she explained that the telegraph operator was her friend, and had informed her in advance when we were due. She would then speed away to a cave in the hills, where she had always had enough food hidden to last her until we had gone.[8]

Anonymous letter-writers provided the authorities with a lot of information, not all of it accurate. In one town, the mayor had ordered that the daughter of a rival candidate be included in the round-up of suspects so that her family would be tainted with the stigma of leprosy. But health officials took care that no one should be sent to Culion without bacterial evidence of the disease. By 1912, Heiser had achieved his aim and 'every recognized leper was in confinement'. There were some 'obstreperous cases', often from 'the criminal classes', who'd had to be taken there by force, but

> most of the patients who were to become the inhabitants of Culion were persuaded rather than compelled to go. Gradually the terror it caused was lost through our educational propaganda, and lepers were lured there by hope of a cure.[9]

Heiser was inclined to gloss over the difficulties of 'leper collecting' for obvious reasons; he didn't want people thinking he was responsible for a deeply unpopular policy. A more realistic picture emerges from the experiences of Sanitary Inspector Lorenzo Taborada, who, in the course of nine years' service in the Bureau of Health, was 'frequently assaulted, knocked unconscious, forced to disarm resisting lepers, shot, stabbed, required to swim for his life, and, after he shot and killed a leper trying to escape, acquitted of murder'. His reward for putting his life on the line so often was a citation, in which he was adjudged a 'very good model of a public servant', whose 'achievements are worthy of emulation by every one of the personnel of [the Philippine Health] Service'.[10]

Ned Langford had reason to think of Carita's brother Sancho at Culion when he was going through some letters from his fiancée Jane and came upon one from the Philippines that he thought he'd destroyed: 'This time I faced it squarely; those weeks in the Nolasco home – Sancho – Carita – those spots on my arm.' In the shower one day he had noticed that there was now more than one numb patch on his arm and he immediately went to the doctor. But neither Doc Windle nor a colleague of his was able to throw any light on his mysterious ailment; all they could suggest was that he consult a big city doctor with wider experience.

Ned was reluctant to do this for fear of what he might find. But when a third spot appeared on his leg, he knew he must go to St Louis. There he was directed to see an army doctor with experience of the Philippines who took a smear and tested it under the microscope. Major Thompson was so absorbed in his work that he yelped with delight on coming up with 'the old Hansen bacillus'. Then he saw Ned's face. He said, 'Oh God, soldier, I'm sorry.' He invited Ned to have a brandy and put an arm round his shoulder. He promised he would support Ned while he digested the crushing information and worked out what to do next, at the same time warning him that he was obliged to notify the Department of Health. He took Ned to a deserted shack beside the Mississippi where he left him, saying he would return the following morning.

Alone and abstracted, Ned wandered upriver, startling some nesting birds into flight and observing a fish leap clear of the water. He rounded a corner and came upon the city dump, a mountain of stinking debris stretching as far as the eye could see. He sat on an upturned crate: 'At last it came to me. Here by this dump I belonged. Refuse, that was Ned Langford.' He walked to the edge of the river and sat on a log, noting how swift the current was out in the middle of the Mississippi: 'If a man were to swim out there and just drift he could go down, down to the Gulf with the drift and the mud . . .' But a small object bobbling towards him at the water's edge distracted him. He was disgusted to see it was a rat, dead, but still moving obscenely in the water. He hated rats, even dead ones, and retreated to the dump, where he resumed his night vigil sitting on the upturned wooden box.

His ordeal had only just begun. Absorbed though he was in his gloomy reflections, he felt something go over his ankle and, looking down, was horrified to see a living rat – not just one but hordes of them. Kicking and yelling, he beat a hasty retreat to his shack, where he found yet more rats, drawn by the meagre supplies the doctor had left him. He tried to frighten them away by banging on the side of the shack, but one great brute remained, 'disputing possession with me'. Cornered, the rat fought like a demon, biting and scratching the hand that eventually squeezed the life out of it and hurled the disgusting object through the window:

> With the sound of breaking glass something crashed within me. Alone, alone for all time: Mother! Mabel [sister]! Tom! Jane! Jane . . . Jane . . . for the first time in my memory I began to sob. I reeled across to the wooden bunk, threw myself down, and wept my heart out.

Dr Thompson – Bill – brought Ned food, took care of his injured hand and discussed his future with him. They talked about Culion, but Bill recommended that Ned go to New York and see a Dr Todd he knew of there before cutting himself off so completely from his roots. The next day Bill brought Tom to see Ned and left the brothers together. Tom was even more upset than his brother and asked what he should say to the family, to Jane. Ned said, 'Tell them I'm dead.' When Tom protested he couldn't do that, Ned came up with a plan; he would make it easier for Tom by faking suicide. Tom was to let him have an old car they had on the farm; he would drive it to New York, and then push it into the river with the windows open, giving the impression that the driver had been sucked out by the current and drowned. Tom could write to him, but for both their sakes not often, and he was to address him as Ned Ferguson, not Langford, a name he would no longer use. He might not actually be dead, but from now on he would be one of the living dead.

The plan worked. Ned had difficulty in finding a sufficiently deserted spot in New York to stage his 'suicide', but eventually he came upon a small dock on the East River near Harlem, where he was able to put the car in gear, release the brake and jump out before it went over the edge – without attracting attention. The next day's newspaper carried a small downpage paragraph about his 'death'.

The professorial Dr Todd, 'with his clipped moustache and tiny goatee', had found him an isolated little house to rent in Greenwich Village, and Ned remained there for almost a year. But it was a life – if life was the word – of unutterable loneliness. As he wrote to Tom:

> You would never believe how alone aloneness is. You have to move, live, breathe, see, hear, in the midst of millions of people, not daring to touch one of them, afraid to speak lest they become friendly – avoiding – avoiding – eternally avoiding . . .

It had its comic side, as when he aroused a streetwalker's ire by spurning her advances. But in the end he could endure it no longer, and begged to be sent to Culion.

His outcast status made the journey a nightmare. First, he had to cross the States to San Francisco, travelling as a kind of moneyed hobo, hiding in boxcars, being chased by railway workers, avoiding over-friendly tramps and begging for food from farm people who looked at him strangely if he offered to pay. Then came the long sea voyage to the Philippines, pacing the little cabin to which he was confined 'like a caged animal', his only visitor the kindly ship's doctor who 'saved up every joke for me', and arrival in Manila Bay:

> That was one of the worst times I put in. Hours and hours passed. From noon to late afternoon, I sat in the stifling heat. I relived my first landing fourteen years before, when I was an eager youngster anxious to do his part in setting the world right. Again I was going ashore to fight, this time without drums or bugles, to fight a foe I would never see.

He was taken to San Lazaro, where he had accidentally sought cover all those years before. Dr Ravino welcomed him, saying, 'As an educated man, you will find San Lazaro a place of interest. For over three hundred years it has been a "sanctuary of sorrow".' The doctor told Ned a story, which Victor Heiser also tells in his memoirs, about how in the seventeenth century, when the Japanese banished foreign Christians from their country, they had dumped more than a hundred leprosy sufferers on the Philippines in the guise of converted Christians.

Heiser's predecessor as Director of Health, a Major Carter, had provoked a diplomatic incident by printing this story. The Japanese had demanded a retraction, and it fell to Heiser to initiate an investigation in the royal archives in Spain. From this he learned there were documents in Seville confirming that the Captain-General of the Philippine Islands had informed King Philip IV in June 1632 that 134 'converted Christians' sent over by the Emperor of Japan had arrived in Manila Bay:

> The Most Christian King had directed that the 'converted Christians' be welcomed with a parade, and that, in addition to the five hundred *reales* already set aside for their reception, two hundred more be expended for their maintenance. In that same year one hundred and thirty of them were admitted to San Lazaro Hospital.

When Heiser passed this information on to the Japanese government, they admitted they had found similar evidence in their own archives and consequently 'withdrew the demand for a retraction'.[11]

Ned's first night back in the Philippines was spent in the San Lazaro Hospital, and his homesickness was so profound that he again contemplated suicide. But he was distracted from his own misery by the sobbing of another new arrival, a nine-year-old boy, whom he went to comfort. The boy snuggled up to him and fell asleep: 'The ice was fairly broken. I had dreaded the moment when I should meet lepers as lepers. But all that was past. We were kin, not strangers . . .'

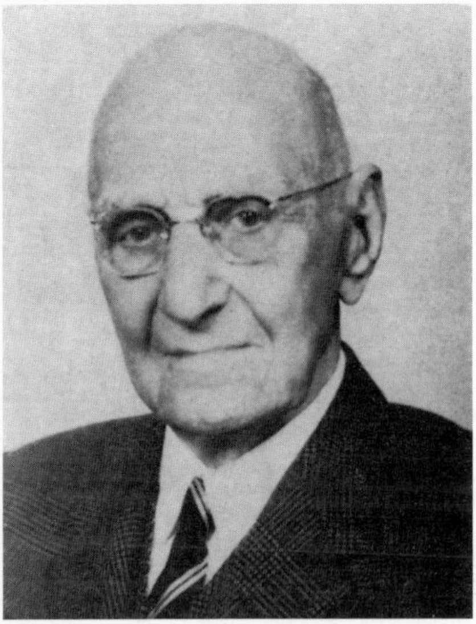
(The Star)

Dr Victor G. Heiser

The next day Ned witnessed yet more anguish when the leprosy sufferers boarded the Coast Guard cutter bound for Culion: both the patients on deck and many of their relations on the pier had to be restrained from jumping into the sea in their reluctance to be parted. Even the tough-minded Heiser found these family partings difficult to endure. He wrote, 'It was an experience to which I never became hardened.'[12]

The United States Director of Health for the Philippine Islands was one of Ned's fellow passengers on his trip to Culion (though Burgess calls him 'James Marshall', not Victor Heiser, and may have taken some fictional license in other ways, too). He is described as a tall American doctor in his late thirties, 'slender and lithe as an athlete', wearing 'a Palm Beach suit and a brown sun helmet'. He befriended Ned and impressed him with his passion for his job and commitment to the well-being of his patients. Ned was flattered that such an eminent man should treat him as an equal, a visiting doctor perhaps, rather than a patient with a dangerous disease.

As they approached Culion, Ned felt someone take his hand and, looking down, saw the boy he had comforted, Tomás, beside him, staring intently at the shore. Knowing just how he was feeling, Ned squeezed his hand and they exchanged a brief glance: 'Suddenly I was glad of that small hand. We were not alone; there were two of us.'

As an American, Ned got privileged treatment. He was met by 'Dr Winton, the Chief of the Colony' (in reality, Dr Oswald E. Denney), and escorted by him to a house set apart, previously occupied by another American, who had died of tuberculosis. Ned expressed his uneasiness about accepting 'special favors', but Dr Winton reassured him, saying the Filipino patients would 'think it strange' if he did not take the house: 'The Filipino is a gregarious individual; he does not want to live alone.'

As for Tomás, 'Why not have him come here with you? He could be your house boy. If you have money you can pay him a little.'

Intentionally or not, the developing relationship between Ned and Tomás, man and boy, master and servant, as told by Perry Burgess, mirrors the benevolent paternalism of the United States towards its dependent, the Philippines – not to mention that of the health authorities, the 'Marshall'/Heisers, 'Winton'/Denneys, priests and nuns of Culion and every other 'leper colony' towards their patients/charges. *Colony* is the *mot juste*.

Culion was, in effect, a colony within a colony. It had its own police force and secret service recruited among the inmates; it even had its own currency. Escape was possible; other islands were within reach; but it was not often attempted and was 'never a source of great trouble', according to Heiser. 'Even those who reached their homes usually gave themselves up after they had satisfied their nostalgia.'[13]

Heiser admitted that 'Life for the staff at Culion was exceedingly monotonous'.[14] But it does not seem to have occurred to him how much more wearisome it was for the patients, who had no hope of curtailing their involuntary exile. Ned at least had a garden, and he resolved to 'find things to do', to 'cheat the empty days' and to 'make beauty'. But first he had a duty to perform; he had to find Carita's younger brother Sancho. He approached the Jesuit Father and learned from him that Sancho was in the island's hospital. He discovered, too, that Carita herself had leprosy; it had manifested itself when she had given birth 'as so often happens,' the Father told him. She was in a leprosarium at Cebu. Ned steeled himself to visit the hospital where the advanced cases were. 'A sweetish, sickening odour came through the open door.' He went in:

> Never in my wildest imaginings had I dreamed of a horror like this. This – this rotting piece of flesh was not Sancho – Sancho the fine-featured lad I had known . . . His eyebrows and eyelashes had gone; his forehead was covered with shiny, reddish welts, some of which were open wounds. The bridge of his nose had fallen in, and the nostrils were widely distended and frightfully swollen with great festering tubercles . . . His lips, like his nostrils, were thick and enlarged and a paralysis of the mouth was beginning, so that it was set in an immobile, open oval . . . his voice was weak and there was a queer and terrifying hoarseness, sepulchral . . . I was being addressed by the dead.

Ned had to leave in a hurry. As soon as he got away from the hospital he threw up into the undergrowth. A few days later he heard that Sancho had died the night after he had visited him.

If he was not to end up like Sancho, Ned needed to undergo treatment. In the past, the only option had been oral doses of chaulmoogra oil but the smell and taste of it were so nauseating that very few patients could be persuaded to persevere with it long enough for it to be effective. Heiser recalled, 'The poor lepers would say, "Doctor, I'd rather have leprosy than take another dose!"' All attempts to make this medicine palatable failed and the doctors experimented with mixing the oil with a camphor-resorcin solution to render it absorbent enough to be injected. They were rewarded with 'the first faint suspicion of eyebrows beginning to grow in again and sensation returning to paralysed areas'.[15] But progress was still agonisingly slow, and Heiser kept pushing for further chemical advances, calling on the eminent English tropical medicine specialist, Sir Leonard Rogers, in Calcutta in 1915 and talking him into postponing his retirement from the Indian Medical Service in order to refine the process.

The new treatment of injecting chaulmoogra oil was optional, but Ned was ready to undergo it: 'No one likes to be punctured with a needle, but I felt little discomfort after it was over' – others became dizzy or had violent fits of coughing. He did get disheartened, though, not so much by the relative ineffectuality of the treatment as by the soul-destroying tedium of enforced idleness once he had got his house and garden in working order. To combat this he came up with the idea of organising a fishing co-operative in the leprosarium. He ironed out the details with the help of a qualified lawyer who was a fellow patient, and the scheme was approved by Dr Winton: 'Here was a new kind of excitement – for lepers; the possibility of achievement and of a chance to make money for themselves and their families . . .'

Another and greater excitement for Ned was the arrival at Culion of Carita, 'a vision of loveliness' unmarked by the disease. They were naturally drawn to one another and Ned, who 'had never associated with any of the women of the island', began to revive his youthful dream of marrying her. But Carita was not prepared to consider marriage without the possibility of children – she was a Catholic – nor would she contemplate having a child who was at risk of developing leprosy. Since the onset of her own disease she had abjured earthly passion in favour of the love of God, and Ned had no choice but to go along with that.

Not every patient on the island was so ready to renounce sexual activity, as Heiser found. On the Governor-General's orders, a new women's block was being constructed behind a high barbed-wire fence. Denney told Heiser that the women fiercely resisted this move: 'Short of a couple of regiments of constabulary we can't do anything with them. If you think you can persuade them, you go ahead and try.' So Heiser called a meeting, climbed on a soap box and delivered his message that it was for their own good, as well as being the instructions of the Governor-General:

> The Filipino women are even better orators than the men. One of them rose and delivered a fervent harangue to the effect that the rest of the world, after having segregated them, had not before seemed to concern itself with their welfare, and why should it take this unpleasant interest in them now? The women of Culion had asked for no protection from the men and did not want any.[16]

More impassioned speeches followed and then the cry, 'Kill him! Kill him!' was taken up. The women snapped shut their parasols and advanced on Heiser with their steel points aimed at his midriff: 'there flashed through my mind a picture of the ignominious fate which awaited me – punctured to death by umbrellas'. He saved himself by giving a solemn undertaking that work on the scheme would cease until he had discussed the situation with the Governor-General. The women relented, knowing they had won and there would be no further attempt to segregate them in this fashion – though separate homes were established for young girls, in the care of the Sisters, who locked them in at night. The point was to reduce the spread of leprosy by preventing propagation, since children were considered most at risk of contracting the disease.[17] Later, when Leonard Wood became Governor-General, an alternative scheme of removing children from their leprosy-affected parents at six months of age was introduced.

As far as Culion was concerned, the First World War might have been taking place on another planet, though when America entered the fray the 'colony' did its bit for the cause by purchasing Liberty Bonds. For Ned there was a more immediate concern: his brother Tom had gone to France with his regiment, and – as he heard from Bill Thompson soon after – had been killed in his very first action. This loss was swiftly followed by another of a different, but no less isolating kind: after a year of testing 'negative' – i.e., bacteria-free – Carita was to be 'paroled', allowed to go home. Ned encouraged her to go, urging her to 'take up the fight for the paroles'. But 'the sacrifice was almost too much for me . . . With her went another dream of real happiness'.

Dr Winton took no credit for these 'cures', claiming that 'the majority were spontaneous recoveries', but they did at least hold out the hope of eventual release. Not in Ned's case, however: his condition was worsening; he had taken to wearing gloves to hide the fact that his fingers 'had retreated to below the first knuckle', though he knew that no one in Culion, of all places, would be fooled. His moment of truth came on Armistice Day, 1918, when he acknowledged that his fight, too, was over; he had lost. He abandoned his false name of 'Ferguson', reverting to Langford, and with it he abandoned 'personal hope'. He still had his work – not just the fishing enterprise, but also an electricity and refrigerating company he had set up – and the power that went with that; he would 'live and work on', but he was 'done with delusion'. 'Then I leaned back, well content. At last I desired to live. I had won my freedom. "He that loseth his life shall find it" – there was a law of compensation and Jesus of Nazareth knew it too.'

The First World War had brought changes to the Philippines, which affected Culion. Governor-General F.B. Harrison's policy of Filipinisation was, according to an indignant American writer, 'rapidly destroying all that America's science and service had accomplished'. An early casualty was Dr Heiser, whose departure meant that at Culion all 'scientific work, whether pathological or alleviative, died down or out'; then, in 1918, Dr Oswald Denney, 'the last American superintendent, gave up his hopeless struggle and left' – he was appointed to run the newly opened US National Leprosarium at Carville, Louisiana.[18]

Ned wanted to go with Denney – or 'Winton'. But Winton pointed out that Ned was still needed at Culion, where his business acumen meant so much. The time might come when he could no longer work, and that would be the moment to consider a move to Carville. Ned, who had momentarily forgotten his personal armistice renouncing hope, accepted that.

There were new arrivals to offset the departures. Huge losses made by the incompetently run Philippine National Bank, set up by Governor-General Harrison in 1916, were just the most sensational example of maladministration brought to light by the Wood–Forbes Commission in 1921 after Harrison had disappeared from the scene.[19] The new Governor-General was Ned's boyhood hero, Leonard Wood, one of the old school, and he appointed Dr H.W. 'Prexy' Wade chief pathologist and acting chief physician of Culion. Wade and his wife Dorothy would remain at Culion for the rest of their lives. Wood and Wade were two of a kind: 'Both had medical backgrounds, were husky, no-nonsense types, and both were completely committed to solving the riddle of the disease of leprosy.' Wood had already made a medical name for himself in Cuba, where he had facilitated Dr Walter Reed's discovery that yellow fever was transmitted by mosquitoes, and he backed Wade to make a similar breakthrough in the fight against leprosy. 'If one was not aware of Wood's other responsibilities,' a historian of Culion writes, 'one would be inclined to believe that he did nothing else but promote the cause of Culion and leprosy.' In fewer than half-a-dozen years he visited the leprosarium no less than seventeen times.[20]

In January 1922, Wade submitted a report on Culion to the new Governor-General. He recommended strongly 'that better living quarters be provided, that the most modern treatment be extended to all the lepers, that more doctors and nurses be employed, and that non-leprous children in the colony be segregated'. Wood gave Wade his head and 1922 became 'a red-letter year in the history of Culion'[21]: the number of physicians rose from two to eighteen; twenty-one trained nurses began work alongside the dedicated nuns, and over 4,000 patients started to receive the latest chaulmoogra 'ethyl ester' treatment hypodermically.[22] By the end of the year, the patient population had reached 5,232, and was increasing all the time as new patients came out of hiding, lured by the prospect of a cure. What was once known as 'the Island of Despair' had become 'the Island of Hope', as Wood would proudly say a few years later.[23]

But Wood's heavy-handed paternalism and readiness to govern 'without the benefit of a cabinet or the active cooperation of the legislature' did not endear him to the Filipino leaders. They took their revenge by focusing on his pet project and turning Culion into a political football, cannily suggesting that the Governor-General was moved less by humanitarian concern than by vanity and personal ambition. A headline in the *Philippines Herald* read, 'Culion is colossal failure. Millions are spent uselessly. Human beings used for experiments to acquire world renown.'[24]

It was true that nearly a third of the total public health budget – 'almost 3% of the entire insular income'[25] – was spent on leprosy, while next to nothing was being done to combat tuberculosis, which was a far more widespread scourge, causing some 30,000 deaths a year in the Philippines. But rather than focusing on that legitimate grievance the Filipino 'Senate Investigating Committee' that (in a parody or neat reversal of the Wood–Forbes Commission of 1921) set out in January 1924 to determine the truth about Culion chose to make *ad hominem* attacks on Governor-General Wood and Dr Wade. An influential politician told the visiting American writer, Katherine Mayo:

> We consider that, in Culion, General Wood is simply making a spectacular demonstration of welfare work, to gain popularity in America, and we are determined he shall not succeed. He is overdoing this Culion stunt and we are going to stop him.[26]

Wood rode out the storm. The only concession he made was to appoint a Filipino doctor as chief physician in place of Wade, who was happy to hand over the administrative duties of the post and concentrate on laboratory research. The high spending on leprosy continued for the remainder of Wood's governor-generalship, though he sought to supplement Filipino government money by undertaking a fund-raising drive in the United States, in which the personable Dorothy Wade, an ex-debutante from New Orleans, played a prominent part. Wood was determined to make Culion not just the largest, but also the most modern leprosarium in the world and no Filipino politico was going to stop him. 'We may fail', he told a convention of provincial governors, 'but we shall have the satisfaction of knowing that we did our full duty, that we did our best to solve this great problem and help these unfortunates.'[27]

Wood's 'strong Puritan devotion to a great cause'[28] may have been a fine thing, but it ignored the deepest feelings of the people he ruled. As a Filipino professional man who steered clear of politics explained to Katherine Mayo, '. . . as to leprosy – you know we are not as afraid of that as you are. We are always, at bottom, opposed to segregation. Family ties with us are strong. We do not consider the disease very horrible and we want to keep our lepers in our own households at home.'[29]

Anti-segregationist agitation in the Philippines remained relatively muted until the end of the Second World War, when a group calling itself the 'Leper Liberalization Committee' organised a march and campaigned for 'a more liberal law which would allow the treatment of lepers in their respective homes without the necessity of segregation'.[30]

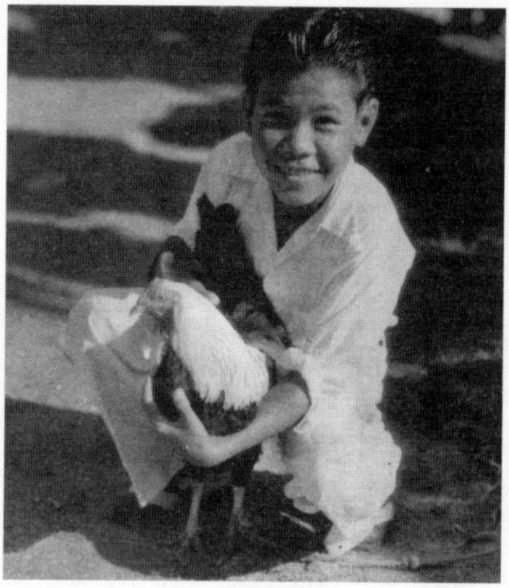
(from 'Who Walk Alone' by Perry Burgess)
Ned Langford's surrogate son, Tomás

Efforts to alleviate the isolation of leprosy sufferers had begun much earlier with the 'paroling of negatives' such as Carita and were pursued from 1928 with the establishment of regional treatment centres where patients, though still segregated, could remain nearer their homes, and the introduction in the same year of 'pass privileges' to allow more outside contact under certain stringent conditions.[31]

Leonard Wood died while undergoing an operation for a brain tumour in the United States in 1927. The American Leprosy Foundation, which he'd been instrumental in creating, was renamed in his honour the Leonard Wood Memorial Fund for the eradication of leprosy.[32] Its Director was Perry Burgess, who would later write Ned Langford's life story. Ned himself remained at Culion. Tomás, who was no longer a child, had fallen in love with a girl called Carmen, whose brother Vicente was 'a dangerous trouble-maker' and instigator of a formal protest demanding 'more liberty between the sexes'. Vicente's group wanted complete freedom to marry and have children. There was wild talk of an impending attack on the staff quarters, which were out of bounds to patients. But Carmen confronted her brother and made him promise not to go ahead with 'this crazy plan to burn and kill'. Instead, Vicente and his gang raided one of the girls' dormitories and each youth carried off the girl of his choice into the hills, where they hid in the jungle. 'It was called The Lepers' Riot, and the newspapers of the world told of it in headlines.'

The authorities were sufficiently rattled to call in the constabulary, but before long the hungry couples began to drift back to the colony of their own accord. Vicente eventually surrendered and was given an indeterminate prison sentence, while the other ringleaders were removed to another leprosarium. Tomás's view of the episode was: 'To carry a girl through the jungle is, I think, most difficult if it is against her will. This unwillingness could have been overcome only with co-operation, I think.' In other words, this was more of a joint conspiracy than a Rape of the Sabine Women.

Relations between the sexes would continue to exercise the authorities. In July 1935, Governor-General Frank Murphy appointed a commission to report on 'leprosy control in the Philippines'. Among its findings was this paragraph on marriage:

> The principal objection to marriage among lepers, namely the resultant birth of children to leper parents, does not outweigh the advantages of family life. However, because these children create problems for the parents, the State, and the individuals so born, the prevention of childbirth by sterilization of the male partners is suggested. This intervention should be strictly voluntary, and it might be made one of the conditions upon which permission to marry would depend.[33]

The committee noted that this was already the practice in Japan (where in fact sterilisation was by no means voluntary), as well as in a missionary-run asylum in Korea. It suggested that two further 'requirements' for marriage be considered: '(a) that the partners should undertake to support themselves, wholly or in part, and (b) that they should adopt and support a leper child from among those in the institutions, which would be advantageous to the families, the children and the State.'[34] So if you had leprosy and wanted to

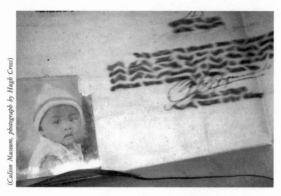

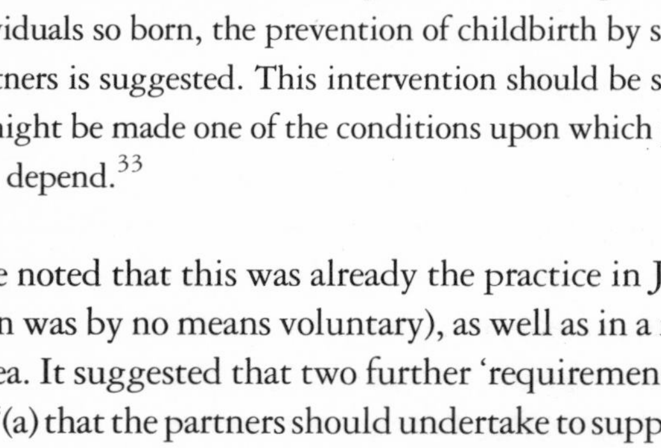

(Culion Museum, photograph by Hugh Cross)

Found among abandoned old Culion documents, this letter certifies that the child pictured 'was released from this Colony on April 16th 1934'

marry, you were to be prevented from having your own children, who might or might not develop the disease, and forced to adopt an already infected child of other leprosy sufferers who had at least been permitted to procreate! And what if a sterilized patient got better, through treatment or 'spontaneous recovery'? The professionals discounted that possibility; they no longer spoke of a cure, only of treatment which at best served to delay the progress of the disease. Leonard Wood would have turned in his grave if he could have read the report of the Philippine Leprosy Commission of 1935: his Island of Hope was reverting to an Island of Despair.

By this time Ned Langford, too, had departed. He had been 'slipping rapidly downhill' and was now 'sick, old, tired'. The doctors had warned him that his heart was failing, and he wanted to go home, if only to die. Others could manage the businesses he had started; his 'son' Tomás had his blessing to marry Carmen (though they could not live together, since she was 'paroled' and he would never be); Carita was back in the normal world, leading a busy and useful life, and their love for one another could anyway never be consummated. There was nothing to hold him in the Philippines. He would go to Carville at last.

He went by boat and train. He didn't have to hide in boxcars on the cross-continental journey this time; he had a compartment to himself, with a health service official in attendance. But as a southern newspaper reported at the end of July 1934, Ned Langford never reached Carville:

> The Federal Health Officer who accompanied him stated that his patient had died shortly after the train entered Louisiana. Langford seemed reasonably well the previous day except that he was greatly excited because the train had passed through his home town and he had seen the house in which he was born. He evidently died because of an overburdened heart, heavily taxed by years of strain.[35]

He was buried with full military honours at the US National Cemetery at Baton Rouge, where he was by no means the only veteran with leprosy to be interred.

Postscript

Culion had seemed to Perry Burgess, when he first visited the place towards the end of 'Ned Langford's' life:

> like a place not of this world . . . The patients had a large degree of self-government, elected the chief of their council and its members, had their own police force, and exercised the right to make regulations as far as their conduct in the community was concerned.[36]

It might be 'not of this world' but Culion was still affected by external events such as the 1930s depression and the Second World War. Its decline began in 1933, when several of the staff were either laid off or relocated to the new regional leprosaria. In 1935 the population of Culion reached a peak of almost 7,000 but, as the less severely disabled patients moved into asylums closer to their homes, the number of patients decreased, and by the end of 1941 there were fewer than 5,000. The privations of the war years hastened the process, so that by the end of 1945 only 1,791 patients remained.[37] The numbers rose slightly in the post-war decade, but fell again when modern sulphone treatment rendered segregation superfluous – though it wasn't finally abolished in the Philippines until 1964.

The Japanese terror of leprosy meant that the occupying forces kept well clear of Culion. Though they cut off supplies to the island, they left the inhabitants alone, even Americans like 'Prexy' and Dorothy Wade. But the lack of food and medicines soon became chronic; the island was far from self-sufficient and though staff and patients cultivated rice on the hillsides malnutrition got worse as the war went on and when it ended the people of Culion were on the brink of starvation. Up to a thousand of the more active patients absconded, with the blessing of the staff; several were active in the resistance movement, carrying messages from the occupied areas to the guerrillas in the mountains, their infirmity for once protecting rather than exposing them.

The most celebrated of these leprosy resistance workers was an attractive young woman in her twenties. Josefina – 'Joey' – Guerrero was not from Culion. Her leprosy was diagnosed only a matter of weeks before the bombing of Pearl Harbor, two years after she had given birth to a daughter. Her husband was a doctor and during the Japanese occupation both were members of the underground. Joey became so adept at mapping military installations under the very noses of the Japanese that she was recruited by the Allied Intelligence Bureau and used as a courier – 'just a little errand boy,' as she modestly put it. Her toughest assignment was also her last: it was to go through the Japanese lines, cross the front line where there was heavy fighting and deliver to the invading American forces a map of Japanese land mines. Her sickness made the two-day journey with the map taped to her back a nightmare, but it also prevented the Japanese who accosted her from carrying out more than a cursory search of her baggage before waving her on. In her bloated face, with its angry red patches, she had 'a terrible passport that would get her through'.[38]

Joey accompanied the US troops into Manila; many were amazed at her reckless bravery, but someone – a doctor – notified the military authorities that she had leprosy. The commander of the military police insisted she be segregated, and she was consigned to the Novaliches leprosarium. This called for heroism of a different order, as Joey recognised:

> During the Japanese regime and during the liberation, the horror, the massacre, the unspeakable devastation and ruin were beyond comprehension. Then I came here to find sick, crippled, starving people lying on pallets, pieces of straw on the floor, everything a filthy mess, the patients moving around like skeletons on strings, bundled or hardly covered with clothing, eating cats and dogs. When I saw these things it took every vestige of courage and stamina I had. I felt like just leaving the place in a great hurry. I had never seen a case of leprosy, except my own, until I went to Novaliches.[39]

Father Forbes Monaghan wrote of it, 'such another God-and-man-forsaken place . . . I hope never to see'. The sick had to do everything, from cooking their pathetically inadequate rations to gathering wood for fires, water for drinking and for washing themselves and their clothes. There was no disinfectant and the wards stank. The patients, the Father learned, 'had become brutalized from despair and the sense of their abandonment'. He was horrified at the thought of such 'a pure, highly cultured girl' as Joey having to go to such a place. But Joey was tougher than she looked; she enlisted the aid of journalists and influential friends such as Aurora 'Baby' Quezon, daughter of the deceased President, Manuel Quezon, in exposing and improving conditions at the leprosarium.[40] Her courage in war earned her the highest award the US government could confer on a civilian, the Medal of Freedom with Silver Palm. But a greater reward by far was her transfer to Carville, where she received a heroine's welcome on 11 July 1948 and benefited from the new sulphone treatment to such an extent that she was eventually discharged and made her home in California.

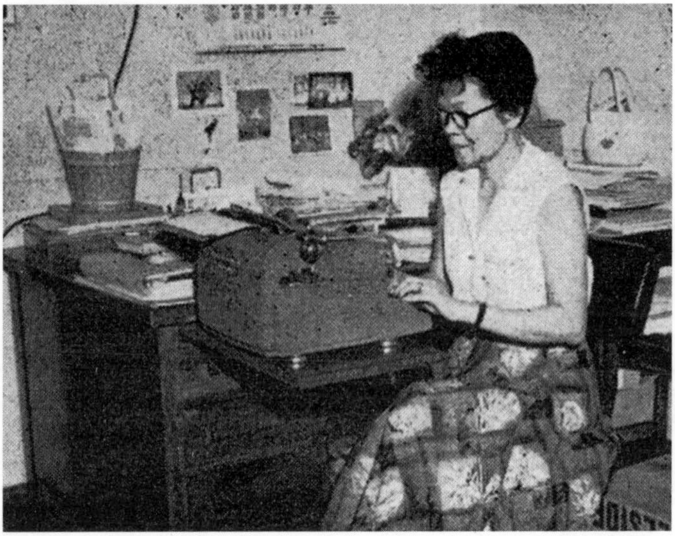
(The Star)

World War II heroine turned staff member of the *Star* at Carville, Joey Guerrero

'Prexy' Wade was also a hero in his way. He made dangerous boat trips to neighbouring islands to obtain food for the starving people of Culion and on one occasion, when the Japanese sank a boat just off the coast of the island, improvised diving equipment and, ignoring the perils presented by sharks that kept others out of the water, managed to salvage some precious food from the wreck.[41] His activities damaged his heart, but he was more fortunate than one of his Filipino colleagues; Dr José Samson suspected nothing when the Japanese called on him as he was often summoned to other islands to treat their wounded. But on this occasion, when he'd treated the wounded, he was invited by an officer to take a bath: 'Then we are going to behead you,' the officer said – and did. Dr Samson's crime was to have written a letter to a friend in Manila welcoming the American invasion; the Japanese intercepted it, and he paid for this indiscretion with his life. A quaint touch was that after the execution the Japanese officer called on the widow, clicked his heels and formally expressed his regret.[42]

From 1931 Dr Wade had been employed by the Leonard Wood Memorial Foundation, rather than the Philippine government, and he had combined his laboratory research with editing the newly founded *International Journal of Leprosy*. In 1946 he was elected President of the International Leprosy Association, but the privations of the war years had undermined his health and though he soldiered on for a couple of decades he never recovered his strength. He might have remained Medical Director of the Leonard Wood Memorial if he had chosen to return to the United States in 1948, but he preferred to remain at Culion as Chief Pathologist. Eleven years later, in 1959, he was officially retired by the Memorial, but still he stayed on, saying, 'I have all of this material here and I am a laboratory worker. I would simply go crazy sitting around waiting to die so I am staying here the rest of my days.' He died in 1968, aged eighty-two.[43]

His widow Dorothy, the one-time debutante who'd 'practically unaided' raised $2 million for the Leonard Wood Memorial Fund during a lecture tour of the United States lasting five years, was now an impoverished recluse. But she, too, refused to leave Culion and died there five years after her husband, at the age of seventy-four. Even before the war she had eaten very little, so it's no great surprise to find that the cause of her death was 'extreme malnutrition from protein deficiency caused by multiple food allergy'.[44] The Carville patients' journal, the *Star*, called the Wades 'true scientists and real people'.[45]

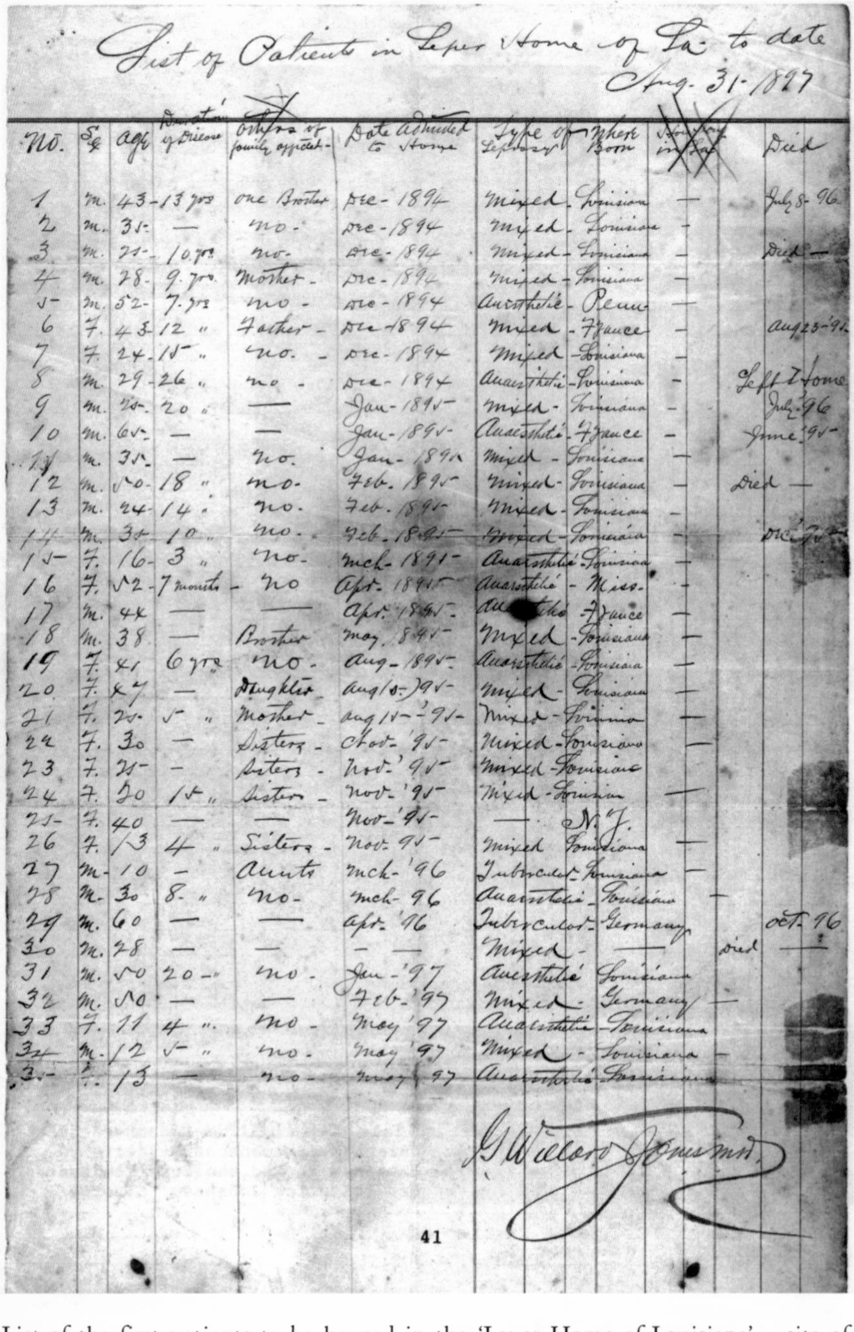

List of Patients in Leper Home of La. to date Aug. 31-1897

No.	Sex	Age	Duration of Disease	Others of family affected	Date Admitted to Home	Type of Leprosy	Where Born		Died
1	m.	43	13 yrs	one Brother	Dec-1894	mixed	Louisiana	—	July 8-96
2	m.	35	—	no	Dec-1894	mixed	Louisiana	—	
3	m.	25	10 yrs	no	Dec-1894	mixed	Louisiana	—	Died —
4	m.	28	9 yrs	Mother	Dec-1894	mixed	Louisiana	—	
5	m.	52	7 yrs	no	Dec-1894	Anaesthetic	Peru	—	
6	F.	43	12 "	Father	Dec-1894	mixed	France	—	Aug 23-95
7	F.	24	15 "	no	Dec-1894	mixed	Louisiana	—	
8	m.	29	26 "	no	Dec-1894	Anaesthetic	Louisiana	—	Left Home
9	m.	55	20 "	—	Jan-1895	mixed	Louisiana	—	July-96
10	m.	65	—	—	Jan-1895	Anaesthetic	France	—	June '95
11	m.	35	—	no	Jan-1895	mixed	Louisiana	—	
12	m.	50	18 "	no	Feb. 1895	mixed	Louisiana	—	Died —
13	m.	24	14 "	no	Feb. 1895	mixed	Louisiana	—	
14	m.	30	10 "	no	Feb. 1895	mixed	Louisiana	—	Dec '95
15	F.	16	3 "	no	Mch-1895	Anaesthetic	Louisiana	—	
16	F.	52	7 months	no	Apr. 1895	Anaesthetic	Miss.	—	
17	m.	44	—	—	Apr. 1895	Anaesthetic	France	—	
18	m.	38	—	Brother	May 1895	mixed	Louisiana	—	
19	F.	41	6 yrs	no	Aug-1895	Anaesthetic	Louisiana	—	
20	F.	47	—	Daughter	Aug 15-'95	mixed	Louisiana	—	
21	F.	25	5 "	Mother	Aug 15-'95	mixed	Louisiana	—	
22	F.	30	—	Sisters	Nov-'95	mixed	Louisiana	—	
23	F.	25	—	Sisters	Nov-'95	mixed	Louisiana		
24	F.	20	15 "	Sister	Nov-'95	mixed	Louisiana	—	
25	F.	40	—	—	Nov-'95	—	N.J.		
26	F.	13	4 "	Sisters	Nov-95	mixed	Louisiana	—	
27	m.	10	—	Aunts	Mch-'96	Tubercular	Louisiana	—	
28	m.	30	8 "	no	Mch-96	Anaesthetic	Louisiana	—	
29	m.	60	—	—	Apr-96	Tubercular	Germany		Oct-96
30	m.	28	—	—	— —	mixed	—		died —
31	m.	50	20 "	no	Jan-'97	Anaesthetic	Louisiana		
32	m.	50	—	—	Feb-'97	mixed	Germany	—	
33	F.	11	4 "	no	May '97	Anaesthetic	Louisiana		
34	m.	12	5 "	no	May '97	mixed	Louisiana	—	
35	F.	13	—	no	May '97	Anaesthetic	Louisiana		

G. Willoird Jones md.

41

(Courtesy of USDHHS – HRSA – BPHC, Division of National Hansen's Disease Programs, National Hansen's Disease Museum)

List of the first patients to be housed in the 'Leper Home of Louisiana' – site of the future National Leprosarium – between December 1894 and August 1897

Chapter 8

VETERANS OF THE SPANISH–AMERICAN WAR, 2: JOHN EARLY AND CARVILLE

John Ruskin Early had little in common with 'Ned Langford' apart from active service in the Philippines and a diagnosis of leprosy. If Langford's life, as told by Perry Burgess, is the story of an honourable man nobly enduring the worst that fate could throw at him, Early's doesn't lend itself to such treatment. According to the celebrated patient activist Stanley Stein, who knew Early in his last years at Carville, the man was 'a religious fanatic, a bigot, an exhibitionist, and, I think, at times bordered on the psychotic'. But in the chapter of his autobiography devoted to Early, Stein paid tribute to 'his long and dedicated fight for the cause of Carville patients' and felt that he – Stein – 'could not claim to be *the* Carville Crusader [which his fellow patients were beginning to call him] as long as John Ruskin Early was alive and kicking'.[1]

Born in 1874, Early hailed from the mountainous western region of the state of North Carolina. He served as a private in the 5th United States Infantry during the Spanish–American war and fought in Cuba, where he suffered badly from malaria, before he was posted with his unit to the Philippines. He was still in the army in 1905, stationed at Plattsburgh, New York.[2] A corporal by then, he was one of a group of soldiers who wandered into a Salvation Army meeting, attracted by the sound of music. By his own later account, this 'big hulking kid, fresh from service, and without respect for anything on the face of the earth except my mother and my flag', was mightily impressed when a 'slip of a girl got up – little bit of a girl she was, only sixteen; she could walk right under my arm. Lord, but she looked pretty in the blue bonnet!' This vision of loveliness mounted the platform and, accompanying herself on the guitar, began to sing the hymns Early remembered his late mother used to sing in his childhood. Early was smitten; and the girl, Lottie, would recall that, as well as ogling her while she sang, he 'testified' that night.[3]

Early lost no time in proposing, but Lottie wouldn't marry a soldier. So Early came out of the army and they got married. A year later their first child was born and they moved to North Carolina. John got a job in a pulp mill, but the chemicals to which he was exposed undermined his health and in August 1908 he had to give up work. Lottie was pregnant again and John decided to go to Washington DC to pursue his claim for a pension for 'aggravated malaria'.[4] His condition puzzled the doctors and it may have been his own suggestion that he had leprosy (Stein reckoned he must have been 'worrying about the sins of his youth').[5] This certainly alarmed the medical authorities, and they claimed to have found bacterial evidence of the disease in a skin specimen they took from his inflamed and puffy face. He was promptly removed to a marshy, isolated spot on the banks of the Potomac River, where a tent had been hastily erected for him.

The first the pregnant Lottie heard of it was when Early's brother came running towards her, clutching a newspaper and calling out, 'John's got leprosy'.[6] What followed would have been farcical had it not been so devastating for the couple caught up in it. When Lottie arrived in Washington DC with her one-year-old son Manly – Emmanuel – she was told she could share Early's quarantine if she wished, but her son would have to be taken from her, as would her baby as soon as it was born. Since Lottie was not prepared to give up either her husband or her children, a compromise was reached. An abandoned old house on the edge of the mud flats by the river was partitioned in two by slapping a brick wall down the middle of it. The divided family was placed under twenty-four-hour guard; a policeman equipped with a strong searchlight patrolled the front porch, his duty being to keep the couple apart. Lottie was appalled by the bareness of the rooms, the cold and the rats that came out and stared at her, terrifying her infant son.

Like the prisoners they were, John and Lottie communicated by tapping out messages on the wall and singing hymns. John had a mandolin, and Lottie had brought her small Salvation Army organ, which she jammed up against the wall so that he might hear her playing. Her mother joined Lottie when the baby was due but the night it was born John and the policeman had gone down to his old tent half a mile away, so Lottie's mother had to seek help from the nearest neighbours.

But they were too afraid to come near, and Lottie's now distraught mother had no recourse but to go out on the porch and give the distress signal by blowing the police whistle.

After the birth of her second child, Lottie campaigned vigorously on John's behalf, writing to President Taft and to a number of eminent leprologists, including the discoverer of *M. leprae*, Armauer Hansen himself. In the meantime, officials in Washington considered shipping Early off either to Hawaii or to the Philippines. As there was as yet no national leprosarium in the United States, they sought legal advice over what to do with him, their preferred option being to return him to North Carolina. Unfortunately for the District of Columbia, this was not practicable, since

> the removal of the leper to North Carolina would be a possible means of introducing or spreading the disease from the District into the States, the very thing which the two [contagious diseases] acts [of 1890 and 1893] were intended to prevent.[7]

A Salvation Army contact brought John Early's case to the notice of the New York dermatologist, Dr L. Duncan Bulkley. Bulkley tried to persuade a Washington colleague to investigate, but this doctor

> wrote me that it would ruin his practice if it were known that he had visited the case of leprosy, so thoroughly alarmed had the public become in regard to the disease with which poor Mr Early had been charged.

So Bulkley himself made the journey from New York and visited Early for the first time on 9 May 1909. He found him 'in fine physical condition', free of all symptoms except for 'a slight redness on the forehead', but in urgent need of a barber:

> His hair had not been cut since his quarantine, and hung very long over his shoulders. The Health Officers had refused to allow anyone from outside to cut the 'leper's' hair, or his wife, but suggested that his mother-in-law cut it![8]

The New York City Health Department, unlike its Washington counterpart, did not regard leprosy 'in this climate' as being 'of so infectious or contagious a nature as to require segregation' and Bulkley's own hospital, the New York Skin and Cancer Hospital, had admitted several leprosy cases to its wards, 'often for considerable periods'.[9] But Bulkley was convinced that Early had been wrongly diagnosed and did not even have leprosy; he could find no evidence of the bacillus in the skin samples he'd removed.

The Washington health officials resented Bulkley's interference and the fact that he ridiculed their diagnosis, but that did not prevent them taking advantage of his readiness to rid them of an embarrassing encumbrance. So on 3 July John Early was bundled into a sealed boxcar and transported to New York, attended by a Salvation Army officer, who was instructed not just to supply him with 'eating and drinking utensils' to be disinfected or destroyed after use, but also with gloves – to 'eliminate all possible criticism from the standpoint of contact on the part of the patient with surfaces or things likely to be handled by other persons'.[10]

Once in New York, Early underwent further examinations and bacterial tests. Neither the director of the New York City Health Department laboratory, Dr W.H. Park, nor the doyen of pathology and bacteriology in America, Dr William H. Welch of Johns Hopkins in Baltimore, could find the slightest trace of the leprosy bacillus in the skin specimens, and after two or three weeks in hospital Early was allowed to join his wife and family in their temporary accommodation in Brooklyn. In August the medical board of the United States Pension Department cleared him – but that meant that his pension was stopped. Later in the year he moved with his family to Virginia, where he found work on a farm. Yet when he went to Washington in early December to collect the back pension he was due, he was arrested and detained in 'his former quarantine quarters on the muddy banks of the river'. A flurry of legal activity resulted in his release and return to New York in a sealed baggage car, which then had to be disinfected – for which he received a bill of $89. He arrived on 11 December, 'in good health but thoroughly disheartened by his long persecution for nearly fourteen months'.[11]

The Washington DC Health Department's trump card was a letter from the American consul in Bergen, Norway, where the Second International Congress of Leprology under the presidency of Armauer Hansen was in progress, reporting that the great man himself 'stated that he had found the bacillus in a piece of skin taken from the American soldier John Early who contracted leprosy in the Philippine Islands'.[12] Since the diagnosis had been confirmed by another eminent leprologist,

Professor Edvard L. Ehlers of Copenhagen, that settled the matter, at least as far as *The Times* of London was concerned. Bulkley continued to assert that Early was free of leprosy; he said he'd had letters from Hansen regarding the portions of skin John Early himself had excised with a penknife and Lottie had sent to the Norwegian:

> in the first he says that there is absolutely nothing to be found indicating leprosy, but in a later letter he says that after a long search he found new bacilli which he thought were those of leprosy.

Bulkley remained sceptical, doubting the reliability of a sample taken 'without antiseptic precautions' and implying that Hansen had been got at by Washington officials.[13]

The medical controversy was disastrous for John Early and his family: whether he had leprosy or not, his notoriety was so great that wherever he went he was hounded – even in New York and Virginia, where official policy towards leprosy victims was more lenient than elsewhere in the States. There was nowhere he and his family could settle openly.

'It is now perfectly apparent to me', his lawyer pointed out when he wrote to the Surgeon General, Dr Walter Wyman, to complain of the refusal of the Washington health commissioners to countenance a private visit by John Early without the prospect of detention:

> that they propose to adhere to their diagnosis in regard to Mr Early – *be it right or wrong*. They have stamped him with the brand of 'leprosy'; he is as a result an outcast in society; using an assumed name; an object to be feared and hunted out for the purpose of being quarantined; such is his status in the *entire country to-day*; and such the treatment accorded an ex-soldier, who was first suspected of having the loathsome disease because he had served his country as a private in the Philippines and Cuba.[14]

The lawyer claimed that the strain on John Early was beginning to tell: 'He cannot stand the intolerable situation longer; but what can he a poor man without money or many friends do?' Early had fled with his family to the west coast, where they were trying to establish a new life and a new identity farming on the outskirts of Tacoma, Washington. By now they had three children and were in desperate need of money, so John applied for the restitution of his pension, thus reactivating the vicious cycle of medical examination, condemnation as a 'leper', exposure and hounding by the local citizenry.[15] Lottie once again appealed to President Taft, and Early was granted a pension of $30 a month. Walter Wyman's successor as Surgeon General, Dr Rupert Blue, came up with a solution to the dilemma of what to do with him. At the quarantine station near Port Townsend, Washington, there was an ex-sailor with leprosy whose disease was so advanced that he required constant attention: what better employment for John Early? He would be out of harm's way and could supplement his pension by $50 a month (minus subsistence).[16] The snag was, he could not take his family with him.

Whatever John may have felt about their parting, Lottie appears to have welcomed it. The stresses of their fugitive existence and lack of money seem to have undermined their previously loving relationship, with John taking out his frustrations on Lottie as though she were to blame for what had happened to him. On 20 May 1912, two months after Early's arrival at Port Townsend quarantine station, the medical officer in charge (whose name, rather confusingly, was Earle) reported that he'd been visited by the local commander of the Spanish–American War Veterans, George N. Tausan, who

> stated that he had been hearing bad reports of Mr Early recently and was afraid that he had sent us a confirmed trouble maker, that he had come to the conclusion that Mr Early is a hypocrite, a grafter, and a notoriety seeker, and had treated his wife shamefully, and that with my permission he was going down 'to read the riot act' to him.

Tausan said that Lottie lived in terror of her husband abandoning the quarantine station and turning up and abusing her, as had become his wont: 'according to her statements, he is little better than a beast in his treatment of her sexually and otherwise and . . . his religious pretensions are simply a mask to hide his animal nature . . .'[17]

Evidently, George Tausan's strong words had some effect. On Dr Baylis H. Earle's next visit to the quarantine station for which he was responsible the previously 'surly and very suspicious' John Early was 'in a much chastened and subdued state of mind, apologising very abjectly for his rudeness to me and others since his arrival'.[18] His contrite mood did not last, however. The following year, when a newly arrived leprosy patient of Italian origin, Dominick Pittori, absconded from the station on 5 July and Dr Earle went to investigate, 'Early was at that time a raving maniac and abused me, personally, the Service, and the Government generally most scandalously'. It was clear that Early had encouraged, if not assisted, Pittori in his dash for freedom, telling him 'that the Service had no right to hold him and that the State of Minnesota had violated law in bringing him here'.[19]

Early's burgeoning sense of injustice was fuelled by his own treatment and the loss of his family – Lottie was now in the process of divorcing him and would shortly remarry. Less than a year later he, too, deserted the station and headed back to the east coast via Canada, intent on 'visiting the House of Representatives, announcing his identity, and demanding redress for alleged mistreatment'. In the opinion of Dr Earle, who was no doubt glad to see the back of him, 'the man is insane and a dangerous character to have at large'.[20]

But there was method in Early's madness. His penchant for publicity took him to one of Washington DC's most fashionable hotels, the Willard, where his fellow guests included the Vice-President of the United States, several senators and representatives, and a host of diplomats. These luminaries were 'thrown into a panic' by the discovery of a diagnosed 'leper' in their midst, and when the city's chief medical inspector, Dr William C. Fowler, an old adversary, got a phone call from Early, saying he was booked into the Willard under the name of E.J. Watson, he 'did not know whether it was someone joking with me or not'. Fowler thought he'd better check it out, so he went to the Willard and found Early holding forth to a group of newspaper reporters. Early told the journalists he'd been planning his trip for months, saving up his wages and his pension so that he could ride in a Pullman car, stay at the best hotels and eat in the best restaurants in order to 'demonstrate how easy it is for a leper to mingle in cities'. When he was asked to what purpose, he replied: 'I knew that if I mingled among the well-to-do and the rich and exposed them to contagion that they would arise out of self-protection and further my plan for a national home'.[21]

How right he was. Congress was up in arms. According to Congressman John Raker of California, allowing Early to wander freely about the country was 'worse than turning loose a band of murderers', while Representative Albert Johnson of Washington was all for banishing Early and others like him to one of the Aleutian Islands, where they 'could be put to gardening and homesteading' even though the climate mightn't be ideal. But

Representative Johnson had reckoned without the delegate from Alaska, who protested furiously at the very idea of a leprosy colony in the Aleutians . . . And so it went.[22] Even though it would take years to achieve, a national leprosarium was now very much on the political agenda and John Early – insane or not – had put it there more or less single-handedly.

The idea of having a national leprosarium didn't originate with Early, of course; he was merely the catalyst. As early as October 1890 the President of the Board of Health in Philadelphia had been urging the Surgeon General to create 'one or more leper stations' to which leprosy sufferers could 'be removed from society and humanely cared for and treated'.[23] In most states, leprosy sufferers were too few and far between to justify the expense of building an isolation hospital especially for them, so it made sense to tackle the problem federally.

In May 1894 Surgeon General Walter Wyman had delivered a paper on 'National Control of Leprosy' to the Congress of America Physicians and Surgeons in Washington DC, in which he'd discussed the constitutional questions involved. One school of thought doubted the US government had the right of national control and argued that

> the end might be met by one state establishing a hospital and being willing to receive into it the lepers consigned from other states, their expenses being paid by the latter, as has been done in a number of instances with regard to jails and penitentiaries.

But another maintained that it was 'quite within the province of Congress to appropriate a sufficient sum to establish a National leper hospital, though the necessity for it must be plainly shown'.[24] Wyman's personal opinion was that leprosy should be under national control, but that before a decision could be reached on the creation of a national hospital a commission should be appointed to report on the prevalence of the disease in the United States.

The advocates of a national leprosy hospital faced two difficulties: one was that many of them, including Wyman, believed that the danger of contagion was slight; the other – not unrelated – was the apparently tiny percentage of the population affected by the disease. A survey at the turn of the century came up with 278 cases of leprosy, and a second survey, nine years later, discovered a mere 139 reported cases (later revised to 146) in the entire United States – as compared with 764 in Hawaii and

2,330 in the Philippines. On purely medical grounds, it was hard to justify the expenditure involved in building and running a national institution for so few leprosy sufferers. As Walter R. Brinckerhoff, who conducted the 1909 survey for the Public Health and Marine-Hospital Service remarked:

> If it were not for the popular dread of leprosy these figures would be of little significance, but when we consider the penalty imposed upon those unfortunate enough to contract the disease we must regard even this relatively small number of cases as a grave condition.[25]

In 1902 a 'Committee on National Leper Homes' had endorsed the resolution reached by the American Public Health Association at a meeting in Indianapolis in 1900:

> That this Association places itself on record as favorable to the establishment of national leprosaria, which may serve not only as a refuge for lepers, but also as a home and hospital, making their lives tolerable so far as possible, furnishing employment to those who are able to work, and giving skilled medical care to all cases, with the intent of possibly curing some, and making the road to death less wearisome and painful than it is now to others.[26]

Despite such laudable intentions, a bill to establish a national leprosarium was defeated in the House of Representatives in March 1905, less on the grounds that it wasn't needed than out of a fear, particularly on the part of those territories battling for statehood, like Arizona and New Mexico, that they were going to be used as a dumping ground for 'such unfortunates'.[27] Yet this merely postponed the inevitable for another few years. Three further bills were introduced in the House of Representatives in 1913 and 1914 even before John Early's dramatic intervention gave the debate renewed urgency.

The District of Columbia health officials must have groaned when they learned that Early was back in town. As the *Washington Times* commented:

> Nobody wants him, and nobody, in the face of the strange, medieval terror inspired by his disease, seems concerned whether he shall be given civilized treatment; to get him away as far as possible and to insure that

> he will not return is the uttermost ambition of everybody and every community that he might possibly impose himself upon.[28]

Washington State would have nothing further to do with him, and after once again toying with the idea of shipping him off to Hawaii – which was not well received at the other end – the health officials of Washington DC had no alternative but to incarcerate him for a third time in the house by the mud flats of the Potomac.

He was still there when the long-awaited Senate hearings finally took place in February 1916, and the conditions in which he was held became the subject of an exchange between the chairman and Dr Fowler. The assembled senators heard that the windows and door of the brick house were barred with steel, and the grounds enclosed with a barbed-wire fence eight feet high, rendering escape all but impossible. When one of them queried, 'You are treating him practically as a wild animal?' an embarrassed Dr Fowler replied: 'Practically, I am afraid; we have to in order to keep him.'[29]

Although it was Senator Joseph E. Ransdell of Louisiana who introduced the bill, arguing that 'in segregation we have a method of protection which, if utilized, is wholly sufficient to prevent the dissemination of the disease',[30] and giving the examples of Hawaii and the Philippines – not to mention the Bible – in support of it, Stanley Stein credited the man he familiarly called Uncle Will with having 'more than a little to do with the movement' to establish a national leprosarium. William M. Danner had been appointed secretary to the American Mission to Lepers (an offshoot of the British parent organisation) in 1911, and his first task had been to raise $15,000 for leprosy missions in India. But he couldn't help noticing the mistreatment of leprosy patients in his own country. He wrote, 'I was horrified at the lengths Christian America would go in treating individual leprosy cases.'[31]

He cited the cases of John Early and Mock Sen, a young Chinese student who had been shuttled back and forth across state lines in a sealed freight car for thirteen days because neither Philadelphia nor Baltimore would take responsibility for him – as Dr Fay F. Schamberg recalled in the 1920s:

> Some years ago the Health Department of Philadelphia asked me to examine a man confined in a boxcar on the outskirts of the city. I found the car surrounded by a gaping herd of people gazing upon a terrified

> looking individual who was eating a crust of bread and drinking water from a can that had been timidly placed near him. He bore upon his visage the tragic insignia of the most shunned of all maladies. The unfortunate man was not permitted to enter the city; the car was shunted to Baltimore, but the authorities there refused to receive the man. For days he was driven from pillar to post, from one state to another, until he died of exposure.[32]

Danner might also have cited the case of George Rashid, a Syrian, 'who died of chagrin and neglect' in 1906 after being isolated in a tent in mountainous West Virginia and threatened with murder by panic-stricken locals.[33] But perhaps he didn't need to. The Surgeon General referred him to Senator Ransdell, 'who gave friendly attention to my story . . . and finally a hearing was arranged'.[34]

Early was a key witness, though he was not allowed anywhere near the hearings. Senator Ransdell had visited him in his prison by the Potomac and asked him, among other things, if he thought there were a sufficiently large number of leprosy sufferers in America to justify a national leprosarium. Early claimed there were 'about 500 known cases in the United States' and that leprosy was spreading. 'To segregate a leprous person is wise and humane thing to do,' he wrote to the senator in his rather stilted English (for which he apologised in a PS: 'I had to write in haste'):

> but to let matters drift on in the present road is another thing. As soon as a leper is found, under present conditions, he finds himself out of a home and absolutely unwelcome in the jurisdiction where he is found . . . Remember we are outcasts of society; yes, with human tastes and feelings.[35]

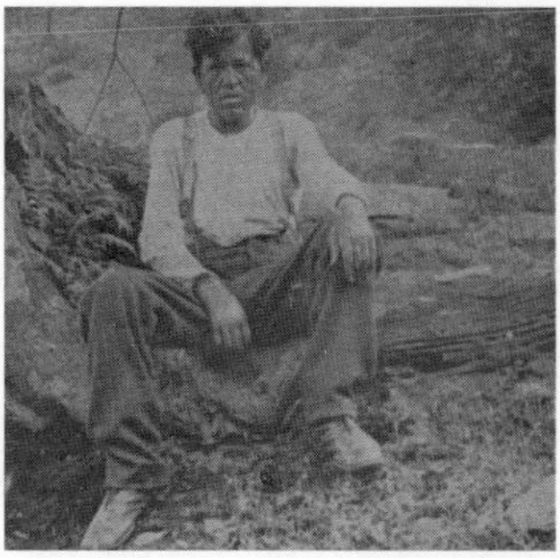
(The Star)
George Rashid

Senator Ransdell's bill became law on 3 February 1917, and an appropriation of $250,000 was set aside for the care and treatment of persons afflicted with leprosy. The timing was significant. In his letter to the senator, John Early had referred to the fact that in three cases known to him the disease had been contracted in the Philippines, and in the year of America's entry into the First World War the authorities were concerned that the experience of the Spanish–American War was about to be repeated, with a number of soldiers serving abroad being exposed to the danger of developing leprosy.[36] It would take another four years before the national leprosarium came into being – four years of argument and fierce resistance on the part of communities targeted as possible sites for it. No one in the United States wanted the leprosarium in their back yard, or within a hundred miles of it.

John Early remained in solitary confinement in his private leprosarium on the muddy banks of the Potomac until November 1918, when the District of Columbia finally got shot of him at the cost of $5,000, payable in advance. His destination: the State of Louisiana's leprosy home at Indian Camp, Iberville Parish – later known as Carville. This was to be a temporary arrangement, pending the creation of a federal institution.[37]

In the 1909 survey of leprosy in the United States, out of the 139 cases discovered in fourteen states, fifty of them were from Louisiana, more than double the number from any other state (next came Florida and California with twenty each).[38] There were at least three theories about the origin of the disease in that state: that the early settlers from southern Europe – Italy, France and Spain – had brought it to the Gulf of Mexico with them; that it was a by-product of the slave trade; and that it was imported into the New Orleans district by the Acadians ousted from Nova Scotia by the British in the second half of the eighteenth century. Dr Joseph Jones, an energetic champion of preventive medicine and public health who would become president of the State Board of Health in 1880, was the first to make the connection between the leprosy in New Brunswick that had necessitated the construction of a leprosarium at Tracadie and the leprosy he was discovering among the French-speaking settlers in southern Louisiana.[39]

Whatever its origins, and however reluctant doctors were to admit it, leprosy had become endemic in Louisiana – the only area of the United States in which it was endemic – and was commoner among whites than blacks. Medical opinion in late nineteenth-century New Orleans, as elsewhere, was divided over whether leprosy was 'infectious and contagious' or 'hereditary and inoculable; in plainer terms . . . transmissible in the same manner, and by the same means as syphilis', but united in the need for rigid segregation of the afflicted 'in hospitals especially erected and set aside for them'. In the 1890s, a decade or more after Joseph Jones had drawn attention to the disease, Dr Isadore Dyer, a New Orleans dermatologist, sought 'to bring leprosy within the framework of science and medicine'.[40]

Dyer did not underestimate the difficulty of his self-imposed task; he wrote:

> Leprosy has always stood as the example of the most fearful of human afflictions. The Biblical estimate of the disease has created a popular horror which even down to modern times has placed the leper as a pariah and a person condemned by his state to abandonment. [It] must be classed among the contagious diseases, not as contagious as tuberculosis or syphilis, but still a menace of no mean importance, when it is considered that its spread is as constant as it is insidious and that its evidences are more horrible than most known diseases.

And he preached segregation, not just to protect the healthy from affliction – 'today, as in ancient times, the "health of the people is the first law"' – but also to protect the afflicted from the healthy. His vision went beyond mere mutual protection, however; for the leprosy sufferer a home had to be as much of a hospital as an asylum, so that isolation 'means more peace of mind, under conditions of existence which make amelioration and even cure possible'.[41]

He actively opposed the attempt by the keeper of the pest house in New Orleans, a Dr J.C. Beard, 'to engineer a bill thru the legislature providing a contract with him for the care of lepers, which was a large bit of graft'. Dyer knew how people fared in the pest house – 'Many of the inmates would jump the fence of the enclosure and come to my clinic at the Charity Hospital for treatment' – and he wasn't impressed. 'Their state was worse than bad', he wrote.[42]

This was also the opinion of a young reporter on the New Orleans *Daily Picayune*, who wrote a series of articles in the early 1890s exposing conditions of 'abandon[ment], neglect, and possible starvation' at the pest house.[43] John Smith Kendall, the author of these anonymous articles, went on to have a distinguished career as war corre-

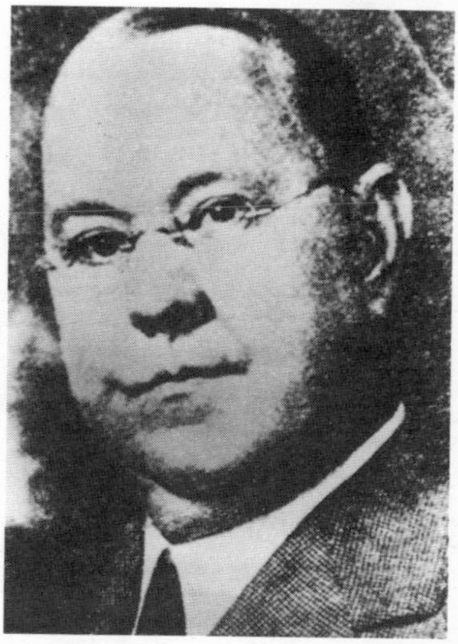

(Courtesy of the National Hansen's Disease Museum)

Dr Isadore Dyer

spondent, university professor of Spanish and historian, and lived to the age of ninety-one. What he remembered in old age was the refusal of his editor to give any kind of prominence to his reports, and the panic occasioned by the very mention of the disease. He recalled a Sunday afternoon in the office of the *Picayune*, when the place was deserted apart from himself and another reporter whose name was Ball:

> The door opened and a shabbily dressed individual came quietly in. He walked over to the ice-water tank in the corner of the room, helped himself to a drink from a tin cup which we all used in common when thirsty, and then drew a chair up beside Ball and said, in a low voice, 'I'm a leper!'
>
> 'What?' yelled Ball. 'Say it again!'
>
> 'I'm a leper. I'm from Dr Beard's place on Broad Street. I read your articles in the paper and –'
>
> Ball jumped from his chair and sought refuge in a far corner of the apartment. Pointing to me, he said, 'That's your man! Don't come near me!'[44]

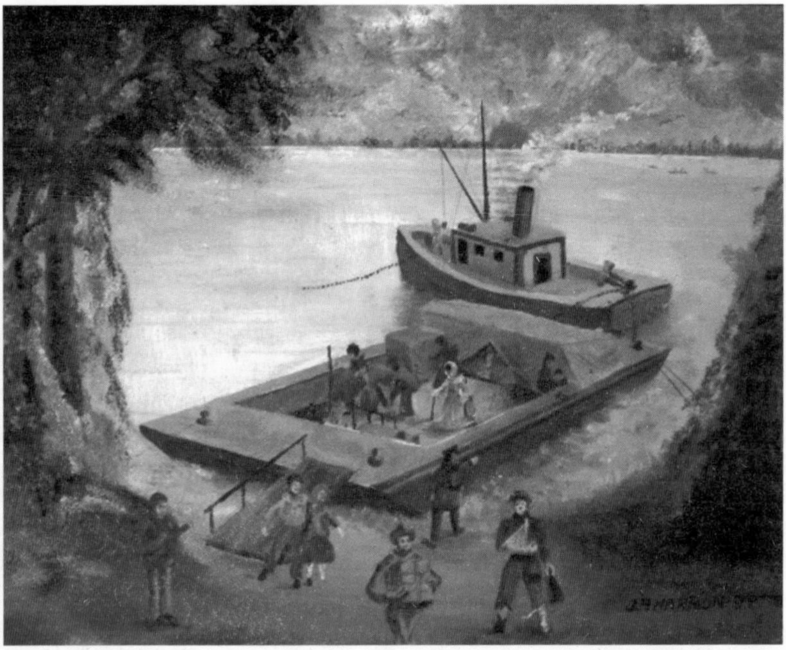

(*Courtesy of Ann Brett and the National Hansen's Disease Museum*)

'Landing of the First Seven Hansen's Disease Patients at Indian Camp Plantation, Carville, Louisiana' painted by latter-day Carville patient, Johnny Harmon

The combination of Kendall's articles and a report prepared by Dyer for the Orleans Parish Medical Society put an end to Beard's 'bit of graft' and persuaded the legislature to create a State Board of Control for the Leper Home in September 1894, with Dyer as its president. The problem was to find a suitable site for the home – just as it would be a quarter of a century later for the national institution. Dyer wanted it to be within easy reach of New Orleans, but no sooner did any location come under scrutiny than what one newspaper called 'the "blocking" game' commenced. The Indian Camp Plantation in Iberville Parish was far from ideal, being about eighty miles by road out of New Orleans, but it had two incalculable advantages: it was isolated, and it was available. Even so, its acquisition initially involved a degree of deception, the cover story being that it was to be used as an ostrich farm.[45]

Secrecy was the order of the day. After dark on the last day of November 1894 seven of the ten inmates of Dr Beard's pest house – five men and two women – were spirited away to a New Orleans wharf. They had no idea of their destination; they were happy just to escape their stinking lodgings opposite a garbage plant. Dr Dyer and a small group of journalists awaited their arrival by cart. They were herded on to a coal barge, prepared for their reception with tarpaulins, beds, mattresses and a mound of provisions for their new home. An observer of their departure remarked, 'This reminds me of the old stories of the floating funerals, sorrow-laden vessels gliding down the Nile to the cities of the dead.' So they went, transported up the Mississippi in a barge, towed by a tug.[46]

The next day, the ten-year-old son of the local postmaster, who was curious to catch a glimpse of the ostriches that were supposed to be arriving, rode his pony to the levee where the barge was anchored and saw a motley group of people shuffling or being carried down the gangplank. His companion, an elderly black man, said to him, 'Lordy, Lordy, little Boss, them's no ostriches – them's sick folks!' The boy did not wait to see the new arrivals settled into the largest of the seven decaying slave cabins at the back of the derelict ante-bellum mansion at the old 337-acre Indian Camp Plantation but hurried home to break the news to his family. Sixty years later, Arthur Carville, who had in the meantime profited handsomely from the proximity of the leprosarium that shared his name, smiled when he recalled the local indignation at the trick that had been played on the community, the petition they all signed and the threats of violence that followed its rejection.[47]

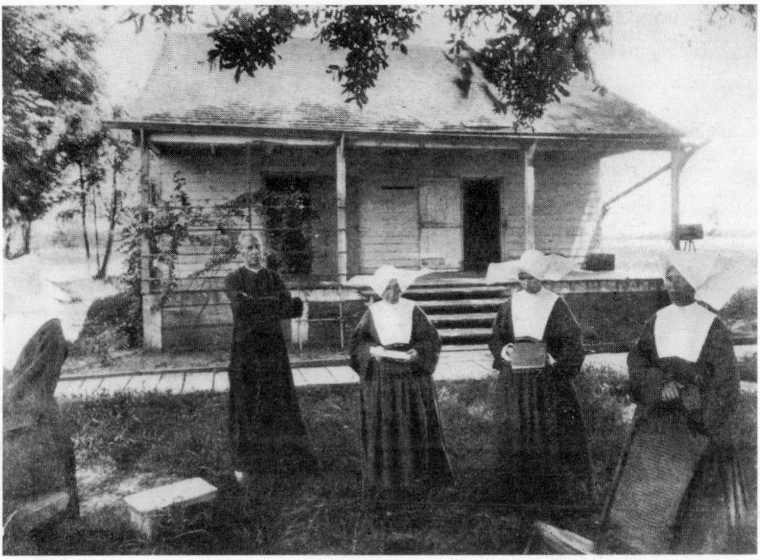
(Courtesy of the National Hansen's Disease Museum)

Carville's first Sisters of Charity with their Catholic chaplain in 1896 outside the slave cabin that served as a chapel

Dr Isadore Dyer, who had accompanied the leprosy patients to their new home, still hoped to find a more convenient location for a permanent state home, but every attempt he made was frustrated, one property being razed to the ground by local protestors rather than handed over to the state for a 'leper home'. At the end of 1905, the state accepted the inevitable and purchased Indian Camp, which up to that point it had been renting at $750 a year.[48]

Long before that, in June 1896, Dyer had resigned from the board of control on an issue of principle, as he later explained at a meeting of the American Dermatological Society:

> The law is explicit and comprehensive in its details, but the Board as it is at present constituted is opposed to the spending of any amount of money in the attempt at cure of lepers, who are looked upon as incurable, and are simply sent to the present asylum to die. On this account, of course, the leper is unwilling to go, and the physician with a conscience is unwilling to have him sent.[49]

Before he resigned, however, Dyer had been instrumental in obtaining the services of the Daughters of Charity of St Vincent de Paul, who were more

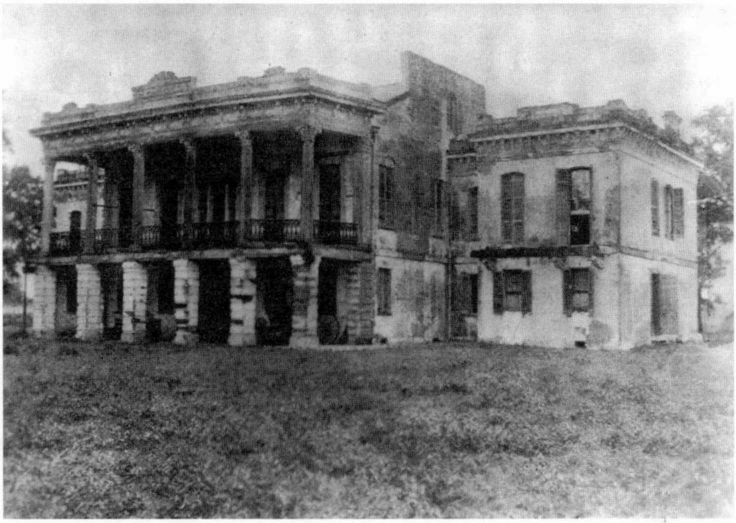
(Courtesy of the National Hansen's Disease Museum)

The derelict plantation house reserved for the use of the Sisters of Charity

commonly known as the Sisters of Charity. Having worked with them at the Charity Hospital in New Orleans, he knew that they would be wholly committed to any task they undertook, and if ever a place and a group of people required commitment it was Indian Camp and its forlorn inmates. The sister who went on a recce on 29 February 1896 was appalled at the conditions there: the place they were expected to occupy was a poky little house on stilts 'like a chicken house', without sanitary provisions of any kind. She reported:

> On the whole, I could not imagine anything so uncomfortable. There is only a single floor and when you are under the house you can see through the crevices. I could not think of letting the Sisters live in this house. They would lose their health . . .[50]

The patients occupied six cabins in about twenty-two acres of land surrounded by an eight-foot-high fence. Four of these cabins housed the patients, two for men and two for women, six to eight persons to a cabin; of the two remaining, one served as a kitchen and the other was empty. For water they were dependent on cisterns, which filled up when it rained, but in dry weather they had to trudge 200 yards to the river to fetch it. The sister spoke to an old man she had known in the New Orleans Charity Hospital and asked him if he had seen a priest. 'Oh no,' he replied, 'none will come here.' In an ominous foretaste of what was to come, the sister noted, 'The worst feature of the place is that there is no segregation of the sexes neither day nor night, and morals, no doubt, are in a deplorable condition.' She recommended that the order insist upon better housing conditions for the sisters before agreeing to take on the work. But she was overruled by the Director of the Daughters of Charity, the Rev. Robert Lennon, who visited shortly after and was so 'moved by the piteous situation' that a contract was drawn up in March and the first four sisters came upriver from New Orleans on the evening of 16 April 1896.[51]

Their home was not to be the 'chicken house' that had originally been intended for them, but the plantation house itself. Its air of faded grandeur could not disguise the ruinous state it was in, as one of a later generation of sisters wrote:

> The walls oozed moisture; the roof admitted torrents of rain; broken floors furnished shelter to rats, while long unused attics and rooms were veritable havens for bats and snakes. It seems scarcely credible that such hardships should have been added to the inherent difficulties of the work. The word 'leper', however, explained everything. Where were to be found carpenters, plasterers and painters who would go into the colony to make the necessary repairs? And it seems rather to have been taken for granted that since the Sisters were willing to make the major sacrifice, subsequent minor ones were not worth mentioning.[52]

There was a visiting doctor who looked after the patients physically and, until the arrival of the sisters, spiritually too. Now the sisters and their chaplain took over the spiritual guidance of the patients, all but one of whom were Catholics; the one exception, according to Sister Beatrice, the first chief nurse, 'seems a little obstinate in the matter of resistance, but still we are hoping he will think better of it, or before it is too late'. The sisters did not neglect the material well-being of the patients, encouraging them to grow flowers, fruit and vegetables, chivvying them into sharing domestic duties and attempting to take their minds off gloomy thoughts by organising games such as croquet, which was particularly popular.[53]

The sisters were nurses as well as nuns and, like Dr Dyer, they wanted the home to have a medical and not just a custodial function; Sister Beatrice, shortly before she died, 'worn out by her labors and frequent attacks of malaria' (with her bed having to be moved 'several times a day to get it out from under leaks in the roof'), drew attention to the physical deterioration and, in some cases, breakdown of many of the more active and helpful patients.[54] But the state legislature saw no point in spending money on an incurable disease; it was enough that its victims were isolated and had a refuge, the presence of nuns ensuring their safe passage into the next world, if not their retention in this one. So as far as the patients were concerned the sisters played an ambivalent role: they were angels of death as well as angels of mercy. Several patients understood the position and voted with their feet. As Dr Ralph Hopkins, who was attending physician from 1901 to 1921, pointed out:

> The hope of being cured is the best antidote to ennui that we have found. If a high stone wall surrounded the home, if its inmates were kept constantly under guard, if they were locked up at night, and if blood hounds were used to trail those escaping, no doubt there would be little or no absconding. But such a method unquestionably would unfavorably affect the number of admission[s,] about one-third of which are voluntary.[55]

For much of its 100-year existence, first as a state 'leper home' and then as a national leprosarium, Carville veered, first one way, then the other, in its attempt to define its role as hospital or asylum. The inmates might not be surrounded by a high stone wall, but they were encircled by a high wire fence, and even if they weren't exactly kept under lock and key, they had no doubt they were prisoners. Dr Hopkins and the sisters did their best to ameliorate conditions and improve the medical facilities, but they were constrained by lack of funds; the chief nurse, Sister Benedicta's report for 1908 tells its own story: out of a total of sixty-one patients, forty-seven were in the home on 1 May 1907, eleven had absconded, two died and one had been discharged as cured.[56] Absconding became a way of life at Carville.

By the time John Early arrived there towards the end of 1918, there were about ninety patients in the leprosarium, 60 per cent of whom were male. The days of the slave cabins were long gone and they were now housed in comfortable cottages equipped with bathrooms, electric light and steam heat, and connected to one another by covered walkways. Most patients had single rooms. They were sexually, as well as racially, segregated; there were separate dining rooms for men and women. There was a Protestant, as well as a Roman Catholic, chapel. According to the superintendent, Sister Edith, the patients

> have plenty of room for outdoor exercise and most of the men have their little vegetable gardens. Raising chickens is one of their chief diversions; many of them specialize in 'fancy' stock. Last year a moving picture machine was presented to the Home and we now enjoy a good weekly show.[57]

Dr Isadore Dyer, who still acted as consultant to the home, outlined the treatment given to the patients (predominantly doses of chaulmoogra oil), but admitted that, with no doctor on the premises, the 'medical care has never been entirely satisfactory'.[58]

The president of the State Board of Health, Dr Oscar Dowling, spoke to Early soon after his arrival at the home and reported that:

> John Early gave a statement to the effect that he was contented and very happy and the Sisters have done as much as his own people [i.e., Protestants] would have done to make him satisfied, and that he expected soon to die and could not ask for better treatment than he is now receiving.[59]

Such an uncharacteristic expression of satisfaction suggests either that this was still the honeymoon period in his relationship with the Sisters, or that he did indeed feel that death was imminent – perhaps both. Needless to say, his restlessness soon reasserted itself and in the first years of the National Leprosarium he was one of the most frequent 'absconders'.

Meanwhile, the committee charged with finding a suitable site for the proposed national leprosarium, under the chairmanship of Dr George W. McCoy (who'd had the responsibility of closing the experimental laboratory at Molokai in Hawaii before he went to Washington as Director of the Public Health Service's Hygienic Laboratory), was still hoping to find an alternative to Carville, which – in McCoy's words – 'had but little to commend it beyond the fact that it would have offered a prompt solution of the question of providing a location'.[60] In the end availability was everything; more suitable sites, in Florida and elsewhere, could not be secured 'on account of the antagonism of the residents'.[61] So in 1921 Carville became US Marine Hospital No. 66 of the Public Health Service, and Dr Oswald E. Denney, who had been director at Culion in the Philippines, was appointed Medical Officer in Charge (MOC). Had Dr Isadore Dyer lived to see the transformation (he died the previous year at the age of fifty-five), his pleasure at this outcome would have been tempered by disappointment that it would take another ten years before the hospital saw fit to appoint its first bacteriologist.[62]

Stanley Stein wrote, 'Dr Oswald E. Denney was not popular with his patients.' But, he conceded, few MOCs were, 'for they represented authority in an institution which purported to be a hospital but whose charges, for the most part, were there by compulsion and lived under what was little short of prison discipline'. When he first met Dr Denney, Stein thought he was 'a cold fish', but as he got to know him better he grew, if not to like him, to understand and respect him more:

> He had a human side and a sense of humor, although he kept both fairly well concealed. I suppose that any man who found himself almost helpless professionally in the face of so much misery entrusted to his care would have to maintain strict objectivity to avoid going mad.[63]

On his arrival at Carville, Denney aroused the patients' ire by hoisting the yellow jack, or emblem of quarantine, next to the United States flag. 'Patients screamed at the baleful quarantine signal', Stein recorded, 'and the most vociferous screamer in Carville history, John Early, made inflammatory speeches and wrote to his congressman.' The yellow jack eventually came down – but not for some years. Another of Denney's innovations was universally applauded, however; that was the removal of the fence the sisters had erected to segregate the sexes. Denney even organised a dance to mark the change of status from 'home' to hospital, and though the patients initially just stood in their segregated groups on either side of the room, uncertain what to do, he and his wife showed the way by selecting partners from among their charges and leading them out on to the floor.[64] Among the staff, the sisters might secretly regret the passing of the era of Catholic control, and some of them undoubtedly resented their loss of authority, but they soon knuckled under, glad of the opportunity to continue as nurses under the new regime.

Denney's most troublesome patients were the ex-servicemen of both the Spanish–American War (John Early prominent among them) and the First World War, who fired off complaints to veterans' organisations. After one such salvo, Denney wrote to the Surgeon General, wearily conceding most of the points raised:

> The allegation: 'The men seem to be very much displeased with their surroundings' is probably, to some extent, correct. It must be recalled that these patients are suffering from a chronic, incurable, contagious disease, which necessitates their isolation from their fellow beings and it is not conceivable that any surroundings, under such circumstances, would be especially pleasing . . .
>
> The allegation that: 'They claim they are getting worse rather than better' is, to some extent, true. It is well known that leprosy is, to all intents and purposes, an incurable disease . . .
>
> The allegation that: 'They claim the place is damp and low and that the water that they have to use is very muddy' is, unfortunately, partly correct. The major portion of the State of Louisiana is practically at sea level . . .
>
> The allegation that: 'The ex-servicemen complain they are placed among a lot of aliens' is, unfortunately, true and unavoidable. Leprosy is not a selector of race, creed, social or economic standing . . .[65]

Denney interviewed the ex-servicemen and found that, when it came to the crunch, none of the World War veterans and only a few of those from the Spanish–American War wanted to be transferred to another hospital. Of those who did:

> One man desired a transfer because, he said, he had once had a 'raw deal from the Sisters'; [and] another said that he desired to be transferred to a soldiers' home in his native state on the grounds that the climate in Louisiana is unhealthy.

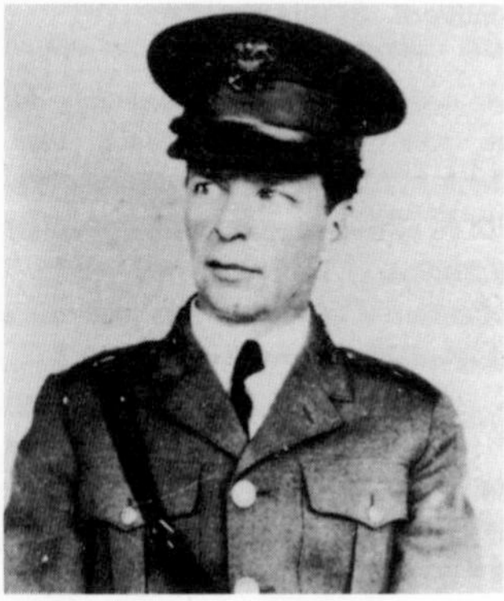

(Courtesy of the National Hansen's Disease Museum)

Dr Oswald E. Denney

A few days earlier, when the hospital was being inspected and patients had been invited to air their grievances confidentially to the inspector, only one person had availed himself of the opportunity: John Early. As the interview was confidential, the inspector could not tell Denney what had passed between them, only that 'the complaints were inconsequential and unimportant'. Denney claimed that much of the dissatisfaction among Spanish–American War veterans was due to their unpopularity with their fellow patients 'for personal reasons'.[66]

Early took himself off to Washington yet again and was unceremoniously returned to Carville, where he was selected as one of the subjects for a psychiatric study designed to investigate the correlation of leprosy and mental abnormality. This was conducted by a Dr L.L. Cazenavette of Tulane University between 1923 and 1926.

> During the time of my first examination, four months after his readmission [the doctor noted], he was at first courteous and affable, though evincing some surprise at my unexpected call, the purpose of which he would not understand, even though explained to him. He gave the examiner little chance to say anything. He was very loquacious, and kept himself much in the center of the stage. At time[s] he was rather hostile and suspicious, and displayed much arrogance in his manner of expression. He was restless and agitated. His emotional reactions disclosed marked fluctuations. He manifested no reserve in expressing his indignation at what he termed the absolute unfairness of the officers in charge . . .[67]

Cazenavette's conclusion, after further 'examinations' of the patient, was that Early's 'querulousness, and the delusions of persecution in which he imagined himself and others at the leprosarium unjustly treated, brought forth a reactive mental disturbance of a paranoid type not unlike the psychotic reactions of prisoners'.[68] This begs the question of which came first – so-called 'delusions of persecution' or a history of actual persecution quite sufficient to induce a psychotic state in anyone.

For Early, the honeymoon period of his relationship with Carville and the Sisters of Charity was over. He masterminded a protest over the employment of Roman Catholic sisters as nurses in a government hospital and signed a petition, along with thirty-two other Carville inmates, eleven of whom were veterans, that was published in the late summer of 1924 in a paper appropriately called *The Menace*: 'We, the undersigned protest their employment in the government's institution, and request their removal, and that trained nurses be employed in their stead as a preventative of proselyting and religious favoritism that is obtaining under their (Sisters') nursing.'[69]

Never mind that the sisters *were* trained nurses. Over the next couple of years the religious controversy rumbled on, involving both the

Protestant and the Roman Catholic chaplains in petty incidents with patients. The R.C. padre tangled with an ex-serviceman over the burial of one of his colleagues, while the Protestant chaplain angered a Catholic patient by his appearances in the patients' dining room during meal times.[70] The tensions reached such a pitch that in April 1926 a formal investigation was held. The hearings lasted two days, during which it became clear that there were 'accentuated factional differences' and that 'the two chaplains were hopelessly divided'. There were 'charges and countercharges of proselyting on both sides' and a number of patients 'stated that if present conditions continue, which they referred to as a war, they would be obliged to abscond'. The investigating officer recommended the removal of both chaplains and their replacement by 'full-time officers of the Service' who would be required to promote 'peace and harmony'. He recognised that the 'presence in this hospital of nurses wearing the dress of one denomination is a source of dissatisfaction among many of the patients' but was reluctant to propose their removal since they would be so hard to replace. Only if the appointment of new chaplains failed to improve the situation should serious consideration 'be given to the removal of the Sisters of Charity as nurses'.[71]

The Protestant cabal, headed by John Early, bitterly opposed the dismissal of their chaplain, gathering nearly a hundred signatories for their 'humble protestation'.[72] But according to Dr Denney, the 'timely appearance of an investigator acted as a safety valve' and succeeded in defusing the situation. Denney's main concern was to lobby against the removal of the Sisters of Charity, whom he praised for their efficiency as nurses, their 'physical and mental stamina' and their readiness to 'personally dress patients in such stages of corruption that the leper orderlies themselves did not care to handle them'.[73]

The Assistant Surgeon General's report on this 'religious war' found 'indisputable evidence' of proselytising on both sides and, on the Catholic side, criticised individual sisters who 'placed emblems of the Catholic faith in the rooms, and even on the bodies of helpless or dying Protestant patients'. But there was 'no convincing evidence' of discrimination against Protestant patients 'in the conduct of their professional work'. On the contrary, 'the nursing service was exceptionally well carried out. All of the sisters are registered nurses. The Chief Nurse is a woman of exceptional ability.'

The report concluded that 'the most difficult situation on the station is

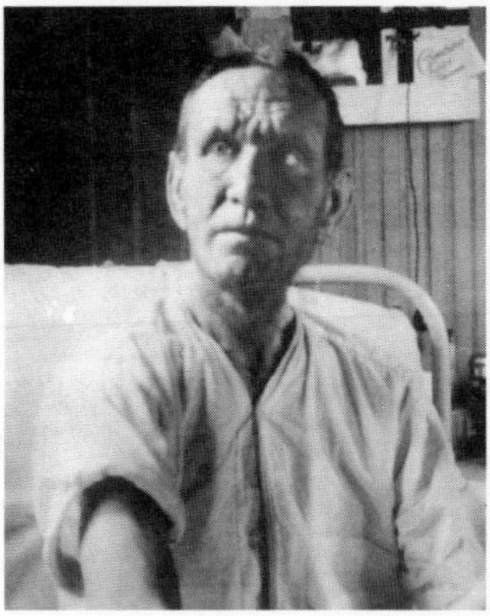
(International Journal of Leprosy)
John Ruskin Early

that relating to the Sisters of Charity'. While everyone agreed that the use of members of a religious order as nurses in a government institution 'was not right in principle', the 'manifest advantages of using Sisters instead of the regular nursing corps were so great as to outweigh the disadvantages'. Apart from the sheer difficulty of attracting secular nurses to the leprosarium, 'a nurse who had served for a period in this hospital would always have attached to her a suspicion which would militate against her securing employment in other branches of the nursing service'.[74]

As for the chaplains, their crime seems to have been that they were both foreigners, or at least foreign born. The Roman Catholic Father, though 'a man of rather pleasing personality', was a German, which did not 'endear him to the ex-service element', and should be replaced by an 'American who is familiar with the character, ideals and prejudices of the sort of population with which he has to deal', while the Protestant chaplain was 'a native of Australia' and 'the fact that he is not an American or an American citizen militates against his usefulness'.[75] The Assistant Surgeon General did not explain how this nationalistic approach squared with the multiracial and polyglot composition of the patient body, consisting of 'Chinamen, Hawaiians, Mestizos, Greeks, Filipinos, Mexicans and whatnot'; perhaps the authorities were only concerned with those who were seen as troublemakers, i.e., 'the ex-service element'.

One of the main troublemakers, John Early, soon absconded again, this time heading for his brother's farm in the mountains of North Carolina, where he hoped to be allowed to remain in 'private quarantine' with the support of the local bigwigs and his brother prepared to stand surety for him.

> This the Public Health Service refused [he wrote], sending marshal, sheriff, doctor and a ham-handed deputy up and in on our blessed mountain retreat and secluded isolation, the last Sunday morning of August, 1927, they hunted me down like I was a desperado, manhandled and lugged me out of my hiding place in the shrubbery . . . brought me

> to Spartanburg, South Carolina, where the health doctor and the ham-handed deputy entrained with me back to the swamp-polluted, mosquito-infested and the then flood-threatened leprosarium where I landed in a concrete jail cell about midnight, August 28, 1927, and in which jail cell I am still locked at this writing, March 6, 1928 . . .[76]

Much of Dr Denney's correspondence with the Surgeon General during the 1920s was taken up with the problem of what to do with persistent absconders. In the year 1927, he wrote, 'thirty-three lepers absconded and thirteen of these were returned, or returned voluntarily. In addition, during the same period, ten lepers who [had] absconded previously, returned to the hospital.' Measures taken to discourage absconding included a short period of isolation and the imposition of bonds of up to $5,000 to be forfeited in the event of re-absconding. Denney sought authorisation to build a proper prison, with at least thirty-two cells, to provide an 'effective deterrent', since all the hospital currently had in the way of detention buildings were 'a small three-room brick structure of unsatisfactory design and facilities, which is used for the isolation of insane lepers' and 'a more modern three-room reinforced concrete jail, occupied by one convicted murderer and two recalcitrant lepers'.[77] One of the latter almost certainly was John Early, whose second initial, R, might have stood for 'recalcitrant' rather than Ruskin.

From a medical point of view, Early's case remained a puzzling one. Bacteriologically, he frequently tested negative, and he was officially discharged almost as many times as he went AWOL. In 1928, Dr Denney described Early's reaction when he suggested he might care to take a look at the notice board, where he would find his name listed among the cases for 'parole':

> He looked at me blankly for a moment, registering no pleasure and grunting 'humph', and addressed me about as follows: 'A complaint I would like to register, if I may be permitted to register a complaint, is that the glare in my present quarters is very great and is blinding the eyes of the well as well as the eyes of the sick.' He had reference to the cement floor in the patio of the new concrete detention quarters. A suggestion has been made that we may have to hog tie a certain gentleman and drag him out of the front gate when the time comes; I assume from past correspondence that you will authorize the use of the caterpillar tractor if dragging is necessary.[78]

Perhaps this is an example of that sense of humour that Stanley Stein said Dr Denney kept 'well concealed'. Certainly Early kept coming back: once in 1930, again in April 1931 – when Stein saw him for the first time, 'a tall, gaunt, hatchet-faced, bug-eyed individual who was preaching hellfire and brimstone to the open-mouthed sinners under the oaks'[79] – and, for the ninth and last time, on 20 April 1934.[80]

Though he still inveighed against 'the nun nurses', whom he refused to address as 'Sister',[81] he was not among the fourteen signatories of a letter addressed to the General Secretary of the American Mission to Lepers, William M. Danner, dated 10 June 1935, protesting against 'the retention of the Sisters of Charity as nurses in this hospital'.[82] Many of the usual suspects among the ex-servicemen signed the letter, but there was a new sharpness to it that belonged to the next, more political generation of Carville patients. John Early was now out on a limb, a part of history rather than an active force for change. So, too, was his old sparring partner, Dr Oswald Denney, who was about to be posted away from Carville. Denney's last letters as MOC there convey a not altogether attractive combination of weariness, detachment and inflexibility that suggests his departure was not before time.

Early lingered on at Carville until 28 February 1938, when he died, apparently of cancer, aged sixty-four.[83] If doubts remain over the original diagnosis of leprosy in his case, there can be no doubt that he came to personify the stigmatised figure of the 'wandering leper' for a generation of Americans. He may well have contributed to his own martyrdom through his publicity seeking but there was a genuinely tragic dimension to his life, and he deserves to be remembered for being the first person in modern times to give the leprosy patient a human face – nodules and all.

Stanley Stein, his heir apparent and the supreme representative of the next generation of Carville crusaders, should have the last word:

> My most vivid recollection of John is the time he called me and another patient to his room to hear the reading of his will. He announced that if there was anything we did not understand, we were free to interrupt. I was the first to interrupt, in the midst of his first sentence.
>
> 'In the event of my death or if I am caught up,' he began.
>
> 'What do you mean, "caught up"?' I asked.
>
> He solemnly explained that Elijah had been caught up to heaven in a fiery chariot, and he was making provision for a similar possibility.[84]

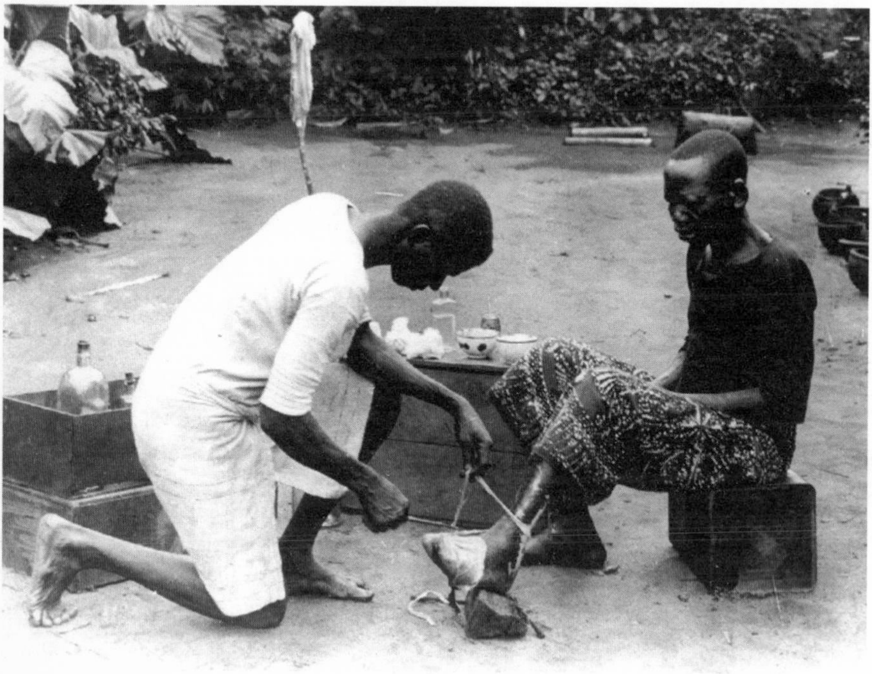

Treating ulcers in Ekpene Obom, Nigeria, 1931

Chapter 9

SIR LEONARD ROGERS AND THE BRITISH EMPIRE LEPROSY RELIEF ASSOCIATION

Major-General Sir Leonard Rogers of the Indian Medical Service (like his American colleague, Dr Victor Heiser, who'd sought him out in Calcutta in 1915 to encourage him to concentrate on the treatment of leprosy) lived to a grand old age. An IMS colleague recalled that he neither drank nor smoked and 'restricted his ration of exercise, recreation, and even sleep, to the amounts essential for maintaining physical and mental fitness'.[1] Rogers did invaluable research on many tropical diseases, but he is chiefly remembered for his work on leprosy, which fell into two parts.

The first was his development of a preparation derived from chaulmoogra oil (or the oil from one of the varieties of *Hydnocarpus*, an Indo-Malayan fruiting tree of the same genus) into an effective treatment for certain types of leprosy, and the second, following his retirement from India and active medical research, was the extension of his practical findings into the field of leprosy control. Approached in his London consulting rooms early in 1923 by the Indian Secretary of the Mission to Lepers, Rev. Frank Oldrieve, with a view to setting up an organisation dedicated to the elimination of leprosy throughout the British empire, Rogers took up the challenge – which amounted to nothing less than instigating a revolution in the prevailing attitude towards the segregation of leprosy sufferers – and together they founded the British Empire Leprosy Relief Association (BELRA).

This was quite an undertaking for a man already well into his fifties. But Rogers was in some respects a late developer. He came of a Cornish family and was born in Plymouth on 18 January 1868. He wrote in his memoir:

> Quite early, I remember, I knew that I was to be a doctor, because in Cornwall it is said that the seventh son of a seventh son is born to be a doctor. I was the seventh son of a fifth son: they thought that was near enough.

His father was a captain in the navy who, having been born in 1824, had seen a great deal of service in sailing ships; he was also skilled at repartee – to judge by his son's account of an incident that took place on a seaside holiday with his brothers at Newquay:

> Once we had walked out to Bedruthan steps and four of us were climbing the difficult Queen Bess Rock. Two of my elder brothers had reached the top and a lady who was alarmed for our safety ran to my father and said: 'Do you see those boys? They will fall and be killed, why don't you stop them?'
>
> Very calmly he laid his newspaper aside and replied: 'It's all right, madam. They are my boys. I have plenty more at home.'[2]

This anecdote notwithstanding, Captain Harry Rogers was a God-fearing man, whose ten sons all grew up to serve in the church, the navy, the army, or one of the Indian services. His seventh son's schooldays were undistinguished and Capt. Rogers did not have very high expectations when Leonard went to St Mary's Hospital, Paddington, for his medical training; so he was surprised and delighted when his son carried off three of the four prizes on offer during his first year there and won a scholarship to ease the financial burden of his education. Leonard's religious upbringing inclined him towards becoming a medical missionary – he was secretary of the St Mary's prayer union – 'but I did not feel altogether fitted for it, partly owing to very great difficulty in learning any foreign language'.[3] Nevertheless, what his biographer calls 'Christian paternalism' guided him throughout his career in India and 'developed almost into a missionary drive with BELRA'.[4]

The science that attracted Rogers most was pathology, but by joining the Indian Medical Service, which was 'primarily the medical department of the Indian Army', he was obliged to undergo some years of regimental service before he could transfer to a civilian department and do the kind of work he liked. He arrived in India in October 1893 but it was not until his thirty-second birthday, on 18 January 1900, that he joined the Bengal Civil Medical Department. In family life, too, he was a late starter, not getting married until 1914 and becoming a father for the first time in 1916, when he was close to fifty.[5]

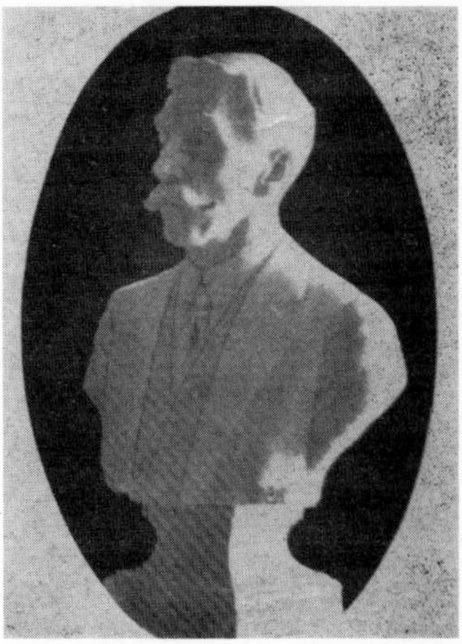
(The Star)

Bust of Sir Leonard Rogers at the Calcutta School of Tropical Medicine

In Rogers' laboratory career, his biographer detects 'a shift of emphasis in his choice of research topic, from diseases which afflicted Europeans and Indians (fevers and bowel diseases) to those affecting Indians in the vast majority of instances (leprosy and tuberculosis)'. At the same time, his promotion in the IMS and involvement in the foundation of the School of Tropical Medicine in Calcutta meant that 'Rogers the researcher gradually became an administrator'.[6]

In February 1920, he attended a conference of leprosy asylum superintendents held in the Town Hall, Calcutta, and addressed the opening session, praising the Americans for their 'splendid work' of segregation at Culion in the Philippines:

> Within ten years the number of lepers has fallen from ten thousand to between three and four thousand. That shows what can be done by go-ahead methods, but there, of course, the problem is easier than in India . . .[7]

What was exercising the Mission to Lepers and asylum superintendents in India (and elsewhere) in 1920, however, was not so much segregation *per se* as the segregation of the sexes within institutions and intermarriage among leprosy sufferers. Rogers regarded these questions as 'of extreme importance' – not least because the notion 'that lepers were largely sterile' had been 'completely disproved by the very extensive figures of Dr McCoy of the United States'. The rationale for the Mission's policy of sexual segregation was 'the excessive danger of contagion to the children of lepers', and McCoy's finding that 'the female leper is by no means sterile' served only to reinforce it.[8]

The question arose at the conference because of a proposal made by Frank Oldrieve (still working for the Mission to Lepers in 1920) for dealing with the increasing number of 'pauper lepers' compulsorily segregated by order of the government: he advocated that, since existing government asylums were all full and the superintendents of Mission-run asylums were reluctant 'to be put in the position of being policemen and having charge, under police powers, of lepers who have been dealt with by the law', they be housed in special 'Leper Settlements' along the lines of Molokai in Hawaii and Culion in the Philippines. The snag was that an official had told Oldrieve that the government would never accept the idea of such settlements 'if you try to keep the men in one place and the women in another'.[9]

The Mission to Lepers was torn over what to do about this. On the one hand, it benefited from working with government and didn't want to lose its predominance in the field of leprosy work; on the other it was reluctant to abandon segregation of the sexes, though this was not practised in all of its asylums. Superintendents worried about marrying couples, many of whose antecedents were unknown. 'If we marry them,' one said, 'and we would surely marry many who are really married people, then we are responsible for that life of sin to a certain extent and for the children brought into the world.' A Dr G.E. Miller protested, reminding the conference that the primary purpose of a leprosy asylum was public safety. Children born there 'could be properly cared for. India was not England or America. Public sentiment was different. If marriage was allowed in settlements it ought to be in Homes. He did not favour absolute segregation'. But his was a minority view, and the conference resolved 'that segregation of the sexes, except under very exceptional circumstances, should be enforced in our Asylums'.[10]

In practice, however, the Mission to Lepers continued to operate a dual policy, allowing cohabitation in some of its asylums – because that had been the arrangement when they were taken over – but not in others; and the debate rumbled on for years. In 1924, the General Secretary, W.H.P. Anderson, accepted the inevitable and proposed that 'Both Policies should be Approved, if not Abused' and questioned the received wisdom of preventing the birth of children through enforced segregation of the sexes:

> It seems to me that it is taking a great responsibility upon oneself definitely to oppose the idea of lepers having children. We know that lepers are not born such. And so long as a Superintendent who allows cohabitation of married lepers makes it clear that children who are born

> must live apart from their parents in healthy surroundings at an early age, it would seem that the birth of children, instead of being a calamity, is rather a matter for rejoicing.[11]

This was a remarkably liberal sentiment for that time.

Segregation of the sexes was an issue in leprosaria run by missionaries or nuns as far afield as Malaya and Fiji. In India, a missionary doctor with whom Leonard Rogers worked closely and collaborated on an authoritative textbook on leprosy, Ernest Muir, called it a 'difficult question':

> In favour of complete separation of men and women there are two main considerations – the tendency of child-bearing to exacerbate leprosy; and the danger to children born of leprous parents. Against separation there is the unnatural life . . . to which patients are sentenced for many years, very often for life.[12]

Rogers himself approved of segregation of the sexes 'in cases that are hopeful under treatment, if only to prevent a healthy partner of a curable case becoming infected'. But with advanced cases, living in asylums, he favoured what he called 'the Panama system of only allowing couples to marry or live together if the male agrees to the simple sterilising operation of cutting the *vas deferens* subcutaneously on either side' and encouraged the missionary Dr Travers to introduce it in Malaya.[13]

The sterilisation of leprosy sufferers was practised in several countries, as we've seen. In the Soonchun colony in Korea in the 1930s, the missionary Dr Robert Wilson pioneered an ingenious scheme in which ten men 'who were considered physically, spiritually and intellectually fit' were invited to select partners from among the women of the colony, to whom they would then be married once they had undergone a vasectomy. But this did not mean they would be childless: 'After the mass marriage ceremony, each of the couples was permitted to choose from among the children in the colony a child whom they would accept.' They were then

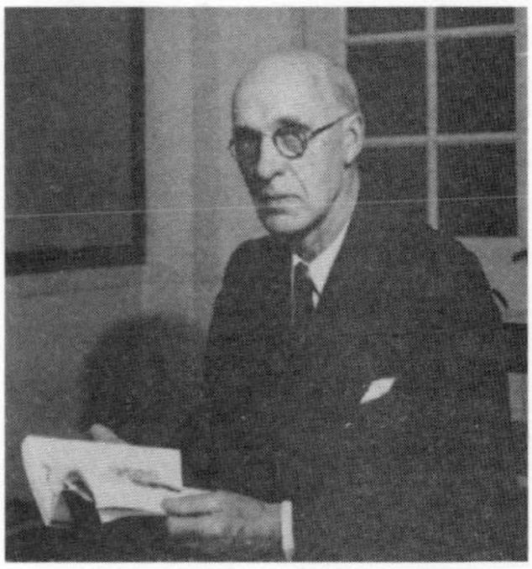
(The Star)

Dr Ernest Muir, co-author with Rogers of an authoritative textbook on leprosy given a small plot of land to farm so that they might be to some extent self-supporting. The missionary instigators of the so-called 'family plan' regarded this piece of social engineering as 'an immediate success'[14] – which others (like the commission appointed by Governor-General Murphy in the Philippines in 1935) would seek to emulate. The American Baptist Mission also operated a sterilisation scheme in the Shan states of Upper Burma, where it sought to replicate village life as closely as possible except in one respect: 'Immorality' was 'more or less universal', but in the 'model villages' run by the mission it was 'dealt with as the most serious crime . . . Public chastisement in the form of a whipping is the expected punishment'.[15]

How the subjects of such treatment themselves felt about it is not recorded in mission literature. But a novel written by a German refugee doctor, A.T.W. Simeons, who became Director of Medical and Health Services in what was then the Native State of Kolhapur in the Bombay Presidency provides a critical counterbalance to the missionary point of view. *The Mask of a Lion* (1952) focuses on a group of leprosy affected vagrants in India and offers a rare insight into how the people the missionaries tried to transform into a Christian vanguard regarded their benefactors and/or oppressors.

Govind is a Hindu tailor who keeps a tin of small change in his shop to give away to a succession of beggars, including 'the inevitable lepers in their unspeakably filthy groups, stinking and wailing in their hoarse voices'. His fastidious distaste for them means that they 'always got more than the others so that they might be induced, as quickly as possible, to remove their air-defiling and obnoxious presence.' The irony is that, even as he is expressing his revulsion for these beggars, Govind is himself incubating leprosy. The first part of the novel charts his growing isolation and descent into penury and, finally, beggary:

> He did not yet feel that he was really begging. It seemed to him that he was merely acting a part, that he was fooling the passerby, disguised as a leprous mendicant. He could not yet fully realise that this was the real thing . . .[16]

At the lowest point of his fortunes Govind considers suicide, but however worthless his life may have become he still feels that 'anything was better than extinction'. In his loneliness he discovers the 'great brotherhood' of leprosy affected beggars, one of whom tells him in no uncertain terms:

> Alone on the road, you are always in danger. You may suddenly get the reaction, the high fever, when your lumps swell up and burst open. One cannot say when that will happen, but if it does when you're alone on the road, then you are helpless.

Bapu is the old beggar who initiates Govind into the mysteries of his new calling, and through him Govind comes to realise 'that leprous vagrancy was a profession that had to be learned, and that on the knowledge, experience, planning and industrious execution depended success or failure'. He also discovers what interests the leprosy fraternity, what subjects they talk about when they get together: 'Prominent among them was the news about the various asylums and leprosaria. What sort of treatment was given, the quality of the food and changes in the senior staffs.'

Bapu is a wizened and deformed little rogue, whose physical frailty contrasts with his mental agility, low cunning, wit and wisdom. These qualities, combined with a cynicism that masks an underlying warmth and generosity of spirit, make him the natural leader of the group to which Govind finds himself attached. Bapu keeps a close eye on his charges and notices when any of them needs medical attention. So one day he addresses Govind, whose turn it is to carry Bapu on his back. 'My Govind', he says:

> 'you see that the rains are coming. You are not well. It is best that for a while we part. You and Premala must go to the big Mission Hospital at Bijabad. The wretched woman will soon go blind. That is a hard time. She will need good care, and only a doctor with lots of useless medicines can give her some comfort and some idle hope. But she will need that until she gets used to it – to the darkness. Then later we will take her back if she still wants to come.'

Bapu prepares his protégé for the ordeal ahead and instructs him on the vagaries of the missionaries:

> '. . . And Govind, they have a big hall where they sing strange songs and pray to their God. They will not ask you to come and join them, but if you

do, they will like it. After you have been there a while, go to their hall, and let them teach you their songs, and listen to the stories they tell you about their three Gods, and they will be proud of you.'

Govind submits to the routine of the leprosy hospital, the punctual meals, regular temperature taking and the twice-weekly injections of chaulmoogra that seem to him 'like pinnacles of activity rising abruptly out of a sticky morass of boredom'. But the 'better he felt physically, the more he suffered from enforced idleness'. Eventually, when he can stand it no longer, he asks the Matron if he can have a book to read. She expresses her delight that he can read and brings him an illustrated book of New Testament stories: 'The stories were full of wonders, and the miracles fired his imagination. He read them as startlingly new mythological tales, innocent of their Christian religious purport.' In no time he has exhausted the hospital's small stock of 'mission tracts, ecclesiastically approved fiction and Church magazines' and the Matron presents him with a copy of the Bible in translation, telling him he must read a little of it every day. 'Govind was proud, grateful and bewildered. He said he would do as she told him.'

An ardent Christian patient called Mr Joseph now takes Govind's education in hand and lets 'no opportunity pass to point out the superiority of his religion over what he tautologically called "pagan idolatry and heathenism"'. Though Govind is happy to accompany him to church, Mr Joseph does not have everything his own way; he finds that, 'in a mild way, Govind could be very disputatious'. Govind stubbornly prefers the 'gaudy lustre of his own [Hindu] pantheon' to the 'too abstract' Protestant concept of divinity presented by Mr Joseph.

After a while Govind hears that Bapu and his troupe are in the vicinity, and he slips out of the hospital to meet them. He is so excited that Bapu, who has come not to take him away but to hand over some money, has to silence him:

'Be quiet, my Govind, *Bapre*! What a chatterbox these missionaries have made out of you. The twenty rupees are not for you, my darling. They are for Premala, so she can buy herself some betel-nut with a pinch of tobacco in it. And, Govind, see that your friends the missionaries don't get hold of it, or they'll buy her their Holy Book to read with her blind eyes or their

> book of songs to sing with her glorious voice that sounds like the unoiled axle of a bullock cart.'

And the little man shakes with laughter at the absurdity of this vision.

Govind fulfils Bapu's errand, but it is no easy matter, given the strict segregation of the sexes in the hospital. The women's quarters are separated from the men's by a high wall and, though married men are allowed to visit their wives twice weekly and walk and talk with them, all sexual intercourse is prohibited 'to avoid the procreation of leprous progeny'. The men return from these visits 'in a storming rage, and lie awake at night, grumbling about the inhuman treatment, which seemed to them a senseless and absurd cruelty . . .'

Bapu's visit has filled Govind with a restless longing for the life of the road again and, after failing to achieve his freedom legitimately – by testing bacterially negative – he turns on Mr Joseph and his Christian God and gives up the job he has been doing as letter-writer for his illiterate fellow patients. He yearns only for the return of the beggar troupe. When they come, Bapu immediately sizes up the situation and invites Govind to accompany them once more. But first he must return to the leprosy hospital to deliver a message to Premala, who in her blindness has decided to stay there, opting for comfort over the wandering life.

> For the last time he looked at the other women, young, old, pretty and ravaged, and once more he sensed that strange, terrifying heat of desire that pervaded the female quarters. He was in a hurry to get away.

Once he has made his escape, he luxuriates in the sights, smells and tastes of the open road; he is ravenous and eats voraciously, relishing the 'strong, earthy flavour' of the food with its 'pungent seasoning', and the 'acrid tang of wood-smoke from the campfire'. 'Women did not seem half as important now as they had in the artificial atmosphere of Bijabad. All that crazy turbulence had somehow subsided. He was calm, contented and happy.'

The novel does not end there, but goes on to contrast Bijabad with a new, relaxed, village-style leprosy settlement in the southern Maratha country, where married couples are free to live together (if a woman has a baby, then it is removed to a children's home where it will be out of danger of contracting the disease) and nobody wants to leave. This 'model hospital-farm' is based on the real-life Shenda Park in Kolhapur State, which the author of the novel, Dr Simeons, helped to create; and Bapu and Govind are based on real patients he encountered there. In reality Shenda Park may not have been quite so idyllic as Simeons paints it – his account is 'true but rose-coloured', according to a woman missionary doctor who knew both the place and the author (a man of 'very large ideas and any amount of drive'), though her view may have been coloured by the book's anti-missionary slant.[17] But it was exactly the kind of place Leonard Rogers envisaged once he'd turned his attention from developing a scientific treatment for leprosy in the laboratory to applying it in the field.

The objective of the British Empire Leprosy Relief Association – what set it apart from the Mission to Lepers – was to tackle the problem of leprosy throughout the British empire; and to do this in a scientific way meant finding and treating early cases, rather than caring for mainly chronic, 'burnt-out' and no longer infectious cases in asylums. But in the beginning, the co-founder of BELRA, dazzled perhaps by the American examples in Hawaii and the Philippines, seemed strangely reluctant to follow the logic of his own insight. In 1923 Rogers was claiming that the British empire was 'doing far less for her lepers than the United States' and that segregation 'ought to be encouraged and undertaken in a more thorough manner' despite the fact that it was responsible for the concealment of early, treatable cases and was anyway impracticable in places as vast as India and central Africa.[18]

It was only with hindsight that Rogers came to see that what was required was 'nothing less than a complete revolution in our 2,000-year-old conceptions regarding the control of leprosy'. By the 1940s it had become clear that, whatever may have happened in nineteenth-century Norway, 'in poor and backward tropical races compulsory segregation has never succeeded in its avowed object of reducing materially the incidence of the disease'. But Rogers was reluctant to admit to any inconsistency in his own thinking, and from his later writings, in which he expressed the 'dilemma' clearly and logically, it would seem that he had always understood the need for 'a complete revolution' in the means of leprosy control:

> The improved treatment was only of material value in comparatively early cases of leprosy. The only method of control of the disease in general operation was compulsory segregation. Under that system early cases suitable for treatment were all hidden for fear of imprisonment for life.[19]

Hence the need for change. Yet at the time he'd been calling for an *extension* of compulsory segregation on the American model and had only gradually come to abandon that idea. The test case for him was South Africa, about whose policy he had a rather acrimonious correspondence with the Health Secretary to the government of the Union, Dr J. Alexander Mitchell.

It is no accident that the two British colonies which introduced the most stringent anti-leprosy laws in the late nineteenth century were South Africa and Australia. The preponderance of white settlers and racial attitudes that would lead, on the one hand, to the development of the policy of apartheid and on the other to the near-extermination of the Aborigines and the introduction of the 'White Australia' policy made compulsory segregation of the overwhelmingly non-white leprosy sufferers – preferably on off-shore islands – inevitable in both countries.

In Australia, as in Hawaii and elsewhere, leprosy was initially blamed on the 'yellow peril', the influx of Chinese during the gold rushes of the early 1850s, and then on *kanakas*, or Pacific Islanders brought in to labour in the Queensland sugarcane plantations. It would have been blamed on the Aborigines had they not been known to be free of the disease before the arrival of these immigrants. Once exposed to leprosy, however, they became the major sufferers and were even more stigmatised than before. It may have been a coincidence, but the Queensland Leprosy Act of 1892, which introduced compulsory notification and segregation of people with leprosy, was passed in the same year that the first Aborigine case of the disease was recorded in that state.[20]

In South Africa the infamous Robben Island had been a dumping ground for 'lunatics, paupers and lepers' from the middle of the nineteenth century.[21] Complete segregation was not imposed until the beginning of the 1890s, though a Leprosy Repression Act had been passed in the Cape Colony almost a decade earlier in 1884. In 1889, the year of Father Damien's death on Molokai, an anonymous article had appeared in *Blackwood's Magazine* exposing conditions there and calling for 'a second Father Damien'. By then there were convicts on the island as well, but the author of the article concentrated his attention on the 130 leprosy patients, an utterly crushed bunch who complained not of pain – they were 'past feeling' – but of cold and hunger. There was never enough to eat and they had nothing to do: no work, no amusements, no games to play, no newspapers or books to read, no access to their families on the mainland. There were two resident doctors on the island, but no nurses, the only relief being provided by less badly affected fellow patients and, in extreme cases, by 'the beautiful angel Death'.[22]

From another report, published in the *British Medical Journal* in the same month and year, we learn that the

> patients lie during the long hours of the day on the ground, clad in shabby, filthy rags, under what shelter they can find from the blazing southern sun. The only forms of existence which appear at all at home are the myriads of flies, which sometimes cover the exposed parts of the diseased creatures' bodies.

The anonymous doctor-writer was *au fait* with social Darwinism and concluded:

> Some will say, But after all these creatures are for the most part blacks; and, as experience teaches us that they, through the process of modern civilisation, must die off before the civilising force, why should we do more to prolong their existence? As members of a profession whose aim and object is to preserve the life of all living beings under all circumstances, absolutely impartial as to the exact form or species with which we are brought into contact, our duty is, primarily, to see to the well-being of the individual and, secondarily, to that of the community at large; and, this being so, we cannot for one moment accept such a short-sighted though possibly patriotic philanthropy . . .[23]

In 1890, as a result of a select committee report to the Cape Colony House of Assembly, Robben Island was cleaned up. Old buildings were renovated and new ones erected; sports and other recreations were introduced, and dances held once a month; and in 1891 a new medical superintendent was appointed.[24] Yet when William Tebb, the author of a polemic linking leprosy with the practice of vaccination, visited the island in February 1892, he noted the enduring miseries (exacerbated by an epidemic of flu) more than the evident improvements and expressed his opinion 'that the lepers and lunatics should be removed to separate quarters, and this barren island should be used exclusively for convicts' – since leprosy and lunacy, after all, were 'not criminal'.[25]

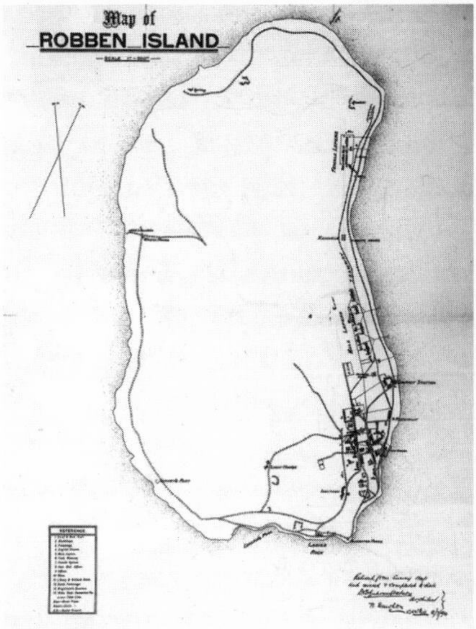

(Supplied by the Mayibuye Centre, Cape Town)

The infamous Robben Island – once a dumping ground for 'lunatics, paupers and lepers'

With the enforcement of segregation that year, leprosy patients began to outnumber the other groups on the island for the first time and even included some whites. Inadequate provision and, in some cases, mistaken diagnosis led to protests: in 1895 a ward was burned down and early in the twentieth century there were demonstrations outside the offices of the administration.[26] The employment of eight female nurses to work in a male ward, also in 1892, caused more trouble. These nurses incurred resentment by introducing such hospital routines as early rising and frequent washing; and because they were women they became a target of the male patients' sexual frustration: 'The lepers threatened to rape the nurses . . . if they were not allowed access to the female lepers, and to strike the nurses with their crutches.' On their side, the nurses soon found the long hours and lack of holidays or even weekend breaks, as well as the ' "repulsive and dangerous" work with recalcitrant patients' who had no hope of a cure, so unrewarding that most of them walked out. By the end of 1893 there were only two left. By contrast, the untrained white female nurses who were introduced on the women's wards in 1895 were so successful in 'managing rebellious situations' that their employment in the men's wards was reconsidered (though male staff remained predominant there until the 1920s).[27]

An off-the-cuff remark by the Secretary of BELRA, Frank Oldrieve, to the effect that the doctors on Robben Island were ignorant of the new treatment for leprosy provided the occasion for the first tetchy letter from South Africa's Dr J.A. Mitchell to Sir Leonard Rogers. In January 1924,

Mitchell wrote that such an assertion was unwarranted and questioned BELRA's claims to have 'found a cure' for leprosy. He said that he doubted the efficacy of any present-day treatment, all of which had been tried in South Africa. Despite Rogers' eminence in the field, Mitchell did not hesitate to reprove him for making claims 'calculated to raise hopes which may be doomed to disappointment and tend to create unrest and dissatisfaction in the Leper Institutions'.[28]

Though Rogers replied that he wasn't responsible for the statement to which Mitchell had taken exception, their correspondence continued to be dogged by mutual misunderstanding. Yet a memo Mitchell wrote for the South African government in 1922 on 'Leprosy Measures and Expenditure' reveals that they were essentially on the same wavelength.

Mitchell was well aware of the ineffectiveness of the segregation policy, citing his experience in the Transkei where 'only one-third to one-half of the lepers are ever discovered and segregated'. He referred to 'old and crude methods of quarantine and isolation' that modern knowledge on the spread of diseases had rendered anachronistic and maintained that it

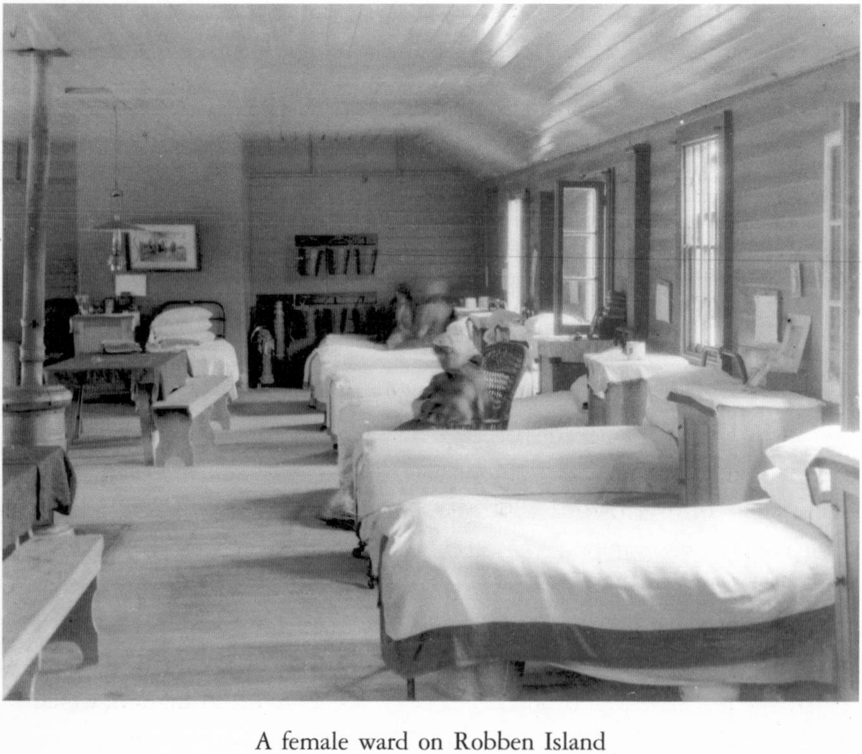

(Supplied by the Mayibuye Centre, Cape Town)

A female ward on Robben Island

was 'only in regard to leprosy that we are still mediaeval'. He wanted to do away with the institutional segregation of 'old chronic anaesthetic lepers' since 'the danger of spread of infection by them, if it exists at all, is so small as not to justify either the cost to the State or the compulsory detention and isolation of the individual'. He hoped to update the 'in many respects obsolete Leprosy Laws' and to transfer the administration of matters pertaining to leprosy from the Department of the Interior, which was the ministry responsible for prisons, to the Department of Public Health. If that were to happen (as it did in 1924), 'we might soon be in a position to convert our present Leper Asylums, which are practically prisons, into voluntary institutions'.[29]

That might have been wishful thinking in a country like South Africa, but one of Mitchell's aims – 'if it were possible to evacuate and close one Institution . . . that Institution should certainly be Robben Island' – was eventually achieved, though it wasn't until January 1931 that the last remaining leprosy patients on the island were moved to Pretoria and their old buildings razed to the ground.

Nevertheless BELRA's sanguine claims continued to rile Mitchell. 'Here in South Africa,' he wrote to Rogers in March 1927:

> we have between 2,000 and 3,000 lepers in Institutions, including a good many persons of education and intelligence . . . If it is proclaimed from the rooftops, on the authority of BELRA – 'A cure for leprosy has been discovered', 'Leprosy no longer an incurable disease', etc., they natually ask – 'Why have we not been cured long ago?', 'If lepers can be cured in other countries, why not in South Africa?' and as a rule they will jump quickly to the conclusion that it is because the Medical Officers treating them are incompetent. I feel sure you will see at once how easy it is to generate in this way acute discontent . . .[30]

For his part, Rogers was piqued by Mitchell's scepticism over the effectiveness of his chaulmoogra preparation, marketed under the brand name Alepol. He wrote in October 1928:

> Many thanks for yours reporting unsatisfactory results from a trial of alepol in five cases . . . in your last report it is stated that your cases are first seen in a large proportion after four, six or more years duration, which is only to be expected under the rigid compulsory isolation laws . . . [31]

In other words, *if your draconian segregation system didn't discourage the early reporting of cases, you might have more success with my treatment*. Mitchell replied huffily and Rogers broke off the correspondence.

There the matter might have rested, if Frank Oldrieve had not undertaken the role of mediator during a visit to South Africa the following year. A mollified Mitchell wrote to Rogers, explaining that South Africa was:

> not a purely Native country like Uganda or Nigeria, but a country where about one-fifth of the population is European . . . The European population, both Dutch and English, still take their ideas of Leprosy largely from the Bible; it is *the* loathsome disease *par excellence* and it will require many years of educative work before the great majority even of intelligent and fairly well-educated Europeans can be got to take a more reasonable view . . .[32]

Rogers responded in a friendly vein but within months they were at each other's throats again, this time over an article published in the Johannesburg *Sunday Times*, in which Rogers was quoted attacking leprosy policy in South Africa – an article Rogers claimed to know nothing about. More mutual recriminations followed and the second break was final. As a closet reformer hamstrung by the prejudices of South Africa's politicians and white population, Mitchell was in an impossible situation; having to defend policies he couldn't really justify probably accounts for his testiness.

The dispute obliged Rogers to define, or redefine, his stance on segregation. He was 'opposed to a rigid system of wholesale compulsory segregation', *but*: 'In countries where much money has been expended in segregating lepers compulsorily, I do *not* advise that this plan should be abandoned for the present . . . ' – only modified.[33] What he meant by this is clear from an article he'd written at the beginning of 1929 for *Leprosy News* (BELRA's house magazine and the precursor of *Leprosy Review*), in which he contrasted South African intransigence with the American system in the Philippines, where:

> recently the policy of compulsory segregation has been modified by adopting the plan, long advocated by Muir, myself and others, of allowing early cases to be treated at hospitals and clinics established near to where the patients live[34]

– something Mitchell had already dismissed as impracticable in South Africa 'as it would be impossible to site such a clinic anywhere in the Union so as to be within reasonable reach of a dozen leprosy patients'.[35] Rogers' ideas, promulgated by BELRA – and the money the organisation raised through Rotary Clubs and by other means – had a far greater impact in other parts of the African continent where there was no institutional segregation.

Back in the 1890s the medical officer of the Hausa Association's Central Sudan Expedition, Dr T.J. Tonkin, had noted that in northern Nigeria 'familiarity with leprosy is a social characteristic':

> The disease is so common that in spite of the repulsive appearance of the sufferers, the general public have, as far as I could make out, no active objection to it . . . Lepers are permitted to mingle freely with the healthy population, engage in business, and marry whom they will. When they live in communities it is not because they are forced to do so, but rather because community of interest acting through long years has drawn them together. Lepers are not subject to any municipal or social disabilities on account of their disease. I have frequently seen them tailoring, selling second-hand clothes, and presiding at provision stalls . . .[36]

Another member of the same expedition wrote that in Kano there were in the region of a thousand leprosy sufferers who had organised themselves into a community, whose headman bore the title of 'king of the lepers'.[37]

But the records of the 'Yaba Lunatic and Leper Asylums' in Lagos for the first decade of the twentieth century, when the colonial impact was making itself felt, tell a more familiar tale of galvanised iron fences, male and female compounds and absconding patients – not to mention break-ins and robberies, and undisciplined, rebellious staff.[38] The prevalence of leprosy in Nigeria, as in India, was so great that enforcing segregation proved impracticable and anyway by the late 1920s, when the Mission to Lepers was beginning to take an active interest in Africa, BELRA's repeated message that segregation 'defeat[ed] its own object by making lepers hide themselves' was having an effect. Dr G.W.St C. Ramsay, who made a study of leprosy in southern Nigeria, found a rather different situation from that described by Dr Tonkin in the north of the country thirty years earlier:

> The natives are able to recognise leprosy very early in its course, and they fully appreciate its infectious nature. They are also very ashamed of the disease, and do not like to admit that their parents have been lepers. But in spite of this, generally speaking, they seem to do little or nothing to prevent its spread among their families and the community at large. They live a very communal existence in small one-room mud huts with the minimum of fresh air. Lepers and non-lepers frequently share the same sleeping couch, the same pipe, the same eating utensils, and even the same loincloths.
>
> In certain districts, however, the natives have a real dread of leprosy, and the unfortunate victims are driven out of their villages and farms, and compelled to live a precarious existence in the swamps and bush. It has even been suspected that occasionally lepers are taken from their homes and secretly murdered.[39]

The problem of what to do with these exiled victims gave rise to an experiment in which the government leased thirty acres of prime land at a place called Itu on the Cross River, about fifty miles upstream from the estuary town of Calabar on the Bight of Biafra in the Gulf of Guinea, and encouraged them to settle there under the direction of the medical missionary, Dr A.B. Macdonald. Macdonald himself wrote of conditions in southern Nigeria in the year the Itu leprosy colony was founded:

> Many of our lepers are friendless, and have been deserted, or driven out of their homes. Leprosy cancels the marriage contract. It is strongly suspected that in many places lepers are got rid of in mysterious ways, and are either poisoned or take their own lives. In going over their individual histories it is astounding to find that nearly all 'contacts' are dead. I have known lepers in the last stage ask their friends to bury them alive.[40]

The Itu experiment was so successful that in next to no time the United Free Church Mission Leper Colony, which was supported by BELRA, had a population in excess of 600. 'All the patients are, of course, voluntary settlers,' Dr Ramsay wrote. 'There is no restriction whatever on their movements, and they are allowed to leave the camp and return at will.'[41]

Over the next two decades it continued to grow: the colony extended to cover four square miles and the patient population expanded to 3,500. An 80-bed hospital was supplemented by an annexe with 100 beds; there was a babies' home, a school, a church, a workshop, a court, a market, farms and farmsteads, residences for European and African staff, five villages known as 'towns', all close to one another and linked by a canal and a network of roads. 'Each street has a headman or, in the Women's Town, a headwoman, responsible for the behaviour of the occupants.' Everyone who was able to work was encouraged to do so, not just to make money but for medical, psychological and social reasons as well. Work was seen as therapeutic in that it increased self-respect, improved muscle tone and gave a sense of belonging, and of contributing to the welfare of the community as a whole. People went fishing in the river and the canal, sang in the choir, or played in the brass band. There were games – football for the young, draughts for anyone – and boy scout and girl guide meetings; children were taught handicrafts and encouraged to sing and dance; and there was, of course, religion: 'When they are able to make words out of letters, they are presented with a Bible.' But the centre of social life was the market, 'the scene of petty-trading, for which all seem to have a natural affinity.'[42]

The patients themselves policed the colony. 'Like all other African communities', Macdonald wrote, 'this has its own Chief . . . an important man, something like the sergeant major in his position. On him depends much of the life and character of the Colony.'[43]

Itu was the first – and largest – such settlement in Africa; it became the model that was followed (with local variations) across the continent, as well as in other regions of Nigeria like Uzuakoli and Oji River. In one remote district in southern Nigeria ostracised leprosy patients themselves had established three 'leper villages', and this gave the doctor in charge of Uzuakoli, J.A. Kinnear Brown, the idea of creating 'a system of dispensaries (local clinics) attached to special satellite villages in which the patients [who were out of range of the provincial settlements] should live'.[44] Kinnear Brown's successor at Uzuakoli, Dr Frank Davey, developed the scheme into a four-pronged exercise, involving investigation, segregation, treatment and control.

First, the size of the problem had to be assessed. Then, since no other method of controlling leprosy was known, some form of segregation was called for: Davey opposed 'the erection of large segregation centres', preferring small hamlets of not more than twenty or thirty people built in such a way as to provide 'a model to the neighbourhood in village construction' – most village chiefs proving more than willing to assist by providing materials 'when lepers are to be removed from the community'. Treatment was essential, not just for leprosy (by the mid-thirties some scepticism about the curative properties of chaulmoogra derivatives had set in), but for its secondary manifestations such as ulcers, since every effort 'must be made to overcome the hopeless outlook of the lepers themselves'. And finally control: a proper census had to be taken and each village resurveyed every two years to determine the success or otherwise of the scheme.[45]

With hindsight we can see that the African leprosy settlement was simply a microcosm of the African colony. But the fact that by and large these settlements were run by missionary societies created a paradoxical situation: on the one hand, they were modelled on the African village and set out to replicate the community from which the leprosy sufferer had been evicted; while on the other a major part of their function was to undermine village *mores*, eliminate the 'primitive' and forge a new – Christian – community. The potential for mutual misunderstanding and resentment was vast and despite the 'voluntary' nature of these institutions riots were far from unknown.

The outspoken Electra Dory, who joined the Universities Mission to Central Africa (UMCA) and sailed to Africa 'under troopship conditions' at the beginning of the Second World War to work at the Likwenu leprosy colony in what was then Nyasaland, was appalled by the 'concentrated misery' of the place. But she knew she must 'refrain from projecting my own emotions into the colony'. After all, it was 'no grim detention camp'; there was no compulsory segregation in Nyasaland; people were free to come and go as they pleased; they were not even outcasts, since there was no stigma attached to leprosy there. Telling new arrivals they had the disease was no problem:

> I never had to resort to the use of any euphemism or beat about the bush. I merely said, '*Nkate*' ('Leprosy'). '*Chabwino!* Good!' was the usual reply, and with no hut tax to pay some thought it a fairly good exchange. I never heard one rave or curse.[46]

So what was responsible for the pervading 'atmosphere of melancholy'? She came to the conclusion that it was not confined to the leprosy colony: the 'sadness extended all over the plain and far beyond'. And if the colony was modelled on an African village, that was not necessarily a good thing because the villages, 'with few exceptions, [were] squalid and insanitary', their people ignorant and superstitious. Dory was shocked to learn, for instance, that the villagers held Europeans responsible for the spread of leprosy because they insisted on burying corpses rather than taking them into the bush and leaving them for the hyenas to devour: 'They thought that burial meant the disease was planted and perpetuated.'[47]

Anthropologists emphasise the significance of death rituals and burial customs in all cultures. In what is now Mali, but was part of French West Africa between the wars, the Bobo people would frequently bury their dead inside their homes; and to be denied burial among 'healthy' dead people, ending up in the bush instead of 'inside cliffs, baobab trees, or termite mounds' was a mark of the 'shame' (*maloya*) associated with leprosy. A recent historian who made a study of the disease in Mali asked former patients at the French-run Institut Marchaux at Djikoroni, outside Bamako, why they'd remained there when they were, theoretically at least, free to come and go as they wished, and was told, 'Here we are one.' The 'sense of community which contrasted with the shame and alienation experienced in their villages' was enough to keep them together, even sometimes in opposition to the colonial doctors and Catholic sisters who ran the institution and made the rules. Thus, as in medieval European leprosaria, the threat of expulsion could be used against recalcitrant patients in the knowledge that they would rather remain where they were than face the rejection awaiting them outside.[48]

By the beginning of the Second World War, on the eve of the medical breakthrough that would transform the predicament of the leprosy patient (albeit slowly), the British, French and American colonial authorities operated a sophisticated system of segregation in which church and state worked hand-in-glove to demonstrate 'the power of colonialism to advance medical control and the power of medicine to return the favor'.[49] Patients no longer had to be dragged from their homes and compulsorily isolated. Instead, they were enticed into 'voluntary' settlements with promises of treatment that, in other diseases at least, had proved dramatically effective; and once there they formed communities, whether in co-operation with or in opposition to the authorities, that gave them the sense of identity that was denied them in their real homes.

With the word 'Empire' in its title, BELRA was unashamedly colonial in its approach, but it tried as far as possible to dissociate itself from the missionary aspect of leprosy work. Its 1930 Annual Report printed an extract from a League of Nations report as an epigraph:

> In some quarters, there may be an impression that the work of BELRA is conducted in an essentially missionary spirit – that is to say, that religious aims take precedence over medical and scientific aims. That is not the case . . .[50]

But it used the same propaganda and fund-raising techniques as the missionary organisations – juxtaposing remarks about restoring the dignity of the individual with the very images that served to undermine it, of deformed, ragged, ill-kempt and obviously poverty-stricken 'lepers' in attitudes of supplication, guaranteed to appeal to Christian 'charity'.[51] Indeed, the Mission to Lepers complained that BELRA was muscling in on its patch and that its own supporters were confusing the two organisations.

Since there was also considerable overlap in the staff they employed – Frank Oldrieve had come to BELRA from the Mission to Lepers and when he resigned as Secretary of BELRA in 1929, he was succeeded by the medical missionary Dr Robert Cochrane, who would later work for the Mission to Lepers – they were able to sort out their differences more or less amicably; but the differences did exist, and BELRA was not above exploiting donors' confusion over which organisation was which. And when the Rev. 'Tubby' Clayton, founder of the Toc H movement, which was designed to carry over the spirit of self-sacrifice so evident in the First World War into peacetime activities, linked up with BELRA at the end of 1933 and sent idealistic young men out to Africa and elsewhere to work on leprosy settlements, that increased the potential for confusion.[52]

But if missionaries more or less monopolised the disease, that was largely because mainstream medicine showed so little interest in it. In its annual report for 1945, BELRA berated the medical profession for its neglect of leprosy, which had acquired the nickname, 'the "Cinderella" of tropical diseases'. Leprosy formed no part of the average medical student's curriculum, and most doctors, instead of rising to the challenge of a recalcitrant disease, were discouraged by the 'comparatively low response to treatment and the nature of the work'.[53] And if this was true in 1945, *after* the discovery of a far more effective treatment than chaulmoogra, how much truer had it been in 1925, not to mention 1885? In the post-war era, the World Health Organization would further the work of secularisation and take the lead in the international campaign to eliminate leprosy, but BELRA deserves credit as one of the pioneering bodies (the Leonard Wood Memorial Foundation was another) dedicated to both these ends.

Of the founders of BELRA, the Rev. Frank Oldrieve, who had settled in what was then Southern Rhodesia, rejoined the Mission to Lepers after the Second World War as Secretary for South Africa and Rhodesia. In a radio broadcast made in Johannesburg on 27 February 1948, he welcomed the new era of sulphone drugs, saying how the cry used to be 'Get rid of the leper' but was now, 'Get rid of the disease'.[54] A month later he was dead. He was visiting a leprosy settlement in Swaziland when he was taken ill, and died the next day in hospital.[55] Leonard Rogers also welcomed the new era, advocating the combined use of sulphones and chaulmoogra in a paper he wrote for the *Lancet* of 3 April 1948; he outlived Oldrieve by many years, retiring to Falmouth in Cornwall and writing the story of his fifty-five years of 'happy toil' in the field of tropical medicine. His philosophy of life, he wrote, was very simple: 'Do your best and don't worry.'[56] It was clearly a recipe for longevity, since he survived well into his nineties, dying in 1962.

A year later the organisation he had founded and cherished decided 'that the abbreviated designation of the Association – BELRA – was unsuitable for publicity purposes' and hit upon the less anachronistic LEPRA as an alternative.[57] Perhaps it was as well that such a stalwart of empire as Rogers did not live to witness the change. Just as with chaulmoogra oil he had taken an old native remedy and westernised it, so his idea of the best way to manage imperial possessions was to westernise their inhabitants. Hence his determination to build a School of Tropical Medicine, not thousands of miles away in London or Liverpool, but in what was still the very heart of the British empire in the first decades of the twentieth century, Calcutta. He may have outlived his era, but greeting him on his ninety-second birthday in 1960, the Carville patients hailed him as 'a trail blazer and a man apparently years ahead of his time'.[58]

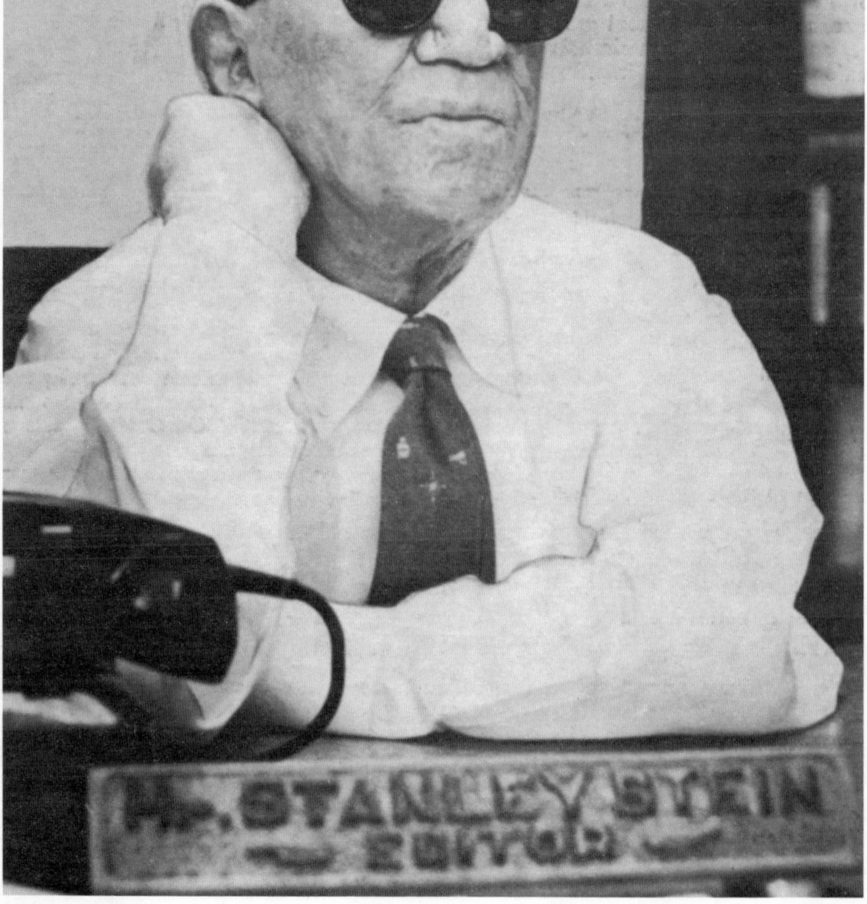

(The Star)

The 'Carville Crusader', Stanley Stein

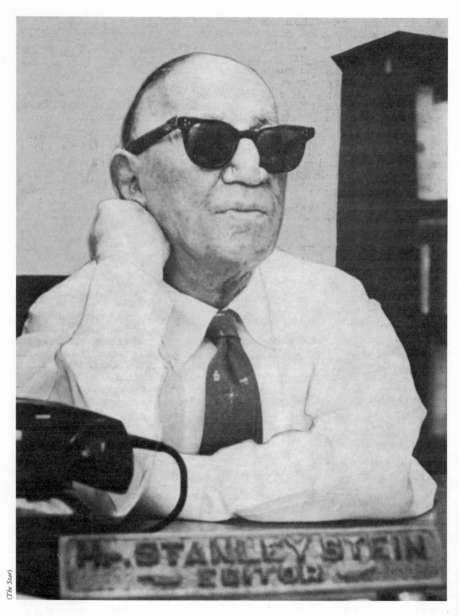

Chapter 10

STANLEY STEIN AND THE MIRACLE AT CARVILLE

At ten o'clock on the morning of Sunday 1 March 1931 a dapper little man in a natty brown suit, camel-hair topcoat and spats arrived from New York at US Marine Hospital No. 66, Carville, Louisiana, clutching copies of the *New Yorker* and *Theatre Arts*. The ambulance ride out of New Orleans along rough roads through desolate countryside was depressing, but the sight of a colonnaded ante-bellum Southern mansion flying the American flag cheered the new arrival – until the ambulance driver told him this was not the hospital but the administration building and he noticed the uniformed guards at the gate and the high metal cyclone fence with three strands of barbed wire running along the top of it. Though he didn't yet fully grasp what it meant, he was about to become an exile in his own country.[1]

Despite his appearance, Sidney Maurice Levyson was not the New York millionaire his fellow-patients initially mistook him for but a Jewish pharmacist from Texas with a passion for amateur dramatics. There was nothing remarkable about his early life except for the fact that ten years before, when he was twenty-one, he had been diagnosed as having leprosy. Unsightly patches on his wrist and leg and trouble with his eyes had alerted a dermatologist in San Antonio to his predicament, and tests established the fact.

> Leprosy! The word was not a diagnosis, it was a pronouncement of doom. My hopes and ambitions were collapsing about me. My future was in ruins . . . What had I done to bring down the wrath of God upon my head? My panicky mind tried to review my life of depravity. It was disappointingly meager. I was not much of a rake, I'm afraid.[2]

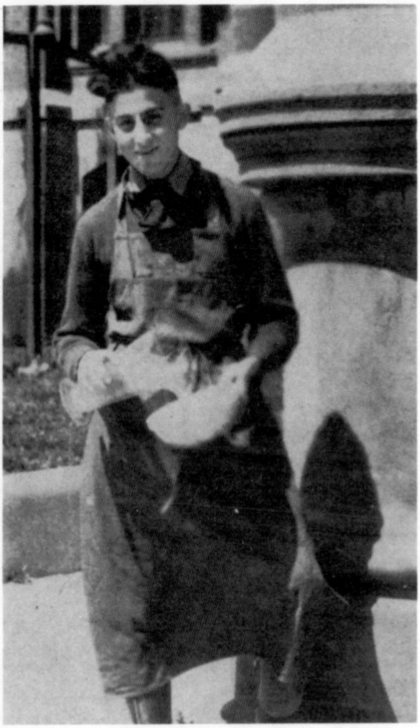

(The Star)

Sidney Levyson as a pharmacy student in Texas in 1918

The San Antonio dermatologist was an enlightened man. He said that leprosy was far less sinister than cancer or tuberculosis, people rarely died of it; and since it was nowhere near as contagious as measles or whooping cough, Sidney was to continue living and working as though nothing were wrong. He, Dr McGlasson, would treat him on a regular basis. For the next decade Sidney did his best to forget the bacteria and get on with his life, but eventually the marks on his face could no longer be ignored and he fled to New York. The dermatologist he had been recommended to see there was a very different type from Dr McGlasson (who had died in the interim) and insisted that Sidney go to Carville, threatening to report him to the health authorities if he didn't.

Among the many surprises that awaited Sidney at the only institution in the continental United States devoted exclusively to the treatment of leprosy was the ubiquitous presence of nuns; he had not expected to find Sisters of Charity in a government hospital. But he was even more surprised when one of them, Sister Laura Stricker, who took down his details on his arrival, asked him, 'Have you decided on your new name, young man?' It was bad enough being reduced to a cipher, Case No. 746, sinking into the 'quagmire of anonymity which society reserves for the victims of leprosy, mental illness, or crime'; to lose one's very name was almost unimaginable: 'Did I have to hide under an alias like a hunted criminal? Could I keep nothing of my old life to clothe my naked ego?'[3]

It took him a while to grasp that he was not just a sick man entering a hospital, but 'a lost soul consigned to limbo, an outcast' and that he must assume a new name to spare his family from any share in his disgrace. Sister Laura patiently explained, 'Perfectly healthy children have been denied the right to attend school because some member of their family was at Carville. Some patients have preferred that their friends believe them to be dead to save their families from abuse and ostracism.' She suggested he choose a name he would one day be proud of.[4]

Sidney Levyson pondered for a time, then (perhaps unconsciously echoing the famous opening sentence of *Moby Dick*) said, 'Call me Stanley Stein' – Stein because it was his mother's maiden name, and Stanley because it retained something of Sidney in the initial 'S' and the final 'ey'.[5] Stanley Stein became the *nom de guerre* under which Sidney Levyson, like French knights of old, rode out to challenge the forces of darkness – in his case, the obscurantist authorities whose attitude to persons affected by leprosy was basically to lock them up and throw away the key. No reverses or adversity, neither sickness nor blindness, could stop his campaign to improve the lot of the people whom fate had cast him among, and when he finally died, in 1967, it was as the celebrated Stanley Stein, not the unknown Sidney Levyson, that he was mourned not just in Carville but throughout the leprosy world.

It did not happen all at once, of course. It took time for Stein to discover his vocation and the means to accomplish it. At first, he was too caught up in his own predicament and the foulness of the only treatment on offer, the chaulmoogra oil that he had first encountered as a child in his father's pharmacy, when he'd helped prepare prescriptions and discovered that this evil-smelling substance was intended for a mysterious veiled woman dressed in black who was rumoured to have been a famous beauty once. This figure had haunted his childhood 'like a recurring nightmare', and it came as a shock when his father's drug clerk had casually told him, 'She's got leprosy.'

> 'She's got what?'
>
> 'She's a leper,' Willie said.
>
> I stared at him, open-mouthed. Leprosy was something out of the Bible, or, at best, the Middle Ages. But leprosy today in Boerne, Texas – unthinkable![6]

Evidence of the ravages of leprosy was ubiquitous at Carville and Stein himself manifested some of them: he had nodules on his face and had already lost the sight in his left eye. But even more debilitating than the physical aspects of the disease was the moral climate he detected at the

National Leprosarium, the hopeless apathy he saw all around him. He detected in his fellow-patients a 'curious combination of rebel and submissive dependent'. The majority of them 'resented being shut away against their will, yet they were complacent about being wards of the Government'. The place might be beautiful – 'if you closed your eyes to the swampy patches':

> The centenarian live oaks, 'bearded with moss like the druids of eld,' the great pecan trees, the yellow-pink brilliance of the rain trees in spring, the colorful profusion of the song birds – no doubt about it, it should have been a tonic to the soul. Except that we were fenced in.[7]

Had Carville been a real prison camp, of course, the observation tower just inside the perimeter fence would have housed armed guards looking inwards, whereas its actual purpose was to allow the more able-bodied inmates to climb up and look out over the fence and the levee and catch a glimpse of the ships going up and down the Mississippi. It was an ideal spot for a lovers' tryst, a place to meet and exchange confidences and dream of a future in the big, wide world beyond the barbed wire, where

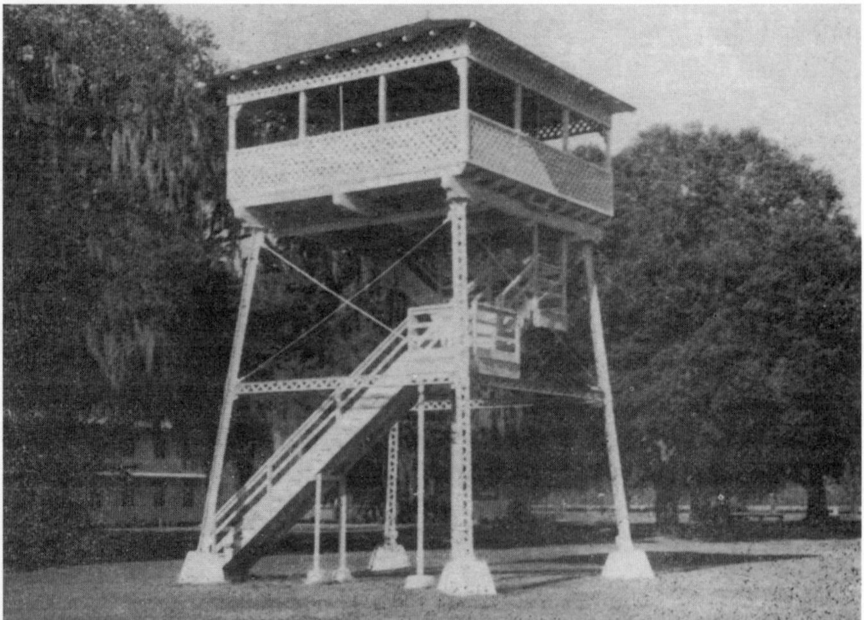

(*The Star*)

The observation tower at Carville

people were as free to come and go as ships along the river. But though its erection was a well-meant gesture, it also served to emphasise the isolation in which the patients were held.

Initially, Stein sought to raise his own and other people's spirits through his favourite pastime of amateur theatricals, to which end he put on a show that made him a known and popular figure in the community. From there he went on to start a newspaper, entitled *The Sixty-six Star* after the number of this particular marine hospital. The first issue was dated 16 May 1931, just two-and-a-half months after the rebirth of Sidney Levyson as Stanley Stein. Though he was unaware of it at the time, Stein had discovered his life's work.

In 1931 and for many years afterwards, there was no post office at the National Leprosarium and all outgoing 'colony' mail had to be sterilised before it left the hospital. There was no telephone until 1936, and even when they acquired one the 300 or so patients had to share a single party line for twelve more years. Marriage between patients was prohibited in either of the two chapels in the grounds of the hospital (until 1952), and patients who were already married were not permitted to live with their non-patient spouses. And just to rub in their non-person, 'living dead' status, Carville patients – 'like convicted felons or Indians living on a reservation' – were denied the vote in either state or national elections.[8]

The first incarnation of the *Star* set about changing all that. The editorial in the anniversary issue of 28 May 1932 pointed to the difficulty of building up a community spirit, an *esprit de corps*, when members of the community were there against their will. But the 'main objective' of the *Star* was to provide a 'single rallying point for all factions and cliques'.[9] In fact it soon went on to the attack and an early article, by Stein's closest collaborator, a patient who had taken the name of David Palmer, angrily challenged the rosy view of Carville as a kind of paradise to which patients were only too happy to return provided by a journalist in a New Orleans newspaper:

> Does society realize why [some] patients ask for re-admission? We'll tell it why! For the same reason that a bird grown old and feeble in the confining captivity of a cage; one whose wings and muscles have become atrophied from prolonged disuse and therefore is no longer able to fly; whose life will – upon release from its cage – be immediately endangered by fellow species-members who hate it by reason of its one-time captivity . . . craves

> only the chance to return to its cage – there to spend its remaining days. Paradise? Yes! Paradise, indeed! But only because of the attitude of those who made competition with them impossible by reason of the manner of life they have forced upon us.[10]

Palmer promised a whole series of articles examining the *status quo*, but they never materialised. According to Stein, the administration bought him off by offering him a paid job, which ceased the day he left Carville.[11] Stein himself was made of sterner stuff; he kept up the fight, exposing the absurdity of the policy of segregation in the following syllogism: 'Isolation is the only method whereby leprosy can be controlled and eradicated. Leprosy is now being isolated. Therefore leprosy is now being controlled and eradicated.'[12] His wit could quickly turn to anger, however, as when he considered the human effect of such a policy: 'the mental – psychic – transformation from a self-respecting citizen to an object set apart from society – leaving friends without warning – without an explanation . . . not even our best friends must know where we are.' And all on account of a word – the word 'leper' that, above all, was responsible for 'the unreasonable dread which in this century of progress still clings to the disease'. Spell it backwards and what did you get? R-e-p-e-l.[13]

But the *Sixty-six Star* overreached itself when it published an editorial attacking the Church for doing 'more to keep the stigma of leprosy alive in the public mind than any other force'.[14] Staff and readers alike melted away. The paper died. Stein, who had been amazed to discover the power of the press – even if the press in this case was 'a barely legible mimeographed sheet published by pariahs'[15] – now had to learn the lesson every crusading editor must learn, that nothing can be

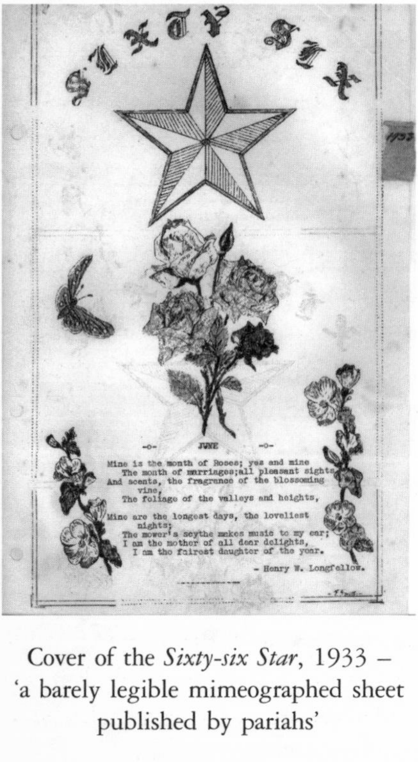
Sixty Six
-o- JUNE -o-
Mine is the month of Roses; yes and mine
The month of marriages; all pleasant sights
And scents, the fragrance of the blossoming vine,
The foliage of the valleys and heights,
Mine are the longest days, the loveliest nights;
The mower's scythe makes music to my ear;
I am the mother of all dear delights,
I am the fairest daughter of the year.
- Henry W. Longfellow.

(*The Star*/National Hansen's Disease Museum)

Cover of the *Sixty-six Star*, 1933 – 'a barely legible mimeographed sheet published by pariahs'

achieved unless you carry your readership with you. It was a lesson he never forgot.

Though Stein was the last person to minimise his own achievements, he recognised that the most significant event at Carville in 1931 was neither the drama productions of his Little Theater nor the foundation of the *Sixty-six Star*, but the formation of an American Legion post there. This came about as a result of the efforts of twenty-odd veterans of foreign wars, the group of patients that included John Early and was regarded by the hospital authorities as troublesome. The backing of such a huge and powerful organisation as the Legion in matters large and small would be critical over the coming decades and in retrospect Stein called the day in June when Sam Jones, the State Commander of the American Legion and future Governor of Louisiana, addressed the little group and advised them to organise a post – 'In union there is strength. You poor bastards here, twenty-three of you, are helpless. But with a million Legionnaires behind you . . .' – a breakthrough. He wrote: 'I hesitate to think what the hospital would be like today if veterans had not been committed here, for it was through the veterans that the national organizations became interested in Carville as a whole.'[16]

Male patients at Carville outnumbered females by two to one, so women, especially young women, were at a premium and they didn't come any prettier than Betty Parker, who later went through the 'hole in the fence' with another patient, Harry Martin (both names aliases), so that they could try and make a life for themselves outside. As Betty Martin, she would become known to thousands of readers as the author of *Miracle at Carville* (1950), the first autobiography to be written by a leprosy patient there, but when Stein first met her she was working as a laboratory technician in the hospital and was described to him by his housemates as 'very French looking, very charming, and very snooty'. On closer acquaintance, Stanley attributed her 'so-called snootiness' to 'partly timidity, partly shock – she came from an old aristocratic Louisiana family – at the tragic separation from her normal milieu, and partly innate fastidiousness'.[17] That tragic separation included a broken engagement with a young doctor boyfriend who went on to become eminent in his field.

As Betty recalled, 'Nothing like Stanley had ever appeared in Carville'. He had presence. 'Sometimes I think none of us knew what vitality could mean till he came.' She writes of his 'low-pitched and memorable voice', his 'fine and beautiful mind, and manner of respectful waiting, as if with the most intense interest, to [hear] whatever you have to say'. Despite the ravages of the disease and its rapid advance in his case, 'Stanley turned Carville inside out and made it shine with possibilities, bringing out the best in all of us'.[18] They became close friends, but no more than that. Betty had Harry and as for Stanley, he told himself that he would never 'become enmeshed in one of these Carville romances'.[19]

But he did, of course. When the comely Texan blonde, Lorene, whom he'd regarded as out of his league, too beautiful for him, made it clear that she reciprocated his bashful interest in her, how could he resist? He knew they were ill-matched; she did not share his intellectual interests and resented the time he spent on the *Sixty-six Star*. But they were both Texans and had plenty of fun together – especially after her hated rival, 'that old paper' as she called it,[20] died and Stanley moved into 'Cottage Grove', the highly desirable collection of self-built but officially sanctioned homes in which the luckier, mainly married, patients lived with a measure of privacy, free from some of the more galling aspects of institutional life.

The romance did not last. Lorene, whose health improved so much that she was discharged from Carville, wanted Stanley to go out with her – in his case, it would've meant going through the 'hole in the fence' – so that they might get married. But Stanley wasn't prepared for that; he knew they were fundamentally unsuited to one another – 'I could not see myself married to a woman, even a beautiful blue-eyed blonde, who went into tantrums every time I opened a book' – and his own health was deteriorating. They wrote one another letters, but by the time Lorene found her way back to Carville, life outside proving tougher than perhaps she'd anticipated, the vital spark was missing. As Stanley slowly and painfully lost the sight in his remaining eye and descended into total darkness, Lorene did her best to be supportive. But she had transferred her affections elsewhere – to one of Stanley's acolytes, a fellow patient to whom she had previously manifested a marked aversion. After testing negative for twelve months, they were both discharged at the same time, got married and had a baby boy.[21]

During this period, the second half of the 1930s, Dr Denney's successor as Medical Officer in Charge, Dr Herman E. Hasseltine – 'a dour Vermonter who carried his rock-ribbed New England Puritanism with him into the steaming Mississippi delta' – made an effort to reintroduce sexual segregation at Carville. He regarded marriage between patients as 'fraught with difficulties', as he wrote to the Surgeon General in September 1939, adding that sterilisation should be a precondition except where the woman partner was post-menopausal.[22] Yet as Stein gleefully recorded, there were probably more children born during his regime than at any other period in the history of Carville: 'Before his five-year term was up, the patients were calling him "Grandpappy".'[23]

Hasseltine made himself equally unpopular with the patients by forbidding the sale of beer in the patients' canteen (spirits were never allowed). He told the Surgeon General that he was convinced that alcohol and leprosy were not 'compatible' and that the patients were much better off without it. He supported his case with figures showing a reduction in drunk and disorderly behaviour among the patients once beer had ceased to be available.[24] But in not seeking the Surgeon General's consent, Hasseltine had exceeded his authority and the sale of beer was resumed.

On another issue, however, Hasseltine and the patients – or at least the Patients' Federation, a kind of trade union or pressure group – were in agreement. An epidemic of malaria at Carville in 1935–6 took a severe toll among the patients; nearly half of them suffered attacks, including Stanley Stein, and forty-two of those were dead within three years. Stein attributed his own clinical regression at this time to the debility caused by malaria.[25] The Patients' Federation agitated for a move to a location with a healthier climate, and Hasseltine approved. 'Here we are situated in the midst of a malaria belt and at a level that is more or less menaced by floods', he wrote. 'Humidity is such that it emphasizes the disagreeable aspects of both hot and cold temperatures.' He did not go so far as Dr G.W. McCoy, who suggested that 'the securing of a better location than is to be found at Carville is but one of the important changes that should be made' and recommended 'important modifications in the policies of health officers, state, local and federal, in relation to the attempts to control leprosy'. Indeed, Hasseltine was so appalled by the latter's idea of 'dealing with every case individually on its own merits' that he threatened to resign – along with 'I'm sure the rest of the Staff' – if such an anarchic and disruptive policy were introduced. Nor was he prepared to fight for a better location once he'd been informed that the prospects of moving were 'nil'.[26]

Since the germs causing leprosy and tuberculosis were so closely related, and TB sanatoria (in pre-antibiotic days) were generally to be found in high and dry situations, there was a strong argument for siting the national leprosarium in a similar location. In 1935, the Leonard Wood Memorial Foundation sent the professor of experimental medicine at the University of Cincinnati, Dr Clarence A. Mills, who had a special interest in the interrelationship of climate and disease, to study leprosy in the Philippines. After this trip and further studies Mills recommended 'that colonies for the segregation of leprosy patients be established in the most stimulating climates available rather than in the regions where the disease spreads most rapidly'. About Carville he would write that 'the long summers of debilitating Louisiana heat reduce disease-resisting vitality' and, therefore, 'it should be moved to the Dakotas where climatic stimulation is high and physical vigor at its peak'.[27]

This unexceptionable argument ignored two practical considerations: the reluctance of many patients who had not severed relations with their families to be moved away from them; and the implacable resistance of local communities in likely sites to having a leprosarium in their midst. A third and decisive factor was that Congress, in response to a campaign by the American Legion, had appropriated five million dollars to rebuild Carville on a grand scale. The Assistant Surgeon General in charge of the Hospital Division, Dr S.L. Christian, who professed scepticism over 'the matter of the alleged disagreeable climate of Carville', told the protesting patients that the plans for Carville were already 'far advanced' and work would begin very shortly; therefore he urged them, in so many words, to quit moaning and 'support the Government in its effort to build a model institution'.[28]

So the campaign for a move eventually fizzled out, but not before a revitalised Stanley Stein, who regretted not having the *Sixty-six Star* 'to carry on a crusade' during this time of upheaval, had given it one last shot. Soon after the revival of the *Star* at the beginning of the 1940s, he latched on to the publication of Dr Mills's book to press for an experimental transfer of a group of Carville patients to the TB sanatorium at Fort Stanton, New Mexico, that was being considered by the Public Health Service. But ingrained leprophobia in New Mexico put paid to that idea.[29]

Ironically, though the Patients' Federation had opposed the grandiose rebuilding plans for Carville, preferring the idea of a move to another site, the 'impressive structures of concrete and stucco' that replaced the old wooden buildings and boardwalks, particularly the superb Recreation Center that was modelled on the ante-bellum architectural style of the original Indian Camp plantation house, inspired the patients. A month after the formal opening of the Recreation Center in August 1941, in Stanley Stein's words, 'the *Star* was reborn'.[30]

In fact, it had been gestating for at least a year and a half before that. In February 1940 Dr Hasseltine forwarded an 'official letter' from Stein to the Assistant Surgeon General seeking permission to publish a paper 'without any censorship'. Hasseltine made his own views plain: Stein wanted the paper

> as a means to propagate his views on abolishing the use of the word 'leper', which is an obsession in his case and I am wondering if he is developing a paranoid trend along that line . . .

As if that weren't bad enough, he was 'also "agitating" in the colony with the aggressiveness characteristic of his race' (by which presumably he didn't mean Texans). Hasseltine opposed any lifting of censorship – not least on account of the fact that patients 'can use their affliction as a means of escaping legal action because most courts will not allow leprous

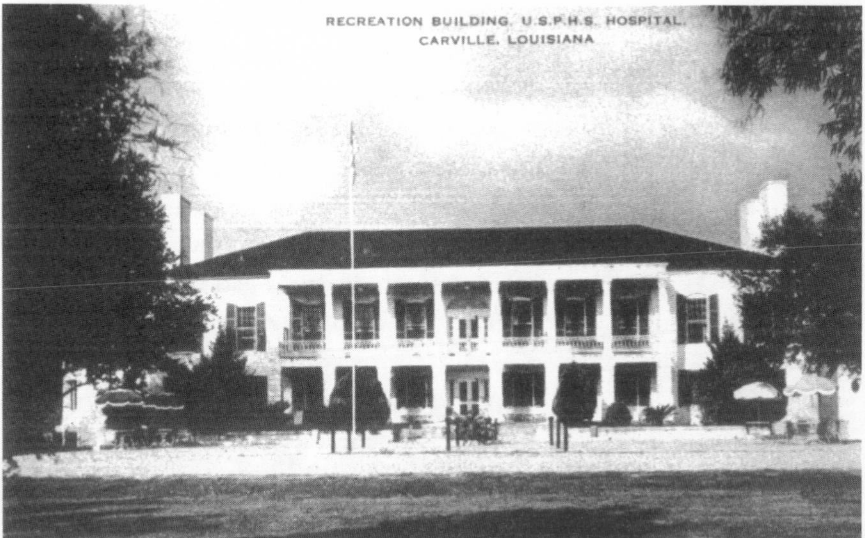

(historical postcard)

Carville's new Recreation Building

individuals to come into their court'.[31] But this was almost his last intervention before he left Carville, to be succeeded as MOC in July that year by Dr Guy H. Faget, whose name is forever associated with that 'miracle at Carville' that transformed the lives of Betty and Harry Martin and countless other patients.

Dr Faget was physically unprepossessing – a little man with glasses and a toothbrush moustache – and his use of such bureaucratic terms as 'paroled' and 'absconded' in official reports did not endear him to patients hypersensitive to demeaning language. In comparison with his two predecessors he had little experience of leprosy; his speciality was tuberculosis. But this turned out to be an advantage when he learned of a drug being used experimentally in the treatment of tuberculosis and wondered if it might not be applied to leprosy. The drug, marketed by the Detroit pharmaceutical firm, Parke-Davis, under the trade name Promin, consisted of glucose sulphone sodium. Sulphone drugs were not new; the compound known as DDS – or diamino diphenyl sulphone, to give it its full title – had been synthesised by German chemists as early as 1908, but its bactericidal possibilities had not been considered until the late 1930s. Parke-Davis were happy to provide the drug for free if Dr Faget wanted to experiment with it at Carville.[32]

Carville patients were used to being guinea pigs. They were so desperate they would volunteer to undergo the most horrendous treatments. Among the worst was 'fever therapy'. This involved a series of five-hour sessions encased up to the neck in a cylindrical cabinet resembling an iron lung, during which the body was subjected to fever-inducing temperatures of 140–55 degrees. The idea was that the fever would succeed where drugs had failed in penetrating the wax-like casings of the leprosy bacilli and destroying them. All very well in theory, but in practice patients suffered all kinds of side effects from delirium and vomiting to 'debility, cramps, loss of weight, and fever blisters'.[33] One volunteer, Johnny Harmon, underwent the first three treatments without any adverse effects, but

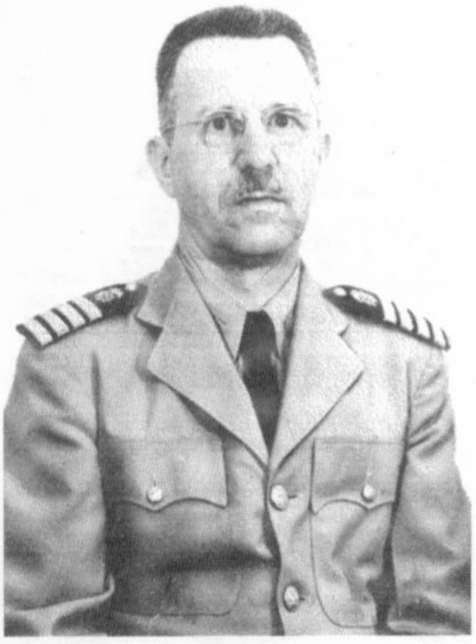
(The Star)

Dr Guy H. Faget

the fourth time, when the attendants may have raised the temperature in the cabinet too high, he 'went hog-crazy and demanded that they let me out of the infernal machine promptly'. He continued to be delirious and then passed out. For the next twenty-four hours, his stomach was so upset he could take nothing but tomato juice. He recovered and, though he did not resume the treatment, not long afterwards he tested negative for the first time and was eventually discharged. In his old age he reckoned that he was the only survivor among those who had participated in the 'fever machine experiment'.[34]

So there was no difficulty in finding volunteers at Carville for the Promin treatment. Harry and Betty Martin, though, were not among the first – in Harry's case it was very much a last resort and in the beginning neither the couple nor the doctors dared hope it would work; there had been so many failed miracles along the lines of fever therapy, and in the autumn of 1941 there was no reason to imagine this would not be yet another. Betty might have survived without it, but for Harry there was, quite literally, no alternative; if Promin had failed he would've died.

Theirs was a touching story – beautiful Betty and handsome Harry, thrown together by Hansen's disease. Their first meeting could hardly have been less auspicious. A malicious typewritten note purporting to be the record of a conversation between the then famous radio duo of Amos and Andy about 'the uncalled-for snobbishness of one Miss Betty Parker, who was no better than anyone else at Carville' had been pinned up on the cafeteria wall. No one had admitted responsibility, but when the typing was checked it was found to match the typewriter owned by Harry Martin, a recent arrival. Harry himself was not under suspicion; someone had borrowed his machine but he was not prepared to say who, even when confronted by an irate Betty. 'If he isn't man enough to own up', he'd drawled, 'I'm not going to tell on him.'[35]

Betty had registered that this twenty-year-old was tall, 'of athletic build, and with a military air', and that under other circumstances she might have liked him, but she was a teacher's pet, the darling of the doctors and sisters, and was unaccustomed to being thwarted. So she stuck her nose in the air and 'chose to ignore Mr Harry Martin'. Gradually, however, she came to admire the 'strong and silent' young man, whom everyone but her seemed to love. Her work in the laboratory brought her closer to her fellow patients and made her less of an 'uppity miss' from New Orleans. But she and Harry were both too proud to make the first gesture and the matchmaking efforts of a third party badly misfired. Eventually, at a Halloween party, the ice was broken and they became friends. There was still a long way to go, however; they were both severely bruised by the failure of their first loves to survive their removal to Carville, and though they confided in one another in the intimacy of the observation tower that deepest of secrets, their real names, and were aware of their growing mutual attraction, they could not contemplate marriage. Marriage meant children, especially to Betty, who as a practising Catholic was not prepared to consider using contraceptives, and to risk having children who might develop leprosy was out of the question. Though Harry was not a Catholic, he professed to feel the same way 'about bringing children into the world'. So they settled for being friends.[36]

This was easier said than done. They were young; they were in love; and though they had leprosy, both had been testing negative for some months and with any luck would shortly be discharged. Then, with freedom almost within their grasp, Harry tested positive and the whole year-long process had to begin all over again. He couldn't face that. So he decided to go through the 'hole in the fence' and begged Betty to come with him. She hesitated, but in the end agreed. If they had to return to Carville, they would be punished, but since they were using false names they could not easily be traced. Their families were supportive and they went to New Orleans where despite the depression – this was 1933 – both succeeded in finding work. The worst part of it was the necessary duplicity; honest as they were, they found deception difficult and lived in dread of being discovered. As Betty wrote, 'There can be no happiness without truth . . . The fear of stigma kept us in a prison.'[37]

More damaging even than fear of exposure was the internalisation of the stigma, which was undermining their personal lives. Harry revolted against their self-imposed limitations and began to put pressure on Betty to marry him, but her anxiety over having children made her resist – tearfully – even though she could see no future without him. It was the same for him: though he threatened to end the relationship, he could not bear the thought of separation. So they struggled on for a few months, together but apart, until fate intervened. Harry's health declined; the disease was tightening its grip and, after a year out of Carville, he started having trouble with his eyes. Betty knew only too well what that meant; she had seen how helpless people became when they lost their sight; and for leprosy sufferers there wasn't even the consolation of Braille because their anaesthesia meant that their sense of touch had gone too (as happened with Stanley Stein, who wrote, 'talking books for the blind probably saved my sanity'[38]). Harry was going to need all the help he could get. He was going to need 'someone who could be close to him – closer than ever before . . . Still, I was just as surprised as Harry when I found myself telling him in a perfectly ordinary tone of voice that we were going to be married.'[39]

Now it was Harry's turn to protest. He told her it wouldn't be fair on her, since she was getting better while he was getting worse, and used all the arguments she had raised against her. She brushed these aside and *insisted* that he marry her, 'thereby placing my gallant Harry in a position where he could no longer refuse'. She had always dreamed of a 'big and beautiful church wedding' but knew this was now impossible; it would be a quiet family affair in the office of the parish priest. On one thing her mother reassured her: she had talked it over with her father and should Betty and Harry have a child, they would look after it.[40]

Happy as any other newly-wed couple, Betty and Harry moved into a small apartment, almost entirely furnished with wedding presents. But how long would they be able to stay there? The shadow of what Carville patients could never bring themselves to name but called 'the disease', 'this package', or 'the gazeek' hung over them, turning the most innocent outing into a nightmare, as when Betty and Harry took a rare holiday trip to Florida and went out in a glass-bottomed boat to look at the fish in the clear waters. Suddenly another passenger pointed to an ugly catfish and remarked, 'That fish looks as if it has leprosy,' and getting no response, kept on, 'What's the matter with that fish? Does it have leprosy?'[41]

What finally drove them back to Carville were the marks on Harry's face, which were beginning to attract comments from strangers. They spent their first wedding anniversary packing up their belongings and tried to get used to the fact that they must also stow away their real names, which they had been using since they left Carville, and get used to calling each other Harry and Betty once again. But paradoxically the loss of liberty and identity they would experience on their return would be counterbalanced by the sheer relief – and freedom – of being able to be themselves: 'Only there, among our own, could we let down our barriers.'[42] In Harry's reduced state, Carville was not so much a prison as a sanctuary.

Nevertheless they had to go through a thirty-day period of detention, Harry in the Carville jail and Betty in the cottage with barred windows set aside for mentally-disturbed patients. Nobody on the staff, least of all the long-serving Dr F.A. Johansen, the patients' beloved 'Dr Jo', wanted to punish them for taking French leave, but rules were rules and they had broken them. To make their separation lighter, it was found necessary for both of them to have hydrotherapy at the same time each day, though Betty seriously doubted the need for it in her case. That way they could also meet their old friends, who soon got to know when they would be in the infirmary and brought them up to date with the news and gossip, telling them who had arrived during their absence, who had succumbed to the malaria epidemic and what changes were afoot.[43]

During a freezing spell at the beginning of 1940, when everyone was getting colds and flu, Harry went down with pneumonia – a killer in those pre-antibiotic days, especially for someone suffering from Hansen's disease – and Dr Jo put him on the latest 'miracle drug', sulfapyridine. For a while it was touch-and-go, but eventually Harry pulled through, as did two other patients given the same drug. If it could cure HD patients of pneumonia, what might it not do against the 'ancient enemy' itself? The problem was its extreme toxicity, but Dr Jo told Betty that with careful monitoring he thought that could be managed. He was just waiting for the arrival of the new MOC (Dr Faget) before seeking permission to begin experimenting. According to Betty Martin, it was Dr Jo who brought the article about the use of Promin in experimental tuberculosis that led to the crucial breakthrough in the treatment of leprosy to Faget's attention in the first place.[44] As MOC, Faget had the ultimate responsibility, but both doctors were deeply committed to the experiment whose spectacular success wouldn't be immediately apparent.

Meanwhile Harry's condition continued to give cause for alarm. Pneumonia had taken its toll and he went from bad to worse; the ravages of the disease were all too apparent on his face and body; he lost his appetite and was sinking fast. Betty got official permission to take him to his aunt's place in Texas for two weeks as a kind of last vacation together (in fact they went to the Ozarks but could not tell anyone because in doing so they had broken the terms of their 'parole'). By the autumn of 1941, when Carville was agog over the opening of the new Recreation Center and the rebirth of the *Star*, Betty's anxiety about Harry

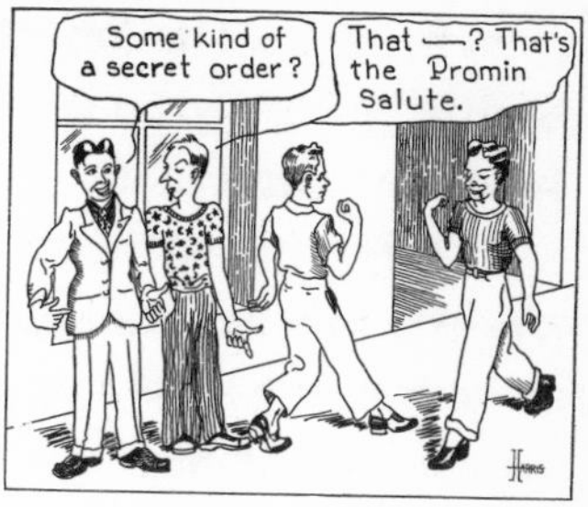
Some kind of a secret order?
That —? That's the Promin Salute.

(*The Star*)

The Star celebrates the Promin revolution in a cartoon by 'Harris', a.k.a. Johnny Harmon

was beginning to undermine her own health. Not for the first time, the sympathetic Dr Jo suggested, 'There's still Promin.'[45]

Betty's 'horror of anything injected into the vein' initially had made her resistant to the idea, but desperate situations required desperate remedies and she and Harry were now prepared to try anything. Soon they were both having daily intravenous injections and, despite setbacks and allergic reactions to Promin, after two or three months they – like most other patients undergoing the treatment – 'began to take a new lease of life'. This was their 'miracle': 'for the first time in all the years we had been sick we felt we were being cured.' When an old friend left Carville and they inherited his cottage, they were able to live together again and their spirits soared: 'On this little plot of land that was not ours, on the rim of a fenced-in reservation we could not leave without red-tape permission, Harry and I found a happiness neither had known before . . .'[46]

Despite the fact that, following the bombing of Pearl Harbor, the United States was now at war, this was a productive time at Carville. The patients supported the war effort by buying war bonds, and Stanley Stein began – or rather, resumed – his 'private war', as Betty Martin called it, on the home front, in the pages of the *Star*, by attacking obsolete rules and regulations in a series of articles entitled 'Carville's Bill of Wrongs'.[47] The new *Star*, he wrote:

> did not abandon its original purpose of being the town crier for our isolated community, but we did adopt as our long-range policy a definite three-pronged objective: 1. To promote an educated public opinion on Hansen's disease [HD, never *leprosy*, which was the other 'odious word']. 2. To furnish vocational training for interested patients. 3. To provide community service.

Of these three aims, the first – 'Radiating the Light of Truth on Hansen's Disease', the motto that was emblazoned across every issue of the paper – far outweighed the other two in the editor's view, if not that of the Public

Health Service. The American Legion provided a printing press and the first issue to be printed on it was published on Stein's forty-fourth birthday, 10 June 1944. He recalled, 'I could not have been given a finer birthday gift.'[48]

Harry and Betty Martin were part of the dedicated group that helped produce each issue of the *Star* and, while Betty regarded it as a 'privilege' to work with Stein because he simply fizzed with ideas, she was under no illusions about how demanding he could be. She took to calling him 'Simon Legree' because he was such a slave driver, thinking up 'more work in a day than any of us could accomplish in a week'.[49] But without his leadership, the social aspects of life at Carville would never have kept pace with the medical progress being made.

Conditions at Carville were certainly improving. For the first time in its history the majority of patients were getting better, and the new spirit of optimism was epitomised in one of the hit songs of 1945, 'Don't Fence Me In', which Carville patients adopted as a kind of theme tune. The down side was what happened to many of them when they did succeed in getting out of the place. As they eagerly anticipated their own release, Betty and Harry Martin were not unaware of the problems they would once again have to face:

> We heard patients returned, well and free, to their homes, to meet on every hand with the cruelty created by fear. Children of patients were asked to leave schools they had attended all their lives. A dischargee was shunned in his own neighbourhood. His barber would not shave him. His grocer asked him to take his trade elsewhere. He was not allowed to ride in the 'white' buses. The old cry of six thousand years, 'unclean,' was still alive.[50]

In the first article she ever wrote for the *Star*, Betty demanded to know, 'Why Am I Not Free?' She questioned society's right to treat HD sufferers in the way it did. To her amazement, her *cri de coeur* met with universal approval among patients notorious for their differences of opinion: 'It was as though I had put into words what was long in the minds and hearts of us all.'[51]

Stanley Stein, who recognised an opportunity when he saw one, seized the moment and 'invented a body to be called the United Patients' Committee for Social Improvement and Rehabilitation, including representatives from the Patients' Federation Assembly as well as the

American Legion post and the *Star* staff. The aim was to challenge the apparent indifference of the Public Health Service to the plight of the patients, and there was nothing like creating a committee to take on bureaucracy. The 1945 National Convention of the American Legion supported the Carville branch and recommended that the Surgeon General appoint a National Advisory Committee on Leprosy in the United States, and Stein drafted a series of proposals and recommendations, which boiled down to a fifteen-point programme. Top of the list of desirable changes was: 'Abolish compulsory segregation, in the light of modern scientific knowledge, and make institutionalisation voluntary.'[52]

The committee, which included a number of influential doctors, met twice during 1946; the first meeting was in May, and the second in December. In between, 'open warfare broke out between our United Patients Committee and the inhabitants of the neighboring villages of Carville, Gonzales, and St. Gabriel, where most of our non-medical employees lived'. The bone of contention was the so-called 'hazard duty pay', which was a salary bonus – of 25 per cent, or as much as 50 per cent in some cases – that Carville workers (like 'fliers, parachutists, demolitionists, and submarine personnel') got as a result of the danger to which they were supposedly exposed in serving in a leprosy hospital. Should compulsory segregation be abolished and the myth of the high risk of infection exploded, then the justification for danger money went too. Stein was at pains to point out that he had no objection to the hospital personnel getting extra money; but he did strongly object to the notion of 'hazard pay' because that kept alive 'all the alarmist, mistaken beliefs about the contagiousness of the disease'.

It was a bitter and dirty scrap, in which the hospital personnel – not one of whom had ever caught leprosy by working at Carville – stooped to scaremongering and outright opposition to patients getting the vote. And when the State of Louisiana voted overwhelmingly in favour of giving patients the ballot in November, the parish registrar got his own back by announcing that they would only be eligible to vote if they gave their actual names and previous place of residence, 'a great shock to those of us who had been hiding behind aliases to spare our families'. Consequently, the majority of patients chose not to register to vote despite the fact they were now free to do so.[53]

The Carville reformers were so taken up with their own situation that when the 'Hornbostel case' broke it took them by surprise. Banner headlines in the Hearst press's San Francisco *Call-Bulletin* proclaimed: 'SAN FRANCISCO WIFE LEPER: Army Mate Begs to Share Isolation for Life'. Gertrude Hornbostel, who had spent the war years in a Japanese concentration camp in the Philippines, had been diagnosed as having leprosy and her husband, Major Hans Hornbostel, a survivor of the Bataan Death March, was campaigning to be allowed to accompany her to Carville, though he himself was unaffected by the disease. What was unusual about their case was that, far from shunning publicity and taking refuge in anonymity – or pseudonymity – the Hornbostels talked openly about their situation and even called a press conference to elicit support for their stance.[54]

The press reacted predictably, spraying the word 'leper' around and playing up the horrors of leprosy in order to dramatise the sob story and give it the necessary *frisson*. For the Carville activists, this was both a disaster – in that this was the wrong sort of publicity, putting about precisely the kind of misinformation the *Star* was at pains to correct – and an opportunity: to enlist the now famous Hornbostels in their crusade to enlighten the public. But what were they like, this couple who had the temerity to break cover and shamelessly court publicity? Stein, the Martins and their friends awaited their arrival at Carville with some trepidation.

They need not have worried; despite their boldness in adversity, the Hornbostels were neither as arrogant nor as pushy as the publicity that had preceded them led the other patients to expect. They were honest, down-to-earth people, who were prepared to learn and keen to help. The tall and upright Major was refused permission to live in the hospital, but he acquired lodgings nearby. He came in every day at 7 a.m. sharp and left by the main gate in the late evening (often sneaking back through the 'hole in the fence' to spend the night with his wife).[55] The buxom, motherly Mrs Hornbostel joined the staff of the *Star* as proof-reader and became a valued correspondent, writing trenchant columns that Stein reckoned contributed as much as the sulphones to her early medical discharge.

> By far the greatest advantage derived from the Hornbostel case, however [he wrote], was indirect. Millions of Americans who had never heard of Carville suddenly learned that so-called leprosy was still a problem in their own country, not some remote Biblical reference or a scene from *Ben Hur*. So in

> the ensuing years, it became much easier to interest newspapers, magazines, and the radio networks in finding out the truth about Hansen's disease.[56]

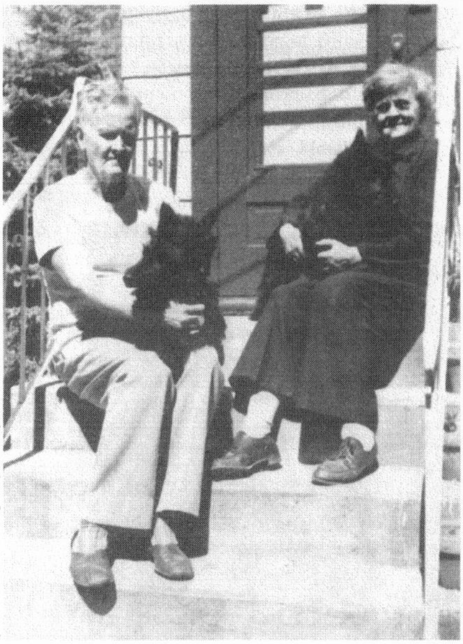
(from 'Alone No Longer' by Stanley Stein)

The redoubtable Gertrude Hornbostel and her husband, Major Hans, a survivor of the Bataan Death March

The liberalisation of the Carville regime was going at a heady pace, thanks to the National Advisory Committee, whose recommendation of a month's leave twice a year for patients brought the biggest cheer at the 1946 Christmas celebrations, and the medical breakthrough represented by the sulphone drugs. Sadly, Dr Faget was obliged by ill health to resign as MOC and died soon after in bizarre circumstances: on 17 July 1947 he was found dead below the open window of his office at the Marine Hospital in New Orleans, where he'd been posted from Carville to a less arduous job. He had been suffering from a heart condition and one possible explanation of his demise was that he had been struggling for breath and had thrown open the window in a desperate attempt to get some air and had either blacked out or lost his balance and fallen to his death. Dr Faget did not live long enough to see the sulphones replace chaulmoogra oil as the 'treatment of choice' at Carville – an event celebrated in the *Star* under the headline 'Goodbye abscesses! Goodbye nausea!' His successor as MOC at Carville, the ever-popular Dr Jo, was very much the patients' choice.[57]

When patients were discharged from Carville, they were handed a certificate – in local parlance, their 'diploma' – at the gate. On one historic occasion, a departing patient had deliberately torn his up in front of the gateman and the Sister who had come to see him off. She'd asked him why, and he'd said, 'Sister, I'm a sailor, and I want to go back to sea. If any shipmate ever found that thing on me, I'd be tossed overboard.' Under 'Class of beneficiary' was written 'PHS Leper'; and under 'Reason for discharge', 'No longer a menace to public health'. In the patients' view, the 'diploma' merely added insult to injury, and the *Star* campaigned successfully for a change. The odious word was excised and the new 'Reason for discharge' was simply, 'No further treatment necessary'.[58] Among the early beneficiaries of this enlightened policy change were Harry and Betty Martin who, for the first time, tested negative for twelve months in succession and were pronounced free of Hansen's bacilli. They departed in the spring of 1947, bursting with hope and plans for the future.

Things continued to improve at Carville. Stanley Stein characterised the year 1948 as 'a period of great social progress'. The hospital got its own post office at last, though the medically unnecessary sterilisation of mail continued for another decade because of the dispute over 'hazard duty pay'. An important symbolic change was the removal of the three strands of barbed wire from the top of the perimeter fence and a practical measure, completed the following year, was the surfacing of the last fifteen miles of road up to the hospital, which immediately reduced the feeling of isolation. But most important of all the reforms was the introduction of 'medical discharge', which allowed patients 'still in the

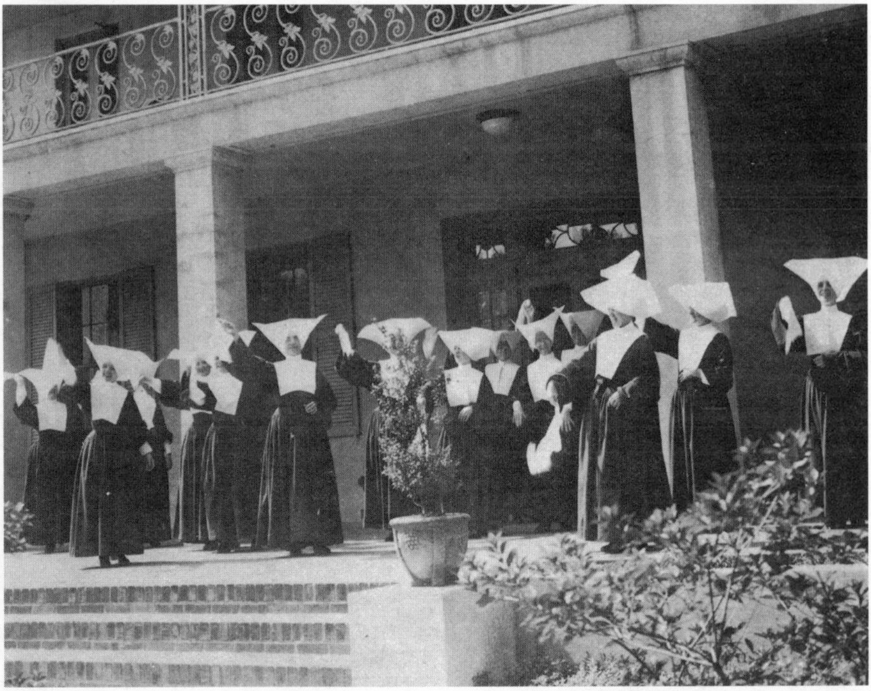

(*The Star*)

The Sisters gather to wave goodbye to a departing patient

so-called communicable stage of Hansen's disease' – i.e., without having to complete the obstacle course of twelve, monthly bacteria-free tests that Harry and Betty Martin had recently endured – to go home under certain, not too stringent, conditions. The *Star* called this 'a crack in the wall of tradition'.[59]

In April 1948 the Fifth International Congress of Leprology was held in Havana, bringing a stream of distinguished medical visitors to Carville en route to or from Cuba. The conference supported the Carville patients in their campaign to get rid of the odious word 'leper' (as did the *International Journal of Leprosy*, published by the Leonard Wood Memorial Foundation), and passed a resolution recommending that it be abandoned in favour of the term 'leprosy patient'. The conference also gave international endorsement to the sulphones as the 'treatment of choice' for leprosy. In May, a National Leprosy Act, sponsored by the American Federation of Physically Handicapped, was introduced in the US Congress. It was the handiwork of a retired army officer, Col G.H. Rarey, whose childhood recollections of leprosy in the Philippines and more recent contact with Carville made him determined to get 'a new deal for HD patients', but though the Act was reintroduced several times between 1948 and 1954 it never passed Congress. What it did, however, was help to keep public attention focused on Hansen's disease.[60]

Though Carville's own Sister Catherine Sullivan had endeared herself to the patients by always insisting that mercy was 'no substitute for justice', not all religious people, or groups, took such an enlightened view.[61] At a Senate subcommittee hearing in 1949, Dr Frank C. Coombes, professor of dermatology at New York University and faculty member of the National Bible Institute, remarked of the hundreds of missionaries he'd taught about leprosy:

> It is surprising how many think that one of their missions in life is to 'care for the lepers,' not in the sense that they would care for an individual with syphilis or tuberculosis. No – leprosy is a thing apart from a purely medical problem. The 'victim' is to be pitied and prayed for.[62]

This was the mentality that Stein and the staff of the *Star* felt they were up against. But though they had the support of outstanding doctors such as G.W. McCoy, some health authorities, including the generally sympathetic Assistant Surgeon General, Dr R.C. Williams, thought they were in danger of overreaching themselves by 'almost denying the fact that leprosy can be transmitted from one person to another'. The disease might not be highly communicable in the sense that smallpox, measles, and whooping cough were, but it was still communicable. Readers of the *Star* might be forgiven for thinking that:

> there are two kinds of leprosy – the leprosy that is communicated from one person to another and the leprosy that is not communicated from one person to another and that all the cases at Carville are in the latter group.

Williams wrote sternly to Stein that 'in your campaign you must confine yourself to scientific facts'.[63]

The more ambitious the aims of the *Star*, the keener the Public Health Service was to rein it in. Letters to Stein from the higher authorities in the PHS came via the MOC at Carville, and many of Stein's letters to influential outsiders were referred to the PHS – and the PHS often referred them back to Carville. For instance, a copy of Stein's letter to Theodore Hayes of the Federal Economic Security Commission elicited some irritated scribbling in the margin, probably from the MOC, Dr Jo himself. Where Stein waxed eloquent about the misery caused by the separation of families at Carville, the annotation reads: 'He should talk. He won't let his mother visit him, to say nothing of going to her.' Against his expressed desire to 'place THE STAR in the hands of every doctor in the United States and in all medical schools and medical libraries', the annotator grumbled, 'Is the *Star* to become the physicians' handbook on leprosy?' And when Stein suggested involving 'someone like [Walter] Winchell' in setting up an International Leprosy Foundation, along the lines of the Cancer Society or the National Foundation for Infantile Paralysis, the commentator snorted, 'He wanted Winchell throttled earlier this year.' (Winchell had angered Stein by using his weekly radio broadcast to publicise the attempt of a Florida 'state police dragnet' to catch an 'escaped leper', giving a detailed description of his clothes and appearance as though he were, in the words of Dr Eugene R. Kellersberger of the American Leprosy Missions, 'an escaped convict from Sing Sing prison'.[64]) But the strongest comment was reserved for Stein's complaint that USO Veterans Camp shows bypassed Carville, and it is the use of the first person here that suggests the writer was Dr Jo himself: 'I had an unofficial agreement for these shows to "come in once in a while". Stein wept to some Legion visitor. She asked for an official opinion and got it – refusal.'[65]

An unsigned and undated PHS report on the *Star* (on internal evidence it must have been compiled in 1948/9) started by complimenting the paper on the 'remarkable job' it was doing. There was no doubt as to who should take the credit: 'The STAR is Stanley Stein and Stanley Stein is the STAR.' But if Stein provided its 'editorial strength', he was also responsible for its 'administrative weakness'. He was an 'unforgettable' character, 'soft-spoken, wistful, sensitive', and seemed to enjoy playing the role of blind editor. He was very impressionable, 'easily influenced by the people he likes' and a sucker for any sort of professional or technical expertise. In 'trying to please everyone he likes and respects' he often found himself pulled in different directions. His sense of time was peculiar in that he would speak of something that had happened eighteen years ago as if it were yesterday, and his thinking had been shaped by how things were a decade earlier. He was also extremely volatile:

> At one moment he is meek dependent – groping for something to cling to. A minute later he snaps out 'big talk', pounds the desk and plunges way beyond his depth into responsibility he can't possibly shoulder, making commitments he can't honor.[66]

The writer of this report had spent 'several afternoons in Stein's office acting as his secretary', but he (the tone of the piece is unmistakably male) was clearly someone with authority since, when Stein said he wanted a full-time secretary, he told him in no uncertain terms that 'he must make do with what he has'. The informality, not to say anarchy, of the editorial office obviously offended the writer's sense of propriety; his sympathies were entirely with the hard-pressed deputy editor, Ann Page, whom he called the 'mainstay' of the magazine. She held things together – as far as possible, given Stein's constant demands on her and his propensity to put off making difficult decisions:

> Stein wants to print everything he has each month and he writes most of it himself. When there is an overage, Ann Page's column on local doings is scrapped. This has resulted in a feeling of inferiority on her part as to her writing ability. Reports have it that, at the last minute, the selective

> process is a mad scramble and that the person nearest Stein dictates what will ride. Since this person usually is Mrs Hornbostle [*sic*], there is a preponderance of her own compositions and of material about her.[67]

The report writer did not share the editor's high opinion of Mrs Hornbostel's talents and described how she ran the proof-reading 'with Prussian might'; her practice might be inconsistent, 'but woe betide the poor fellow brought up on Websters who would make a single change after the royal signature is affixed in witness that all is correct'.

What the writer principally objected to about the *Star* was that it was unrepresentative of Carville and the patient body as a whole. The report criticises Stein for trying to have it both ways, for wanting to educate 'professional people and the masses' on the one hand and claiming to be the voice of the patients on the other: 'In an attempt to blend the whole gamut of purposes, the STAR actually accomplishes none and this is probably the cause of its unevenness.' Easily said, but how might the *Star* be improved? 'This writer discussed the feasibility of thinking of the STAR in terms of a company organ.' That remark, and his enthusiastic endorsement of the admittedly admirable MOC, Dr Johansen – 'Even in the gripings at which [they] are expert, his patients recognize that the MOC has at heart their best interests' – indicate where the writer's sympathies lay.[68] A PHS man through and through, he mocked the nonconformist patients for their pretensions and condemned what a genuinely independent observer might have applauded: namely, the attempt of a small, possibly unrepresentative but dedicated group of activists to revolutionise social attitudes to leprosy in the same way as the sulphones had revolutionised the treatment of the disease.

Even the fact that Stein had been in the hospital for the best part of two decades was used against him. According to the report writer, he hadn't 'been outside in so long' that he didn't realise how much of his mail came from 'screwballs'.[69] But it wasn't a screwball who wrote in July 1949, 'Your journal goes on from strength to strength . . . I left my copy [of the current issue] with my doctor who enjoys reading them very much . . . We need you and your journal very badly. At last a leper speaks.'[70] It was an English ex-technical civil servant who had contracted leprosy in Malaya and was now living quietly in the countryside near Liverpool. Peter Hall had done time in the leprosarium at Sungei Buloh, outside Kuala Lumpur, so he knew from inside what motivated Stein and his band of Carville activists. He would have dismissed with contempt the notion that they should have been producing something as banal as a 'company organ'.

As a result of the public interest aroused by the Hornbostel case, a radio broadcast of the programme *We the People* in 1948 came from Carville and one listener was particularly struck by 'a character called Stanley Stein, blind editor of the hospital publication'. She thought he sounded remarkably like her long-lost cousin, Sidney Levyson. She thought she recognised his voice. In fact, she was so convinced it was he that she aired her suspicions at a family Thanksgiving dinner in Detroit, suggesting they write collectively to the editor of the *Star*. The letter began: 'Dear Mr Stein: We don't believe you are Stanley Stein at all; we think you are Sidney Levyson . . .' It went on to relay all the family news and gossip and to say how proud they all were of him – if indeed it was he. Stein was overwhelmed. In his reply he told them 'how pleased I was to find out, after years of believing that I was the skeleton in the family closet, that I was now considered a hero'.[71]

His pleasure at re-establishing contact with his favourite cousin Trudie was matched, if not eclipsed, by a long-distance phone call he received in 1950 from New York, which marked the beginning of one of 'the wackiest, dearest, and most exhilarating friendships of my life'. As a lifelong theatre groupie, he 'almost fainted' when he picked up the receiver and 'heard that vibrant, thrillingly husky voice saying, "It's Tallulah, darling."' Unable to use his eyes, he had long been in love with Tallulah Bankhead's voice and now, through the intercession of mutual friends, he could listen to it to his heart's content. Tallulah phoned him not once but several times and then, to his amazement, invited him to New York. Caught between his longing to meet his idol and his fear of venturing into the outside world after two decades of virtual imprisonment, Stein prevaricated. When he told her he needed someone to take care of him, she volunteered to fly down to collect him; but no, that was not what he'd meant: he needed someone to help dress him – to which the irrepressible Tallulah replied that she did, too. 'Bring anybody you want', she said. His health, like everyone else's, had improved with sulphone treatment (though in his case it had come too late; the damage already done was irreversible) and after several months of testing negative he took the plunge and went to New York, where he was fêted by all and sundry, not just the wonderful Tallulah. From there he flew (for the first time ever) to Chicago and back to New Orleans, arriving at Carville – in the words of an African-American employee there – 'journey proud' and ready for the critical twelfth consecutive skin test that, if negative, would release him from the hospital.[72]

It was negative. He drew up plans for the future of the *Star* following his departure, listened to offers from patients to buy his cottage, which he'd named Wits' End, and awaited his discharge papers. Three weeks after the test they still hadn't come through. Then he was summoned to see Dr Jo, who told him apologetically that the clinical director, Dr Rolla R. Wolcott, was insisting on a medical board examination in his case and was within his rights to do so. Wolcott was a dedicated doctor and a deeply religious man, whom Stein had really wanted to like, especially after Wolcott had come to his cottage to treat his beloved Boston terrier, Bing, for convulsions. But they were at odds personally and ideologically and their relationship was 'icy'. Wolcott himself conducted the examination and sat for two hours (twice as long as usual) peering into the microscope in search of bacilli. Though five of the six scrapings were found to be free of bacteria, the sixth showed 'a small number of *M.*

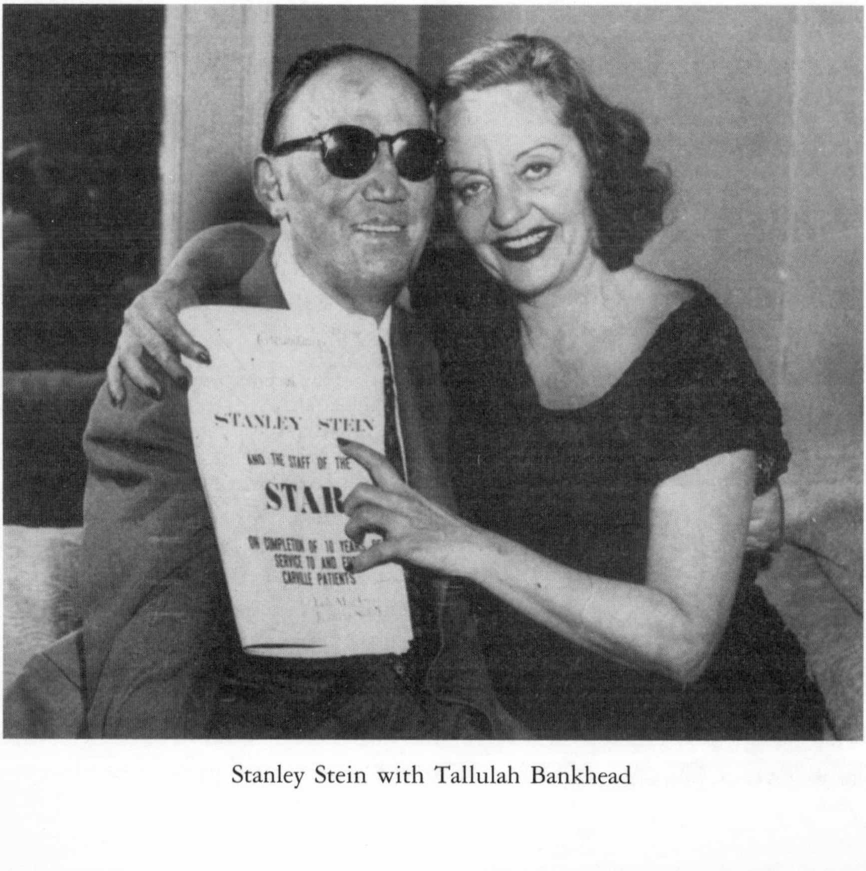

(*The Star*)

Stanley Stein with Tallulah Bankhead

Leprae'. Verdict: discharge denied. The report was dated 15 January 1952.[73]

Worse was to follow when Dr Jo's term as MOC was up and Dr Edward M. Gordon, who had no previous experience of Hansen's disease, replaced him. Stein's relief that at least it wasn't Dr Wolcott was short-lived. The closure of the jail – the 'local bastile' – on 6 February 1954 was welcome, but some of the other changes Dr Gordon was introducing gave cause for alarm. The price of the success of the sulphones was that there was mounting pressure on patients, 'some physically able, some not', to leave the institution, which – in the view of the PHS – had become just a little too cosy under the benign regime of Dr Johansen.[74] Dr Gordon – no doubt under instruction – set about transforming the place from a sanctuary, as it was for many of the patients, into a leaner, meaner government hospital, intent on treatment and research. The emphasis on discharge, which was ironic in view of Stein's bitter experience, might have been welcomed by patients had it been accompanied by a rehabilitation programme that prepared them, psychologically and vocationally, for life outside the institution. But that was not part of the plan. As far as the PHS, in its new, tough stance, was concerned, leprosy was now a treatable disease and the sooner patients were discharged the better. Dr Gordon contended that 'if you had no active germs you were not sick and you should get off of Uncle Sam's gravy train and go to work'.[75]

A corollary of this was the new regime's plan to demolish 'Cottage Grove' and rehouse married patients in hospital apartments without kitchens: 'No more raw rations. All must eat in [the] dining room.' This struck at the heart of the community feeling that had been building up over the years of progress from both a medical and a social perspective. The aim was to make Carville 'an institution again, instead of a liberal hospital community'. The notice of visiting hours at the main gate was removed; no visitor under twenty was admitted (the previous lower age limit had been twelve, which was recognised as a sensible precaution given the apparent susceptibility of very young children to leprosy); and fraternisation between patients and outsiders through sporting events and entertainments was actively discouraged.[76] The *Star* itself was rumoured to be under threat and, though this was officially denied, a PHS memo to the Surgeon General confirms that 'the MOC at Carville did recently recommend to the Hospitals Division that publication of the

STAR be discontinued, and that the recommendation was turned down'.[77] Patients could no longer hold inside jobs and were replaced by hospital personnel, whose anxiety to preserve their hazard duty pay meant that they enthusiastically endorsed Dr Gordon's non-fraternisation policy.

However, the PHS miscalculated if it reckoned it could put the clock back without provoking a patients' revolt. Carville patients were not prepared to give up their hard-won gains without a fight. They hired a lawyer, briefed an influential Congressman and kept the press abreast of what was going on, since in Stein's view the PHS had 'a healthy respect for two things: the Congress, from which it gets its annual appropriation; and the press'. Eventually, under political and media pressure, the PHS backed down, Gordon was posted away from Carville, Dr Edgar B. Johnwick was appointed MOC and 'the climate at Carville changed overnight'. In contrast to his predecessor's policy of divide and rule, Johnwick brought all the contending factions together and gave the following undertaking: 'No one should be discharged from this hospital against his will. No one should be kept in this hospital against his will.'[78]

The patients' victory was not without cost for one of its chief architects. The fate of Cottage Grove was still undecided and, though the government agreed to buy out the owners and to build and maintain new cottages for married couples (and provide kitchens in the planned married patients' apartments), Dr Johnwick was powerless to prevent the eventual eviction of Stanley Stein from his cottage. 'So they were going to raze Wits' End, my home for a quarter of a century, and put me in House 25, a dormitory for the sightless,' he wrote in an outburst of self-pity.

> Nobody cared that Segundo, my private orderly, would be blocks away in House 22, or that I would have to sacrifice my most precious possessions – my privacy and my little dog Bing, who was barred from the dormitories. I couldn't blame the MOC who was busy reorganizing his staff, and yet . . .[79]

By good fortune, he managed to be relocated in House 22 along with his orderly Segundo, though Bing had to be kennelled elsewhere and did not long survive the upheaval, dying a few months later. By a further stroke of luck, Stein was then offered the one old cottage to have escaped

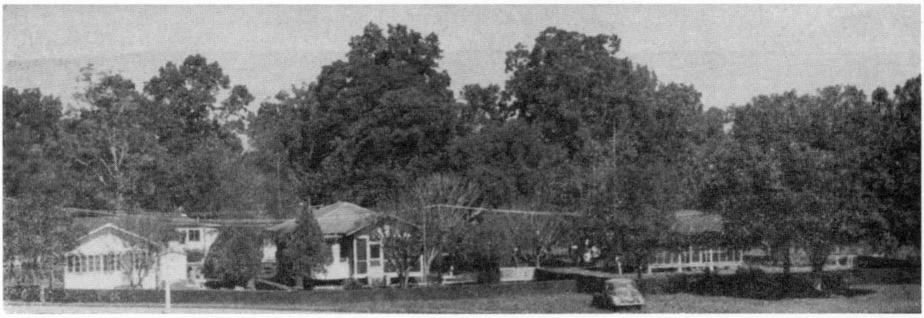

(The Star)

End of an era – part of the condemned Cottage Grove, May 1959

destruction, the home of his one-time deputy Ann Page and her husband Hank Simon, who had built it 'with their own hands around what had once been a chicken coop'. Since he knew his way around it, he was delighted to accept the offer and, to complete the picture, he soon acquired a successor to Bing, a 'precocious pug' he called Beau, 'who, I am afraid, was not quite a proper Bostonian'.[80]

Old patients returned to Carville for treatment. During the 1950s, both Harry and Betty Martin spent some months there – separately – Harry for reconstructive surgery on his hands and Betty when her health deteriorated and positive tests revealed that the disease was reactivated. She was impressed by the changes that had taken place in her ten-year absence: 'Carville was no longer a place of refuge where the victims of a mysterious disease were kept hidden until they died. Carville was now a great modern hospital in every sense of the word.'[81] Plastic surgery had been introduced, to correct such unsightly deformities as collapsed noses, for instance, as well as reconstructive surgery for hands; there was an increase in both specialist medical staff and visiting consultants; and there was a new emphasis on research and rehabilitation. For years, as one writer puts it, 'the federal government had tried to get people with leprosy to come to Carville. Now the problem was to get them to leave.'[82] Dr Gordon had tried to achieve this goal by 'administrative fiat' and failed. Dr Johnwick, with his softly-softly approach, favoured rehabilitation as the means of encouraging patients to go of their own free will.

But that took time and, though the open conflicts of the Gordon era had ceased, there were tensions between the clinical and the rehabilitation members of staff over the handling of patients:

> The stance of the medical branch was that patients should be encouraged to leave once the staff had determined that maximal hospital benefits had been received. The rehabilitation branch, on the other hand, argued that psychosocial considerations must also be weighed in planning for discharge.[83]

One outsider, a young journalist called Jim Duncan who worked on the *Star* for the best part of two years in the early 1960s, had no doubt that Carville needed a 'thorough' rehabilitation programme: 'What already exists is fine, but more is needed – particularly in the area of vocational rehabilitation.' There had been moves in that direction; but in Duncan's opinion patient employment still tended 'to benefit the hospital, not the patient'[84] despite the fact that it was now 'perceived as having "therapeutic" or "rehabilitative" value'.[85]

The difficulty was that rehabilitation meant different things to different people. The sociologist Zachary Gussow, who conducted studies at Carville during the Sixties, found that:

> most members of staff spoke in very general terms: restoring 'the individual to his highest possible potential' or 'helping the individual to adjust to his handicaps.' Few mentioned returning patients to society, and one member, in fact, saw rehabilitation as an adjustment to Carville.[86]

This was the crux of the matter. In most hospitals, even those dealing with other disabling and chronic illnesses such as polio, the aim of rehabilitation was to equip patients to cope in the outside world; at Carville, for so long an isolation hospital, there was a deep-seated ambivalence among both staff and patients over its proper function. Neither long-term staff, like most of the Sisters of Charity, nor long-term patients (also in a majority) questioned the notion of stigma or the need for patients to be protected 'from the trauma of social ostracism'. Indeed, it could be said that by insisting upon it, they colluded in keeping it alive.[87]

When Gussow and a colleague, George S. Tracy, conducted a survey of public attitudes towards leprosy 'in a southern metropolitan area' – presumably New Orleans – they found, among other things, that the public ranked leprosy in 'about the middle of ten diseases in terms of the seriousness of the disease both medically and socially', and that it was 'generally viewed with less anxiety than either mental illness or cancer'. This was because 'most people do not see leprosy as a threat – it is something that exists somewhere else'. So the sociologists concluded that there was 'a discrepancy between what the public expresses and what destigmatization theory asserts – i.e., that leprosy is categorically stigmatized'.[88] They use the phrase 'career patients' to characterise those who, like Stein and even Betty Martin, took upon themselves the 'peculiarly "American" ' role of educating the public and demythologising leprosy, a role the sociologists describe as 'the only legitimate one the leprosy patient has available to him for life in open society'.[89]

Martin's *Miracle at Carville* had ended on a high note, as she and Harry set out in April 1947 in search of a new life. The book elicited great praise for its sympathetic portrayal of leprosy patients and was translated into several languages. (In England it was adapted for radio and broadcast on the BBC; a recording found its way to Carville, where the patients were tickled to hear themselves speak with British accents.) Its sequel, *No One Must Ever Know*, is, as the title suggests, a more sombre book. It charts Betty and Harry's subsequent quest for their own Eden, which in a physical sense they found in California but in other respects was marred by their continuing fear of exposure as Hansen's disease sufferers.

Published in 1959, *No One Must Ever Know* got a muted response, not least in Carville, where various members of staff commenting on the book in the *Star* grappled with the notion that while you might take the patient out of Carville, it was a much tougher proposition to take Carville out of the patient.[90] In a curious inversion of the norm, Betty and Harry could not admit to their aliases, since 'Betty Martin' was now famous; only their real names gave them the anonymity they desired. 'We are not alone', Betty wrote in the final paragraph of her book. 'We belong with the secret people. There are thousands like us, who for one reason or another must walk carefully, that no one may know we walk in a secret world'.[91]

A sad conclusion, compared with the optimistic ending of *Miracle at Carville*. But as 'career patients', both Betty Martin and Stanley Stein were themselves ultimately trapped in the myth they made it their life's work to expose. They were of a generation that, having been subjected to the full force of the prejudice against 'lepers', could not throw off the conviction that they were still enveloped in it. Both of them were aware that the post-Promin generation of patients (following in the footsteps of such courageous individuals as Gertrude Hornbostel and the Filipino war hero Joey Guerrero) was demanding that the world outside – family, friends and workmates – accept them on their own terms, as people who happened to have had Hansen's disease but were in no way disqualified by that from pursuing a full and normal social life.

Stein wrote admiringly of his former secretary, Julia (née Rivera), whose marriage to a fellow patient was 'one of the first to be celebrated in the Carville chapel after the old unwritten ban on marriages between patients was forgotten' and who, when she was discharged, found a job in a nearby city entirely through her own efforts and 'made a point of revealing her background not only to her employer, but also to the girls who would be her office colleagues'. To Stein's surprised delight, they 'all accepted her without reservation'.[92] And Betty Martin, on her return to New Orleans after a ten-year gap, was staggered to find 'old friends who were living openly as former Carville patients':

> The new sulfones, the new home treatment and the more lenient laws, and above all, the widely publicized news of these changes, had brought about a change in attitude in Louisiana. Harry and I were amazed by it. A tolerance and understanding was given the discharged Hansen patient that had been unknown in our day. In turn the patients had learned to accept life on normal terms.[93]

Harry and Betty could observe and admire the new openness of Carville's ex-patients, but they could not emulate it. As one newspaper article put it, 'their secret past remained a heavy burden'.[94] They continued to live in California, returning to Carville periodically for treatment. In 1990 they moved back there for good. Harry, who might have died in 1946 but for the miracle of Promin, finally died in 1996, a full fifty years later. Betty lived on into her nineties (when the present writer and his wife dropped in on her in her hospital room in Baton Rouge in 2001, they were astonished at how beautiful she still was and the care she took to maintain a coiffured appearance). Now she, too, has gone.

Stanley Stein did not survive the 1960s; he died in the week before Christmas 1967. But his legacy, the *Star*, still exists. Across the corridor from its offices is a small room in which there are books and albums of photographs, a sculpted head of Tallulah Bankhead, more photographs,

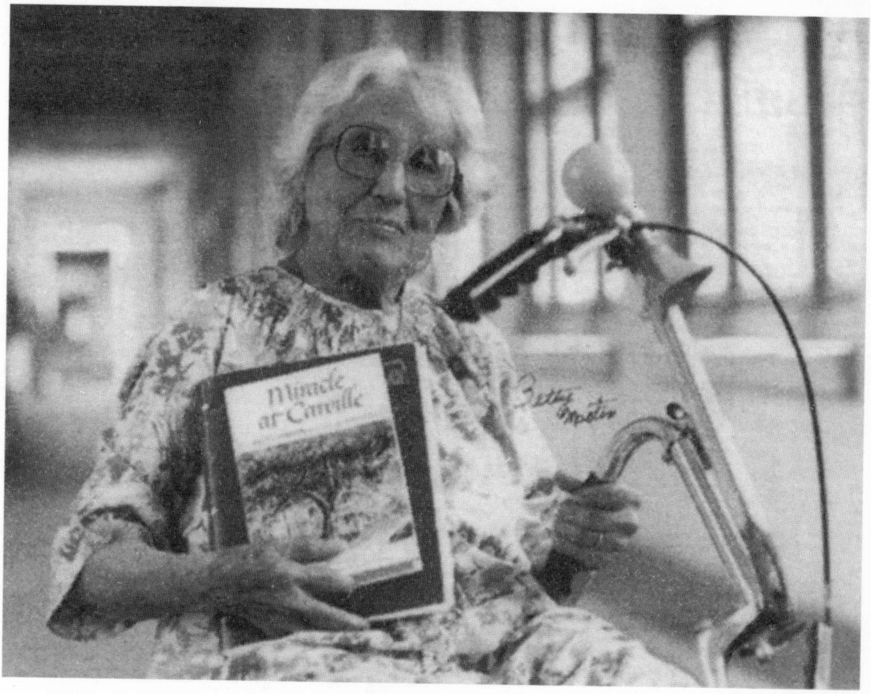

(©Tanya Thomassie)

Edwina Meyer, better known as Betty Martin,
author of *Miracle at Carville* – photograph by Tanya Thomassie

framed and hanging on the wall along with the scroll of the Damien–Dutton Award (named after Father Damien and his acolyte Brother Dutton and given annually for an outstanding educational, scientific, or humanitarian contribution to the relief of Hansen's disease), the first ever to be presented. This is the Stanley Stein Room, a shrine to the memory of the Jewish pharmacist from Texas who did more than any other individual to revolutionise social attitudes to the disease he refused to call leprosy, a 'career patient' who gave his life to improving the lot of his fellow patients and found fame and fulfilment in the process. Institutionalised for close on four decades, blind for nearly three of them, the man who was once called Sidney Levyson died, if not happy, at least secure in the knowledge that, as Stanley Stein, he had done exactly what Sister Laura had suggested thirty-six years before and made a name he had every reason to be proud of.

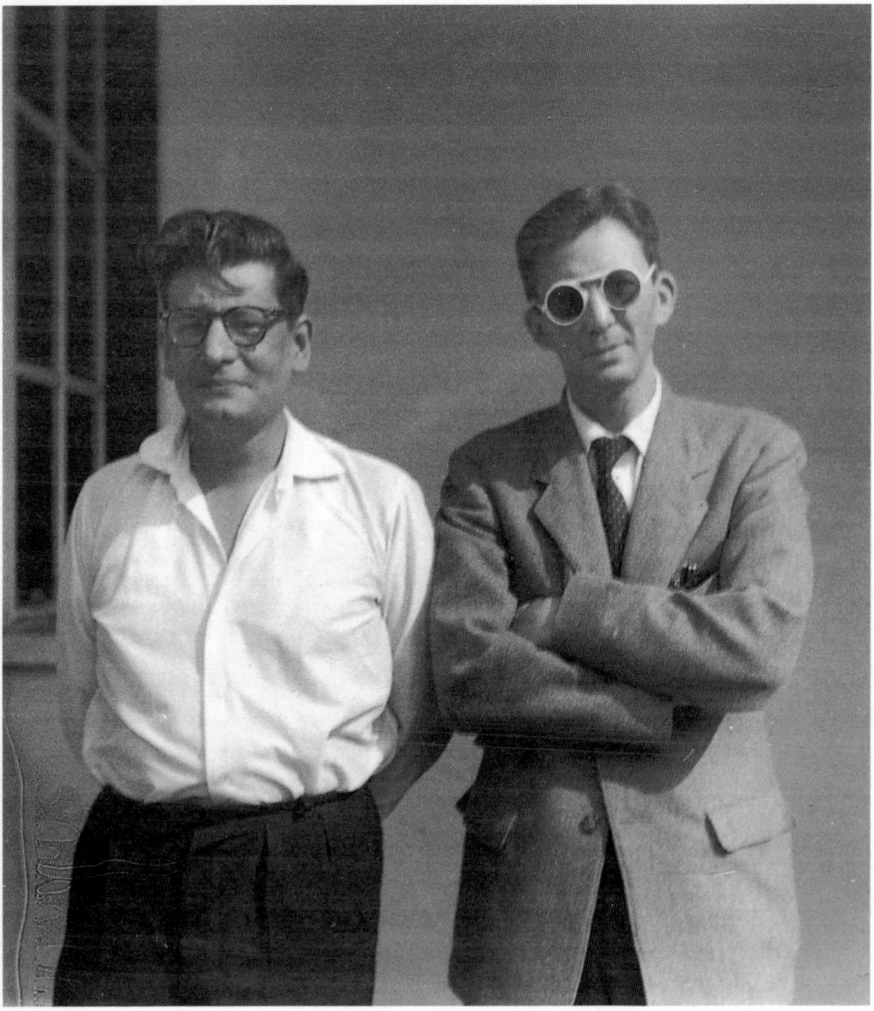
(Courtesy of G. Les Parker)

Peter Greave (*right*) with his friend and fellow patient,
G. Les Parker, at St Giles, Essex, in 1959

Chapter 11

PETER GREAVE AND THE HOMES OF ST GILES

There were two dates Gerald Peter Carberry, aka Peter Greave, would never forget. One was 11 August 1939, the day on which he was diagnosed in Calcutta as having leprosy and as a result went into hiding in Kipling's 'City of Dreadful Night'. The other was 15 September 1947, which he likened to 'a tower in the rushing water of my consciousness, or a boundary stone, marking off one part of my life from the other'.[1] A week earlier he'd arrived in Liverpool after a lonely voyage from Bombay. He was nearly thirty-seven years old and British by nationality, but this was the first time he'd set foot in England.

On that September day Greave was driven across England from an isolation hospital in Liverpool to a 'home' for leprosy sufferers in a remote part of Essex. His driver was taciturn, volunteering no information, but it struck Greave as odd that they should pass through no towns along the way until they reached St Albans. Then it dawned on him that this had nothing to do with the driver's ability to negotiate heavy traffic, but was on account of himself and the need to 'keep this journey, the very fact of my existence, as secret as possible'. By the time they reached St Albans it was getting dark, so there was less risk of his being noticed – this thin, tall, sallow and oddly dressed individual, with his tropical suit and wide-brimmed hat, bloodshot eyes and livid marks on his face.[2]

Soon after leaving St Albans the driver pulled up on the highway opposite a brightly lit café and pondered for a moment before switching off the engine. Greave sensed his dilemma: they'd been on the road all day and they were both hungry; but the driver must have been under instructions not to lose sight of his passenger. When he did get out of the car he avoided looking at Greave but said that he'd get him something to eat. At last Greave could relax: 'It was an indescribable relief to be alone, to know that it was no longer necessary to keep my face twisted into a poor mask of courage and resignation.' All he wanted to do was to rest, 'to slump back in my seat and enjoy the peace of being myself', but his instincts as 'a hunted animal' made him aware that this was his last chance of escape. If he stayed in the car, he was doomed to a life of virtual imprisonment – however benign – in a leprosy home.

There were two other options: he could let off the brake of the car, which was parked on a slope, and it would gather speed and plunge off the road at the first bend, and that might be the end (but what if it wasn't?); or he could open the door and slip away into the night, returning – once the car had gone – to the bus stop he'd noticed on the far side of the road. He could then make his way into the first sizeable city the bus went to and, 'with my strange facility of becoming invisible, disappear into the crowd, and live like a phantom among men'. But well before the driver returned with a mug of tea and a tasteless sandwich, he knew he couldn't do it. He told himself:

> This is one assignment that you can't evade; a problem that can't be solved as you solved the others – by running away from them. What chance would you have? So sick you can hardly walk; so blind you can hardly see. And, worse than either, so filled with terror and uncertainty that every movement gives you away.[3]

For Peter Greave, this was the moment of surrender, the end of an eight-year struggle to maintain his independence against the odds. He was a phantom in more than one sense; though a tall man, he weighed just eight-and-a-half stone. How could he possibly survive on his own in this strange and alien land in which he found himself? As the small Ford nosed its way into the night, Greave resigned himself to his fate. It did not help that when the driver stopped to ask some men the way to the 'convent' one of them said, 'Convent . . . I reckon what you mean is the Leper Homes down Shadley?' The word was like a slap in the face: 'I felt as I suppose Cain felt when he was branded, so that every man's hand was against him.'[4]

It was pitch dark when they arrived at their destination. The silence was broken only by the hoot of an owl nearby. A nun who'd been waiting up for him showed him to his room. It was, Greave wrote, 'as if I had entered the country of the dead.'[5]

There could hardly have been a greater contrast with the extraordinary vicissitudes of his early life. His account of his highly unconventional childhood and youth, *The Seventh Gate*, the last and by far the best of his four books, is reminiscent of *Kim* – of Kipling the artist who celebrated the rich diversity of India rather than the imperialist who preached on the theme of the 'white man's burden'. Greave's father was a businessman, who made and lost fortunes; but though he was a handsome and imposing man there was something not quite right about him, a guilty secret that had nothing to do with any shady business deals in which he might be involved. Like his son, but for a different reason, he always seemed to be on the run. The family was constantly moving, criss-crossing the Indian subcontinent and going overseas to southern Africa and the United States. Only gradually did Greave discover his father's fatal flaw: he was a compulsive 'flasher'. Marriage made no difference; he would encourage his wife to play the piano, pretending to enjoy her performance but intent on keeping her occupied while he stood out on the veranda exposing himself to the woman next door.[6]

Greave's mother put up with her husband's erratic behaviour, probably because she had no alternative, and continued to love him despite his terrible obsession. She was Irish (Greave's father was also half Irish, though he hailed from Manchester), 'a fervent, though unusually broad-minded Roman Catholic' and the stabilising force in the family. She died when Greave was sixteen and the family fell apart 'like an old trunk eaten by white ants'.[7]

A decade earlier, when his parents had left India on a business trip that took them across war-ravaged Europe and into southern Russia, Greave and his brother, who would never be close (a much loved sister was born later), had been packed off to Darjeeling in the charge of a Eurasian nurse called Sophie – 'tall and unusually dark for an Anglo-Indian, with the flat nose and thick lips that might have been due to traces of African blood'. For young Peter, this was a kind of expulsion from Eden. He was the first-born and up to that time had basked in his mother's love, enjoying the comforts of a big Calcutta house with a sunlit garden. His father was at the zenith of his business career and the family wanted for nothing. Suddenly separated from his parents for no reason he could fathom and transported to a strange mountainous place, Peter also found himself the object of his nurse's sadistic attentions; Sophie would beat him with a long-handled hairbrush so hard and so frequently that even the nuns at his nursery school became aware of the cuts and bruises on his back and arms and remonstrated with her:

> I heard later that when Sophie was confronted by the evidence of her neglect and cruelty, she would burst into a flood of tears, swear to mend her ways, and assure the credulous sisters that she would hurry to confession the next morning and be absolved from her sins.[8]

The beatings became more and more frenetic, and at the end of one particularly violent session Peter fell and impaled his chin on a rusty nail, letting out a howl of terror. Soon two nuns appeared and though Sophie tried to pass it off as an accident the evidence was against her; the hairbrush, which she'd dropped on the floor on the veranda, was smeared with blood. The police were called, and Sophie was sufficiently frightened not to lay a finger on Peter again; instead she professed to be ill and took to her bed. Now Peter started to feel guilty, as though he were to blame for reducing her to such a state. Sophie had never beaten his brother Michael, so the beatings had somehow made their relationship special, and though he found them both frightening and painful they also gave him 'a curious sense of pleasure and excitement'. Later he came to believe that Sophie was responsible for arousing in him lasting masochistic desires. Worse still, she may have been the one to infect him with leprosy, the disease being notorious for its long-drawn-out incubation period. In *The Second Miracle*, which was his first book, he wrote: 'The doctors say that quite probably I contracted it while still a small child, from a Mauritian [*sic*] nurse with a swollen leg, who had charge of us for a time when my parents were in Russia.'[9]

One morning Peter was outside the cottage playing with his brother when he looked up and was startled to see a well-dressed and beautiful woman approaching. Her voice seemed vaguely familiar, but he barely recognised his mother. He kept quiet about the beatings but when she saw the dirty bandage on his chin and heard that Sophie was in bed she knew at once that something was wrong. The boys were told to wait outside while she went in and summarily dismissed their nurse. Only then did they go with their mother to her hotel, where they washed and changed their clothes and hugged her in an ecstatic reunion. Peter felt as though he'd 'escaped from a nightmare'.[10] The next day they were back in Calcutta.

But they didn't enjoy the old life for long. Greave's father quarrelled with his employers and lost a lawsuit they took out against him, leaving him bankrupt. That was when the family's travels – and travails – began. At first they sought their fortune abroad but after some years in New York they returned to India, where their father, not for the first or last time, deserted their mother, going off in search of work and somehow failing to return. The boys were sent back to Darjeeling to a Catholic boarding school that catered mainly for Anglo-Indians; but Peter had become accustomed to the free and easy ways of America and didn't take kindly to the strict discipline imposed by the Irish Christian brothers of St Theobald's. After a few months he ran away. He couldn't hope to get home to Bombay, so he headed for Calcutta, where – after some days of Kim-like adventures – he was picked up by the police and put in the custody of an older boy who was returning to St Theobald's. But during the train journey he managed to give this boy the slip and headed for Assam, where some American friends of the family took him in and looked after him until his parents, now reunited, reclaimed him.[11]

He didn't have to go back to Darjeeling but attended, along with his brother, a number of different educational establishments (including – for a brief but blissful time – a senior girls' class in a Roman Catholic convent school) as the family resumed its peripatetic existence, chased out of place after place by his father's 'private demon', his propensity to expose himself no matter how damaging the consequences. It was this obsession, Greave believed, that led his mother to an early grave; when she could no longer stand the shame of it, she succumbed to cancer and gave up the ghost. Her six-year-old daughter Mary was whisked away to a convent, and the boys were left with their father until mutual dislike drove them apart. Greave returned to the house late one evening to find it empty. There was a note from his father, which said: 'I've got to get out of this bloody country. Here is 50 rupees. Best of luck.'[12] At sixteen, Peter was on his own. For the next several years he drifted, from place to place and job to job. He lived 'like a nomad, moving from one city to another, existing in seedy hotels or in shoddy rooms' but never stopping for long. He didn't think of himself as a failure or a misfit; he was perfectly content to 'read, dream, make firm friendships, and implacable enemies, while I explored the vast, unpredictable labyrinths of India'. He was 'obsessed with sex', but a stranger to love: 'I was satisfied to respond to the fugitive, short-lived adventures of the road, and these were not particularly difficult to find, either by luck or the simple expedient of disgorging a few rupees.' He got into drunken brawls, was thrown out of dance halls and brothels, sometimes losing his job as a result. Yet he never doubted that a dazzling future awaited him.[13]

After some years his father reappeared, cutting a sad figure, both down in the mouth and down at heel. He had been in Australia and then in Rangoon, but success had eluded him in both places. Neither Greave nor his brother welcomed the return of the prodigal father and he soon slunk off again. So it was with some surprise that, months later, Greave received a letter inviting him to come to Calcutta, where his father had started a new and successful business and was living with Mary (who, at seventeen, had left her convent) in a 'small flat overlooking Dalhousie Square'. Peter accepted his father's offer to support him for a minimum of six months but made the mistake of joining him in a dubious business venture involving an unseaworthy vessel that had to be brought from Chittagong to the Calcutta docks. As the owner's representative, Peter was to supervise the voyage, and he and a hastily assembled crew narrowly escaped drowning in the Bay of Bengal before the captain, with Peter's hearty concurrence, turned back to Chittagong. After that, Greave refused to have anything more to do with his father's business schemes.[14]

He stayed in Calcutta and resumed his shiftless ways, but a new person had entered his life: 'Her name was Sharon, and despite her splendid red hair, her jade green eyes, and the pallor of her smooth white skin, somewhere deep inside her was the dark colour of India.' She was illegitimate and her European father's identity remained a mystery. Greave was convinced that, 'like a kitten reprieved from drowning', she owed her life to her extraordinary Nordic beauty:

> Had she been born with dark hair and a coffee-coloured skin, I think she might well have been left to die in a ditch, instead of being brought up by her aunt, when she was discarded by her feckless gypsy mother. I now know that her life was an example of the debris left in the trail of the British Empire. She was one of the losers, a casualty washed up by the great tides of colonial expansion.[15]

What started off as a casual relationship in which Greave came and went as he pleased, selfishly expecting Sharon to be waiting for him on his return, grew into an obsession on his part when she showed an independence of spirit that more than matched his own. He was stunned, but also enslaved, by her changeability, 'her capacity for destruction, her genius for involving herself with the most unsuitable men'. He admitted that he loved her 'not so much in spite of her intransigencies as because of them'. Sexually, she was the dominant partner, but he had the intellectual edge:

> Once we were above the level of passion, of glandular reaction, I could control and sway her far more than anyone else. She respected my judgment and trusted me; I could say things to her that would have resulted in an immediate and final break if said by anyone else. It may sound foolish, but I am certain she loved me in her fashion, though not as completely and utterly as I loved her.

Sharon is a crucial presence in all Greave's books and (as Jessica) is central to his novel, *The Painted Leopard*, but he admits to finding it 'almost impossible' to write of her objectively.[16]

In *Young Man in the Sun* (where she is known as Jobina) he describes his role in her 'feckless life' as 'a mixture of lover, bodyguard and poor relation' – he could make her laugh and because they both 'belonged to the poor white trash' they had the same outlook on life. In *The Painted Leopard*, he writes: 'She was my weakness, my blind-spot, my perpetual hunger . . . my vice was this thin, feckless girl, with a small, self-willed mouth, and greedy, restless hands.' He thought of her as 'the destroyer, because she built nothing, valued nothing, understood nothing'; she was 'lazy, slipshod, a liar, a bully, and, when necessary a thief'; she was also 'unpunctual, greedy and revengeful', yet 'there was more generosity, warmth and love in her than in anyone I have ever known'. One moment she would be all over him, the next 'a hard, brittle shell, facing me with implacable hostility'. Greave blamed her background: 'That crippling sense of insecurity, that heritage of "not belonging", with all the cheap evasions and subterfuges it entailed, was responsible for the flaws and unrest of her tempestuous nature.'[17]

Sharon encouraged Greave in his first awkward attempts to become a writer. But far more important was her spontaneous and unstinting support in the crisis that threatened to overwhelm him in 1939, when he was diagnosed as having leprosy. Until he could arrange for a doctor to come to him, he had to go to hospital twice a week for treatment:

> I had become afraid, shrinking from leaving my room, dreading the long uncomfortable journey by tram to the hospital gates. I am quite sure that I would have given up even the pretence of attending the clinic had it not been for Sharon's unfailing courage and sympathy. She would accompany me on these journeys, chattering loudly to distract my attention, threading her arm through mine when my footsteps faltered as we approached that sinister objective. I do not doubt that without her presence I would have succumbed to the temptation of suicide which, in those early weeks, constantly obsessed my thoughts.[18]

Sharon continued to give him practical support, at one point allowing him to share her room when he could no longer stand the cockroach-infested hovel he'd been living in, though discovery would have resulted in her instant eviction. This arrangement lasted only a few weeks, until Greave's father, hearing of his predicament, gave him a monthly allowance of 300 rupees. ('This', Greave writes, 'in view of our prolonged estrangement, was indeed generous, and it is only fair to record that he continued to support me for the next eleven years.') Yet the emotional roller-coaster of his relationship with Sharon went on unchanged, becoming, if anything, more extreme as the years passed. Then, when the war was nearly over, Sharon got engaged to a sea captain, a much older man who had amassed a fortune – through smuggling heroin, it was rumoured – and promised to take her to England: 'It was as though she had suddenly become aware of all that she had missed in a material sense during the years that lay behind, and was now determined to get her share of life's luxuries.' Alas, she didn't have long to enjoy them. Three months after a tearful, passionate parting from her, Greave received news from his sister Mary, who had also left India, that Sharon was dead: 'it appeared that the car in which she was a passenger was cut down by a tanker, somewhere on the outskirts of Birmingham.'[19]

By this time Greave's own predicament was becoming critical. His room was in a Muslim part of the city and in the midst of the communal riots that provided a lurid backdrop to the birth of independent India and Pakistan his (Hindu) Bengali doctor no longer dared visit him to administer chaulmoogra injections. In a sense this was a relief; he dreaded the doctor's weekly visits and found the injections a form of torture:

> In my case it was the face that was chiefly affected, and every week I received somewhere in the region of a hundred stabs, most of them grouped around the forehead, nose and eyes. Each jab – the needle had to penetrate quite deeply – increased the burning torment, and after seventy or eighty of them I would begin to jerk my head from beneath the doctor's hands or even make an effort to catch at his wrists.
>
> When at last it was finished, my face would be bleeding copiously, covered with red puncture marks from forehead to chin, swollen and disfigured, while I was a nervous wreck, shaking in every limb.
>
> But my greatest torment, far outweighing the physical pain, was the fear that I should be discovered while all this was taking place, or that the horrible, distinctive smell of the oil would betray me.[20]

Yet the doctor's defection, though perfectly understandable – why should he risk his life by entering a Muslim quarter of Calcutta when the patient might, with less danger, come to the hospital? – was the last straw for Greave. Sharon had gone; so had his sister Mary, and his father was planning to follow her; even his Indian servant boy had deserted him; he was already blind in one eye, and the other eye was severely infected and so painful that he couldn't sleep at night; his room had been looted and ransacked twice in a single month; bloodthirsty mobs roamed the street, setting fire to buildings and smoking out victims whose screams rent the air as the crowd closed in on them and hacked and beat them to death; and 'the vultures became gorged with their diet of human flesh'.[21] (In a bitter memoir of that time, the British general responsible for Eastern Command in India, Lt-Gen. Sir Francis Tuker, describes how troops clearing the dead would look back when they reached the end of a street only to see two or three fresh bodies, which had appeared during the brief time they'd been engaged in their grisly task.[22])

Then, when he'd abandoned all hope of rescue, Greave received an airmail letter from a doctor in London he calls Riley, but whose real name was Ryrie, the Medical Secretary of the British Empire Leprosy Relief Association: 'In some inexplicable fashion he had heard of my plight, and was now writing to press me to come to England, where, he assured me, I could depend on both treatment and care.' At first Greave was unable to take in what he read, it seemed so unlikely, but gradually 'hope returned like a long-lost friend'. He realised that this was his one chance of escape and he'd better make the most of it. He knew it wouldn't be easy. Even without his medical history, it was almost impossible to get a passage to England when so many people were trying to leave India; and first he had to cross the country by rail to get to the port of departure at Bombay.

Ryrie had asked for his medical notes, which showed to his satisfaction that Greave was 'completely non-infectious' and therefore free to travel in the normal way. But Greave couldn't afford the fare. In desperation he wrote to his father, whom he hadn't seen for years, and suggested a meeting. His father agreed to see him but when they met tried to discourage him from making the journey: 'I mean, what do you expect to achieve by travelling half way across the world in your condition?' Nevertheless he eventually pulled out his cheque book and, however reluctantly, provided the money:

> I remember that after I had thanked him I caught a fleeting glimpse of his face as I walked quickly towards the door. He was staring after me with impassive concentration, as though he never expected to see me again, and I still do not know whether pity or mere boredom lay behind that blank, unrevealing gaze.[23]

Back in England, Greave's father married again. In the late 1950s, when the *Evening Standard* quoted the aged writer and *grande dame* Edith Sitwell saying, 'I have *everything* infectious except leprosy', his second wife wrote her an indignant letter denying that leprosy was infectious and telling her she ought to be ashamed of herself for stirring up prejudice against its sufferers. A chastened Sitwell sent an emollient reply and there ensued a lengthy correspondence in which the 'Leper's Stepmother', as Sitwell called her, poured out her troubles in daily – sometimes twice-daily – letters. Prominent among these was the havoc caused by her husband's compulsion to expose himself, to which the police responded by periodically carting him off either to jail or to a lunatic asylum. Though fascinated by the story, the ailing Edith Sitwell eventually tired of the correspondence and got her doctor to put a stop to it, but not before she'd written to her secretary, 'The leper's stepmother is pursuing me at every turn. Her husband has undressed publicly again. He is seventy-eight and has taken a job as a night watchman. They have, in toto, £12.' It's sad, if fittingly Indian, that Greave's father should end his roller-coaster career by becoming a night watchman.[24]

Edith Sitwell, incidentally, provides a textbook example of leprophobia, putting on gloves to read the 'Leper's Stepmother's' letters and initiating a hunt in her bedroom for a missing envelope 'stamped with the Leprosarium's special stamp in addition to the ordinary one' that the woman had 'thoughtfully' sent her, for fear of infection. When she heard that her old friend Graham Greene was intending to visit 'leper colonies in the Congo' (see next chapter) she remarked to another friend that adventurousness could 'go too far', and was extremely nervous about meeting him on his return:

> I shall just have to say to Graham, 'My dear boy, I could not be more pleased to see you, but if, by any chance, you should want to sneeze, then please go to the window and sneeze out of that.'[25]

In 1911 the President of the Local Government Board, John Burns, received a dignified and moving letter from a former officer of the Indian Woods and Forests Department, who described himself as 'the unfortunate victim of the worst malady that afflicts humanity . . . and which had been described as a living "death" '. He was blind and his hands and feet 'were reduced to mutilated stumps'. He was sixty-four years old and totally dependent on his seventy-three-year-old wife, who had nursed him for years; but now her health had broken down and she was unable to continue. What was he to do? He had tried to get into 'some Hospital or Home for Incurables but without success' even though he was prepared to pay. He appealed to the minister to use his influence to get him into an institution that would care for him, adding: 'It is also perhaps in the public interest as well as my own that I should be located as I desire.'[26]

Further inquiry revealed that this was just one of six similar sad cases, all living within a few miles of one another in London suburbs. There was a former Indian Police officer, also tended by an aged wife; a 'professional gentleman from Ceylon'; two well-educated Mauritians, one of whom had worked at the Greenwich Observatory; and a young Polish Jew who had trained as a dentist, but had sunk into such a depression on contracting the disease that 'the only available shelter for him was the lunatic ward of a workhouse'. Sir Arthur Downes, the Senior Medical Inspector for Poor Law purposes, knew of 'some 25 cases in all' across the country, but suspected the true figure to be double that number. Statistically, this might not amount to much, but the prospects for these individuals were truly appalling:

> As things now stand the popular horror of this disease is such that these poor people have no security even of shelter other than the workhouse, the last place into which they should go if we are to consider the feelings of other unfortunates who have also to be received there. The hospitals will not keep them; none will knowingly let them house or lodging, or even serve them with necessaries. In one of the cases listed above, a kind-hearted doctor who has attended to the patient has been discarded by other patients.[27]

A 1916 trial reported in the *British Medical Journal* highlighted the leprosy sufferer's predicament. Mr Humphreys, a Bayswater lodging-house keeper, filed a case against a Miss Miller – who'd lodged in his house along with her leprosy-stricken father from July 1914 until the latter's death in December 1915 – and Dr Harboard, the physician who'd treated Mr Miller. Humphreys argued that once he discovered that the deceased Mr Miller had had leprosy, he'd been obliged to destroy all the furniture and could no longer hope to let the lodgings. The case hinged on the question of whether or not leprosy was an infectious disease. The doctors giving evidence for Humphreys took the line that it 'was contagious though "not highly so"'; Sir Malcolm Morris, the specialist speaking on behalf of the defendants, said that in England at least 'he had never known one person catch the disease from another'. The jury had no doubt that Miss Miller and Dr Harboard were guilty of 'fraudulent misrepresentation' and found against them to the tune of £250 damages, but the judge overturned this decision on the grounds that Dr Harboard had 'genuinely believed that leprosy was not contagious in England'. Humphreys took the case to the appeal court, where it was also dismissed. The trial provides a striking instance of the huge gap between popular prejudice and informed opinion.[28]

The authorities' dilemma was whether or not to make leprosy a compulsorily notifiable disease – as tuberculosis became in 1913. This, too, hinged on the question of contagion. If leprosy was indeed contagious, then the public needed to be protected from the risk of catching it. By making leprosy notifiable, the authorities would become better informed as to its prevalence and would be in a position to take steps to prevent its spread. But there was the rub. Leprosy was incurable and the approved method of prevention was compulsory segregation. To introduce that in Britain, where (as the 1916 trial would demonstrate) popular prejudice against the disease was already strong and its contagiousness unproven, would not only involve huge expense but would further stigmatise its victims. Another official worry was that 'public provision would tend to attract to this country alien cases which should properly be cared for in other lands or in their place of origin'.[29]

'When in doubt, do nothing' might be a government motto. But it was harder for officials like John Burns and Sir Arthur Downes and their medical colleagues with first-hand experience of the problem to ignore it. So in 1913 a handful of these public-spirited individuals held a meeting at which they resolved to raise funds to provide a refuge for British nationals unfortunate enough to have contracted leprosy. An immediate difficulty was the need for secrecy if public suspicions were not to be aroused: it is hard to raise money without publicity and funds were slow to come in. Then – in the words of one writer – there 'occurred a series of strange "coincidences"'.[30]

First, some of the group got lost driving in the Essex countryside near Chelmsford. They stopped at a remote and dilapidated farmhouse to ask the way. The farmer invited them in for a cup of tea and enquired what had brought them to that part of the country in 'their new-fangled motor car'. When they said they were looking for a property to buy, he told them he wanted to sell his place. So almost without trying they acquired 'a site of 27 acres, with a small house, in a secluded country locality within convenient reach of London' for £1,500 (£1,000 of which the vendor allowed to remain on mortgage).[31]

Shortly after this stroke of good fortune a meeting was held in London to discuss the now urgent need for more money and the ex-President of the Local Government Board, John Burns, volunteered to make the journey to Scotland to sound out his friend Lord Strathcona. When he arrived, Burns found the old man was so ill that it seemed tactless to raise the subject of money. But Lord Strathcona was not too far gone to discover the purpose of his visit, or, once he knew it, to summon his solicitor and dictate a codicil to his will, leaving John Burns the sum of £5,000 to be used for the benefit of leprosy sufferers in Britain. Twenty-four hours later Lord Strathcona was dead.[32]

So far, so good. But despite the secrecy surrounding the project, word inevitably leaked out about what was happening, and the local press carried a story of plans to 'establish a home for chronic disfiguring diseases and lepers' at Moor House, East Hanningfield. At the instigation of the local parish council a public meeting was held on 6 July 1914 and a resolution passed expressing 'detestation and alarm' at such a development. But it was too late: two nursing sisters from Guy's Hospital had been there since April and the first leprosy patients had already been smuggled in. And when, less than a month later, war was declared and East Hanningfield found itself in the 'second line of defence', a possible target for German bombardment, the arrival in the vicinity of a handful of blind and/or severely disabled leprosy patients did not seem quite so much of a threat after all.[33]

We get a glimpse of life at St Giles in the early days in a letter to Wellesley Bailey, the founder of the Mission to Lepers (which contributed funds), from someone who worked there. The Hon. G. Scott wrote to Bailey about the four patients in residence in March 1916, two British and the two from Mauritius mentioned above. 'Daddie' was an old man who had served in the Indian Army but was now 'blind and crippled, both hands and feet', and was looked after by his equally old wife. Bishop was a young soldier in the early stages of the disease; he was the institution's driver and helped look after the other patients. Both the Mauritians were scientists. Monsieur Rampal, who was 'very clever at chemistry', was 'our pet'; he was in a very advanced stage of the disease, completely blind and dependent on morphine; though he had a 'young and charming' Belgian wife, who had nursed him devotedly for almost a decade, he prayed only for release. Monsieur Giraud was the astronomer who'd worked at the Greenwich Observatory; he also had a young wife, who was half French, and before they found refuge at St Giles, the couple had been 'literally turned out into the streets by the authorities'; Giraud was less disabled than his compatriot, but was nearly blind and suffered from severe depression. All except for the soldier contributed financially according to their means.[34]

Each couple lived in half a bungalow, with two rooms, bathroom and scullery. Bishop, the only bachelor, occupied one of the common rooms separating the two halves of the bungalows. The other common room was used as a meeting place; it contained a gramophone and Scott had just acquired a piano for it. His work consisted in reading aloud to the patients and looking after the garden. He lived in a cottage ten minutes' walk away and often invited the wives, or the nursing sisters, to tea there. He loved the work and found the religious life, which 'occupies a good deal of our time', a 'great help'.[35]

Monsieur Rampal did die, as expected, in 1916 and – according to an article by Dr J.M.H. MacLeod, a dermatologist at the Charing Cross

Hospital and medical adviser to St Giles – his Belgian widow, who up to the time of her husband's admission to St Giles 'had taken no precautions to avoid infection', subsequently developed the disease. Hers was one of a clutch of 'indigenous cases' (she had married Rampal in England) that MacLeod had encountered in the course of his work and brought to the attention of the Ministry of Health, whose doctors were relieved to find he agreed that 'it would be a calamity to such patients if public attention were drawn to them by making the disease notifiable in this country'. At that time St Giles did not admit women patients (in general the demand for places outweighed the very limited supply) and MacLeod was hoping for a subsidy from the ministry to enable it to expand so that it might take in patients like this poor woman, who was 'morbidly fearful lest the nature of her illness be discovered in the boarding house where she lodges'. Although the ministry proved reluctant to become officially involved, MacLeod succeeded in getting Madame Rampal back into St Giles in 1925, as one of the first two female patients ever to be admitted.[36]

The ministry's anxiety that any 'Government provision for lepers might become known and bring lepers flocking to this country' was reinforced by the case of Joseph Attard, aged twenty-seven, who came to London from Malta in 1930 and made his way to Cardiff, where he was admitted to the Isolation Hospital that October. Two-and-a-half years later he was still there, maintained at the expense of Cardiff City Council, though his presence among acutely sick patients was beginning to cause friction. At first he had been on his best behaviour, grateful for the privileges accorded to him. He had 'his own wireless, an ample supply of newspapers, and complete freedom within the hospital grounds'. He was allowed 'a bottle of beer a week' and was kept in cigarettes by the hospital employees. All he had to do in return was make his bed and keep his room tidy. In June 1933 a doctor in Cardiff's public health department wrote to the controller of the Welsh Board of Health:

> He has lately been refusing to do these things and on Friday, 26th May, he threw his dinner out of the window and since then has refused to take off his clothes, spending the night on the floor of his room. He has threatened more than once to take his life, and to murder the staff, and patients in his ward . . .
>
> It is obvious that some special arrangement must sooner or later be made for this man. He is upsetting the normal working of a whole hospital.[37]

Attard was moved to St Giles, where the same pattern repeated itself. He worked as a gardener, which he'd done in Malta (where he'd been employed at the Governor's residence), and at first showed himself 'amenable to the discipline of the place and clean in his personal habits'. But a year later the general practitioner responsible for St Giles, Dr Ivor Pirrie, wrote to the Ministry of Health complaining that Attard was 'not a satisfactory patient'. He was of 'a different type and race to the others' and, once the novelty of his surroundings had worn off, he'd become 'surly and rude to the Sisters'. He refused to do work that he was perfectly able to do – and would have received 'pocket money' for doing – and was generally a disruptive influence. Dr Pirrie wanted to know if he might be repatriated 'without obtaining his consent' – since he certainly wouldn't go willingly, especially as he was 'likely to be segregated on his return'. Life at St Giles was luxurious compared to that of a labourer in Malta and Attard had probably left the country in the first place '*because* he knew he had leprosy'. But it seemed 'illogical that he should remain here – and an expense to some one or some public body – indefinitely'.[38]

Ministry officials had already tried to have Attard repatriated when he was in Cardiff. The government of Malta had made no objection to his return, but no shipping company had been prepared to take him and the cost of flying him there would have been prohibitive. So they thought of military transport and had actually persuaded an Indian Transport vessel to take him, though it involved a diversion to Malta. All that was needed was the patient's consent. Both Dr Shaw, from the Ministry, and a Cardiff medical inspector who thought he 'could handle Attard' had visited St Giles, but neither could move him. So the ship had left without him. The bottom line was: 'Attard is a British subject, and there is no power to force him to leave this country against his will.' According to the Homes of St Giles records, Joseph Attard was still in residence in July 1947, the year of Peter Greave's arrival there.[39]

Since the mid-1930s the nursing care and day-to-day running of St Giles had been in the hands of the Community of the Sacred Passion, an Anglican order based in East Africa (their Mother House was in Tanganyika – now Tanzania). This arrangement suited both the governing body of the Homes and the nuns: St Giles acquired dedicated nurses at minimal cost, and the sisters procured a rest house in England where they could both recuperate after their labours among leprosy sufferers in

Africa and train novices for the work they would be doing when they, in their turn, went out to Tanganyika.

Peter Greave was not a religious person. Despite his mother's devout Catholicism, he'd 'always held organised religion in considerable suspicion and had little respect for Convent life'. When he arrived at St Giles, he was terrified of the sisters: 'the very sight of their long-robed figures induced a kind of a paralysis of the brain, so that every idea departed from me and I could do nothing but goggle at them helplessly'. But their humour, tolerance and humanity soon won him over. He was impressed by their goodness and unselfishness, which – far from making them 'colourless and stereotyped' – gave them 'character and contentment'. The fact that 'they succeeded in being tremendously happy' was, in his opinion, 'their greatest achievement'.[40]

Though he continued to hold the sisters in awe, it was a different matter with the novices. The patients saw much more of them, since they were the ones who brought trays to their rooms and cleaned and tidied up for them, and 'they had as yet gone such a little distance along their long and difficult road that they seemed less important, and nearer to us'. One novice in particular, to whom significantly – in view of his earlier attachment in Calcutta – Greave gives the name Sharon, attracted and repelled him in almost equal measure. A 'tall, graceful girl, with long legs' – an important point for Greave – 'and narrow hips', she had a 'small, petulant mouth' and brown eyes that were 'set a little too close together'. She also resembled her Anglo-Indian namesake in her unpredictability: 'One moment she would scratch without warning, the next appear meek, pliable and tender.' Older than the average novice, she came from a wealthy and socially well-connected family, had been 'expensively educated' and had worked as a model and an MP's secretary, as well as in welfare in the slums. She had also travelled widely. All of which made it difficult for 'this spoiled, self-assured girl' to knuckle under and live the life of 'hard work and unquestioning obedience' demanded of a novice: 'She had a gift for organisation and a real dexterity in handling facts and figures; but her long, graceful fingers became all thumbs as soon as she was asked to lay a fire or sweep a room . . .'[41]

After reading of Peter Greave's combustible relationship with this intelligent, aspiring, awkward and troubled girl who, at the end of *The Second Miracle*, prepares to leave for Africa along with two other novices, it comes as no surprise to learn that an actual relationship with an educated novice would lead the young woman to renounce her vows – no doubt much to the disapproval of the sisters – and marry him. Though this must have seemed like a miracle to Greave, it had nothing to do with the 'second miracle' of his book's title; nor is this title a reference to Betty Martin's or Carville's miracle, the sulphone drug treatment that, in the oral form of Diasone or DDS – diamino-diphenyl-sulphone – transformed Greave's life, too. No, if the first miracle was the unaccountable arrival of a flimsy airmail letter that precipitated his rescue from strife-torn Calcutta, the second miracle was that the 'defeated animal brought to a cage' expecting nothing but 'captivity and death' found instead a 'fuller and more satisfying life' than any he had previously known.[42]

DDS was, of course, an essential ingredient of this 'second miracle'. The treatment, which had only just been introduced at St Giles when Greave started taking it on 22 September 1947, postponed for many years the onset of the blindness he dreaded. It did something else, too:

> Those small white pills changed the whole mental outlook. As soon as the efficacy of the drug became widely recognised, the new generation of patients bore none of the horrors of a life sentence. They did not suffer physically or mentally to anything like the same extent as we had done in the past. Gone too was the stabbing sense of being an outcast, of self-loathing and disgust. Now that they knew their cure was only a matter of time, they mostly settled down philosophically – indeed, at times with what seemed to us old-timers an almost sacrilegious lightheartedness – to their period of treatment.[43]

The British, as is their wont, had initially responded sceptically to Carville's miracle; they distrusted what they saw as the naïve enthusiasm of the Americans. BELRA's annual report for 1948 asserted that:

> the sulphone drugs, hailed as the absolute answer to leprosy, have not yet shown themselves to deserve this description; their cost is as yet prohibitive for universal use, and while they have proved successful in a large number of cases of the infectious type treated, their effect on other cases – perhaps three quarters of the total – is not yet recognised as superior to the older treatment.[44]

In other words, though the sulphones might work in cases of lepromatous leprosy, they were no more effective than chaulmoogra in curing non-infective tuberculoid leprosy.

The following year, however, in BELRA's twenty-fifth anniversary report, Greave's rescuer, Dr Gordon Ryrie, at least, adopted a very different tone: 'It is difficult for anyone who has not worked in the pre-sulphone era to realise the immense change made by the sulphones.' He recounted how in 1907 an obscure German chemist had discovered 'a new chemical substance' he'd named diamino-diphenyl-sulphone, but for which he had no practical use. It wasn't until thirty years later that the success of the drug commonly known as M & B had alerted researchers to the healing powers of the sulphonamides. Now, the year 1948 had seen 'what is probably the most important development in the treatment of leprosy up to date'. The problem with the sulphones – apart from their cost – was their toxicity, as the Americans had discovered. But British research (in which Dr Robert Cochrane played a leading role) had

> found that by going back to the original [DDS], the drug could be used in doses too small to be of any effect in human tuberculosis, but which proved to be of marked efficacy in the treatment of leprosy . . . at a cost of about 15/- a year.[45]

Dr Gordon Ryrie became an adviser to the Ministry of Health on matters pertaining to leprosy early in 1947, when he was appointed medical secretary of BELRA in succession to Dr Ernest Muir. Ryrie was well qualified for the role. For thirteen years from 1928 he had been Medical Superintendent of the Sungei Buloh leprosy settlement in the Malayan Federation in charge of 2,500 patients of all races. During the 1930s he'd caused a brief flutter of excitement when an experimental treatment he'd developed, consisting of injections of trypan blue, an aniline dye, had been hailed as 'a cure for leprosy', a claim which – like so many others – turned out to be false. Ryrie had acknowledged his failure and he was still at Sungei Buloh in January 1942 when the Japanese overran Malaya and he had to make a decision whether to follow the advice of the British authorities in Singapore and leave immediately, or listen to his patients who begged him to 'leave his light on during the night to give them courage'.[46]

Like 'Prexy' Wade in the Philippines, he stayed on, but at considerable personal cost. He recalled:

> I was in the hospital when the Japs came. They left us alone for two and a half years because of their great fear of the disease. We had 2,600 patients when

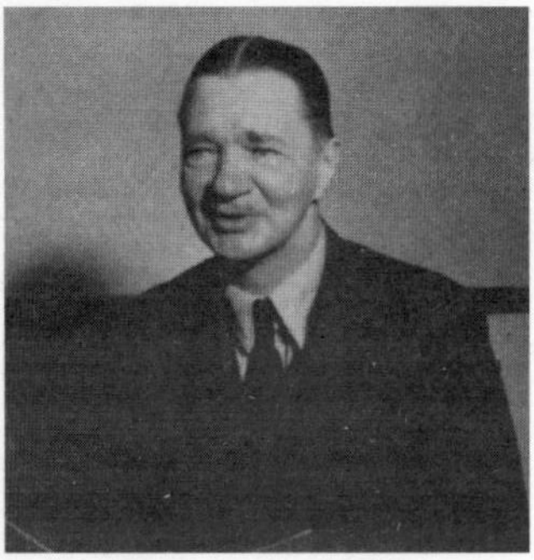

(The Star)

Dr Gordon Ryrie

> the Japs came, but on VJ day there were only 600 left. The rest had died of starvation and diseases. It was terrible to see ten or twelve die daily . . .

He took part in the underground resistance movement, giving medical treatment to wounded guerrillas until the Japanese caught him and sent him to Changi concentration camp in Singapore. By the time he was liberated, he was so severely weakened by repeated attacks of malaria and dysentery that he was forbidden to travel. Nevertheless, he made his way north of Kuala Lumpur to Sungei Buloh, where he found nothing but desolation: '. . . the hospital wards were empty, for no one was left able to care for the sick. Like wraiths over the untended paths, the patients came out of their houses with uncertain eyes and wavering gait, to welcome their liberators.'[47]

But Ryrie's own health had been undermined by the privations he'd suffered, and he was obliged to return to Britain.

During the war there had been some discussion at the Ministry of Health of a possible increase in the number of leprosy sufferers among troops and civilians serving in areas where the disease was endemic. This was not expected to exceed forty or fifty cases and at first it was hoped that the Homes of St Giles might be expanded, with government help, to cope with such an increase. But the case of a Polish ex-soldier with an English wife and a child, living across the Mersey from Liverpool in Wallasey, put paid to that notion.

This man had lived in Brazil for sixteen years before coming to Europe in 1940 to join the Polish Army. Two years later he was medically discharged, but leprosy was not diagnosed until 1947. By then he was 'a chronic alcoholic' and it was doubtful that 'he would remain in hospital even if he could be persuaded to go' – and some isolation hospital were prepared to accept him. The Fazakerley Hospital already had one Chinese leprosy patient who was causing trouble and upsetting staff so much that they were threatening to leave, and another had recently committed suicide there, so it was reluctant to admit a third.[48]

The obvious solution would have been to repatriate the man, but the fact that he had an English wife and a daughter precluded that. Though the child was at risk of infection with her father living at home, he could not be forced to go into a hospital or any other institution against his will so long as leprosy was not statutorily notifiable. And even if he were prepared to go, the only suitable refuge, St Giles, could not take him, (a) because it had no room, and (b) because it was 'legally precluded from taking non-British subjects':

> It thus becomes necessary to consider forthwith, in anticipation of the National Health Service, the setting up of a small institution under the Ministry's control for the care of lepers for whom such provision cannot otherwise be made, this action being all the more urgent because of the necessity of dealing at once with the Wallasey case . . .[49]

The Polish soldier was eventually taken into the Infectious Diseases Hospital, where he came under the care of Dr A.R.D. Adams of the Liverpool School of Tropical Medicine, a specialist in leprosy. To begin with, all went well. Then he developed a rash and became very depressed. In addition to suffering from a leprosy reaction, it was found that he had pulmonary tuberculosis and Dr Adams recommended moving him to another hospital with better facilities. The patient didn't want to move, and – in what the doctors considered to be more of a theatrical gesture than a serious attempt on his life – slit his throat. He was stitched up and moved anyway. Though his throat soon recovered, his general condition deteriorated, due to the TB. He refused treatment and, to the considerable relief of the authorities, died on 3 September 1948.[50]

But the need for a home run by the newly founded National Health Service and without the entry restrictions of the privately financed St Giles remained. Dr Adams was in favour of having a colony for leprosy patients along the lines of the Papworth Settlement near Cambridge, which was a kind of model village for tuberculosis sufferers. In such an institution they might live ordinary married lives – as long as any children were removed at birth for their protection – and could be offered employment, particularly such therapeutic outdoor work as farming and gardening. They should not be confined to the settlement, but allowed to venture out, and the public, including doctors and nurses, must be educated to recognise that they represented no more of a threat – less, in fact – than tuberculosis patients. He thought that 'to isolate a patient completely so that he had no contact with the outside was medically and psychologically wrong'.[51]

Adams may have been influenced by one of his own patients, the *Star*'s 'British Correspondent', Peter Hall. Isolated up on a mountain, in despair and going blind, Hall had had a vision of the good life: 'Somewhere down there in the pleasant valley there was a garden, with plenty of flowers, a few animals, a greenhouse, all tended by me, who had no previous experience of such things.' In December 1946 he found his garden on Merseyside, in the village of Melling. He had an acre of land, but after years of neglect it grew nothing but weeds:

> In the first few months of 1947, the land was frozen hard. Blindness came, so did mutilation of hands and, so they told me, disfigurement. My very good doctor and friend [Adams] said nothing, but I sensed the grimness in his voice. The good lady who cares for me, coming as she does from a long line of German pastors, never faltered. My one contact with the outside world was the radio.[52]

One Sunday night he heard a programme about what churches were doing for leprosy sufferers and wrote to the broadcaster. The reply – from the Mission to Lepers – was prompt and helpful. Hall learned about the new drug that was rumoured to be so effective and was given the address of the American Mission to Lepers (which was less financially stretched than its English counterpart). Dr Adams got hold of the sulphone drug and started treating him with it: 'Soon my eyesight was restored, ulcers healed, lesions vanished and now there is no sign of disfigurement.' The American Mission to Lepers was equally prompt in providing him with a small tractor and some implements, and he set to work clearing his land and making it productive. He planted fruit trees and kept a few geese and pigs and a 'nice mongrel pup'. Every night he went to bed exhausted but with a 'song in my heart', and every morning he woke to 'the cackle of geese, a friendly welcome from Strulch [the dog], and Sonia [one of the two pigs]'.[53]

Unlike Peter Greave, who had reason to be grateful to Dr Ryrie and BELRA for rescuing him from Calcutta in the nick of time, Peter Hall regarded both with a jaundiced eye. He lost no opportunity of questioning BELRA's activities and expertise, and compared Ryrie unfavourably with Adams. 'I place Dr Adams of the School of Tropical Medicine, Liverpool, streets ahead of any other [leprologist]', he wrote to the Minister of Health, Aneurin Bevan, in 1949, 'and you can throw Ryrie in the list . . .' He had been in Ryrie's care for some months in

1941, just before the Japanese invasion. He had been working as a technical civil servant in Singapore when he was diagnosed, not by any doctor he went to see but by his Chinese servant, as having *marfu* – leprosy. He was eventually sent to Sungei Buloh, and when he arrived there the doctor (Ryrie) made him strip: 'There in the open for all to see I was told I was a leper and would come under the law of forcible segregation.' He called the settlement 'Totalitarian Valley' and wrote of his predicament there:

> Apart from the Medical Superintendent, his lay assistant and the Matron who lived apart in more senses than one, I was the only European dwelling within the fenced area of the law. I was an outcast among outcasts. A leper among lepers.[54]

Ryrie's treatment of a fellow European, who was still in a state of shock over his misfortune, may have been lacking in tact. While Hall wrote chatty letters, full of charm and generosity, he could be prickly in his dealings with officialdom. Those who had regular contact with him seem to have warmed to his quirky personality, but a welfare officer who visited him in the 1960s described him as 'a very embittered man'. Such bitterness probably stemmed from his experience of isolation in what was known in Malay as the 'Home of the Rotten Men', to which the afflicted were conveyed in a 'specially designed leper truck, very like a cattle truck'.[55]

Even before he'd left Singapore for Sungei Buloh, Hall had learned 'how true "Shunned like a leper" could be':

> I was distressed to discover how many of my large circle of friends quit. Where fear and ignorance might have been excusable, I found the opposite. The heathen Chinese stood firm, the civilised European walked on the opposite side of the street. I had looked for succour in the wrong places.[56]

On his arrival in 'Totalitarian Valley', Hall had been assigned a hut next door to a Eurasian sergeant major – Tam was 'a kind of Major Domo to the Colony' and used his power to enrich himself and lead a comfortable life. As a European, and the only paying inmate (he paid three Malay dollars a day), Hall had the best accommodation, but that wasn't saying much. He inherited 'a stinking mattress' from a previous tenant with a passion for chaulmoogra, or hydnocarpus oil, and to begin with he just lay on it, hypersensitive to any noise – including the slithering sounds of a python that had made its home in his loft:

> These intrusions I never resented. On the contrary I rather welcomed them for somehow I had a bond with Norman as I christened him. He too was lonely and despised, but he had his freedom to come and go as he wished, which was one up on me.

Hall worried that Norman might end up in a cooking pot, as some Chinese believed that 'a diet of dogs and snakes will affect [*sic*] a cure'; his tacit understanding with his unseen companion was that neither would disturb the other: 'If he has not fallen foul of the Japanese atrocity machine, [or] a native's machete, and the hut still stands, he may be there still, which puts me one up on Norman.'

Hall eventually forced himself to go out and join a group of people who'd just been watching an outdoor movie. These film shows took place every two or three weeks and afterwards there was always a lively debate at which Hall, once he had earned the others' trust, picked up 'views and information of what centuries of fear, ignorance and neglect had done to cause so much distress to lepers'. He learned all about his fellow patients. At one extreme there was Hadji, who had contracted the disease as a child: half Malay, half Arab and a brilliant linguist, he was, in Hall's opinion, 'the finest man East of Suez'. At the other, there was a young Chinese who was rumoured to be a millionaire and was certainly a successful businessman, owning two shops, a zoo and a poultry farm, and planning to build a private swimming pool on the premises:

> Altogether, one way or another, he must have employed thirty or forty patients. From a good-looking young fellow he had advanced in the disease, his face [had] assumed the dreaded leonine look, and he bore the sign of the clutching hand. Often at night he would smuggle his car out, ostensibly to visit his sister, but rumour, ever a lying jade, had it that he hit the high spots. He must have had considerable protection.

Hall had been promised employment in the so-called 'technical school', which was little more than a covered yard with an old and unserviceable van 'in some stage of undress' standing at its centre; but neither that nor any other means of occupying himself materialised. He was, however, allowed to go into nearby Kuala Lumpur – 'providing I steered clear of hotels, cafes, cinemas, or anywhere I was likely to be identified, which would mean the ringing of telephone bells, and the warning a leper was at large'. As for treatment, the Medical Superintendent (whom Hall never names in his memoir) soon disabused him of any such expectations:

> The law does not say you must have treatment. The law simply says you are a danger to others and must be separated from contact with healthy people. Neither the RAF [his employers in Singapore] nor health authorities care very much what will happen to you if you are found temperamentally unsuitable for Sungei Buloh. They will just sling you home and drop you.

It's clear that Ryrie and Hall didn't get on. Hall bitterly resented his loss of freedom and admits that he found the atmosphere of Sungei Buloh 'dictatorial, as all one-man governed states are'. He was aware that others might feel differently, that what was 'a living hell' for one person might be another's 'home from home'. And his rebelliousness served him well, as it enabled him to escape from Sungei Buloh and Malaya just before the Japanese came. His 'way back to normality' was via Scotland, where he was held in an institution in a ward full of children – of all unsuitable places – until he absconded five weeks after his arrival and headed for

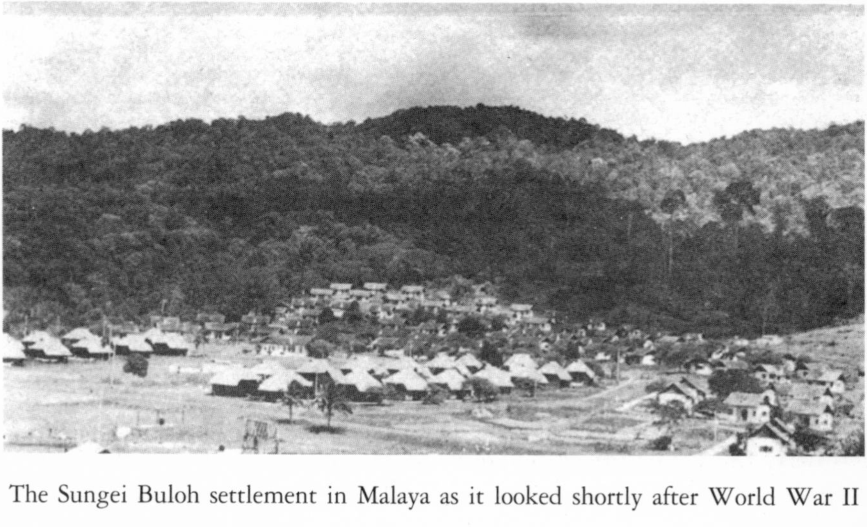

(The Star)

The Sungei Buloh settlement in Malaya as it looked shortly after World War II

Liverpool. Since then he had been living 'a semi secluded life, happy and contented' under the watchful eye of Dr Adams until he read in a newspaper of a move to include leprosy in the list of statutorily notifiable diseases. This was what had prompted him to write to Nye Bevan.

In his letter, he contrasted his treatment in Britain, where 'enlightened civil servants at high level gave me every chance to live a normal working life' – though 'less enlightened individuals made life a little difficult' – with his experience of legal ostracism in Malaya and pleaded with Bevan as Minister of Health not to introduce compulsory notification.[57]

For his *bête noire* Dr Ryrie, in his capacity as government adviser on leprosy, this was just one of a number of measures needed to combat the disease, the most urgent of which was to open an NHS leprosy home. The government's favoured site was the old Reigate Isolation Hospital outside Redhill, which, suitably adapted, could function as an annexe to the Hospital for Tropical Diseases in London (where active treatment would be undertaken). But Ryrie took against the Ministry's preferred option:

> Reigate struck me as one of the most dismal places I have ever seen. I can, of course, suggest lines of adaptation, but I think it would be just as cheap to make a fresh start. We cannot expect any really scientific work of interest in Reigate.[58]

(He'd visited Carville en route to Havana for the 1948 International Congress of Leprology and had been mightily impressed by the extent of its medical staff and scientific facilities, compared to which St Giles, 'the only place in Britain for the care of lepers', hadn't 'even a microscope'.[59])

The government ignored Ryrie's objections to the Reigate Isolation Hospital and plans went ahead to convert it into a long-stay facility for about twenty leprosy sufferers. Conveniently, perhaps, Ryrie resigned as BELRA's medical secretary when his health finally broke down soon after this; he was the same age as the century and died in 1953. Dr Robert Cochrane replaced him, taking on the job for the second time and also becoming the government's consultant on leprosy. Like Ryrie, Cochrane favoured some form of notification, regarding it as essential to have exact information on the number of cases in Britain, but they both shared Ministry of Health officials' – and Peter Hall's – anxiety not to expose leprosy patients to obloquy. So when the Notification of Leprosy became law in June 1951, local medical officers of health were bypassed – much to their chagrin – and the Ministry was to be informed directly, in order to maintain 'strict secrecy'. The government recognised that the public had 'an exaggerated horror' of leprosy and urged people

> to learn that it is an ordinary medical disease, not highly dangerous or infective, and extend to the person who has been unfortunate enough to contract leprosy, generally in the service of the Crown, that sympathy and understanding which he deserves.[60]

Even Peter Hall acknowledged that 'the Ministry [had] been very wise, considerate and sympathetic', particularly in refraining from introducing statutory powers to remove leprosy sufferers to hospital. Commenting in the *Star*, Stanley Stein wrote, 'Verily when we compare the British law with our own, we American citizens shall have grave doubts about our right to boast that this is the "land of liberty".'[61]

In addition to introducing notification regulations, the government announced the opening of the Jordan Hospital (as it was to be called) in Reigate. Inevitably, there was local resistance to having a leprosy hospital in the Reigate area and 'more particularly about the patients being allowed to move in and around the town'. In an attempt to defuse the situation, the mayor and corporation of Reigate were invited to the Ministry of Health to meet senior officials, including Dr Cochrane, in December 1951. The government officials reassured the local authority, saying that while 'it would be inexpedient to impose complete restriction, even if it were practicable, on the patients at Jordan Hospital, because this would cause them to leave or others to refuse to come to the hospital, thus defeating the whole object of the Ministry's efforts to deal with the problem', they had nevertheless 'taken steps to see that patients . . . were enjoined to exercise every care, to avoid frequenting the town as much as possible, and to refrain from visiting restaurants or public houses'.[62]

Fear and loathing of leprosy were so ingrained that not even the family of the physician in charge of the Jordan Hospital was exempt. Dr William H. Jopling recalled that he had been in residence three years before 'any local children were allowed by their parents to visit the doctor's house', even though two of his four children were at a local school. If it hadn't been for an enlightened and highly respected local medical officer of health, who spoke up for the hospital at public protest meetings, it would have been harder to carry the project through.[63]

The Jordan Hospital accommodated twenty-four patients in separate flats, each consisting of a bed-sitting room, kitchen and bathroom. There were twice as many men as women there. In the seventeen years of its existence, the bulk of the patients came from India (they were mostly Anglo-Indians whose families had been cold-shouldered out of the country after independence), with a sprinkling of Greeks and Maltese. Jopling had become interested in leprosy when he was a government medical officer in Rhodesia before the Second World War. He looked like – and in his youth had been – a rugby player, and was 'a lifelong socialist and humanist (and campaigner for nuclear disarmament)', a keen naturalist, fisherman and musician. His senior nursing sister throughout the Jordan era, Jean Cooper, became his second wife.[64]

The memories of patients there (four of whom have talked to the present writer) are mostly happy ones. One said he 'loved it at Jordan'; there were a lot of Anglo-Indians – 'which is how I am classified' – both men and women, and several Indians: 'Hindus think [leprosy is] a curse from the gods, a matter of shame, and some tried to commit suicide . . .' Yet you couldn't hope to find a happier bunch of people: 'Most of it I put down to the staff, who helped us to keep a sense of proportion and a sense of humour; they treated us as another human being.' (He should know; he married the cook there and they were still together forty years later!) For another, a young Jewish woman who had grown up in Calcutta and was for some time the only member of her family in England, Dr Jopling became something of a father figure; she would turn to him when she encountered racial prejudice among the other patients (and staff): 'Dr Jopling was so good to me, he put his wing over me.' A third, who was there a decade later, in the early 1960s, remembered Dr Jopling playing tennis with the patients, but said that his family – 'he had two daughters' – kept to themselves. Wisely, perhaps, in view of the fact that this Anglo-Indian ex-patient 'found it easy to date the nurses, they were so full of religious fervour' and 'even used to visit the nurses' home at St Pancras'.[65]

But another Anglo-Indian, Patrick M, who first went there in the mid-1950s, 'rebelled against the system' and 'got off on the wrong foot with Dr Jopling'. Patrick had grown up in Bombay, where his father worked in Customs & Excise, and came to England as a young man with his mother and two older sisters in 1951. He was conscripted into the army for National Service in 1953 and joined the Royal Inniskillen Fusiliers in Northern Ireland, where he completed ten weeks of basic training. Before being posted to Korea, however, he had to undergo a medical examination and it was then that a sharp-eyed doctor spotted a rash on his left thigh and took a skin biopsy, which revealed that he had leprosy. He spent several weeks in isolation at the Military Hospital at Waringfield, where the staff took care to avoid him; when they brought his meals, they knocked on the door and left the food outside for him to collect. He soon became restless and the army doctors feared he would abscond. So in the end he was sent home, pending further treatment, and arrived in Chiswick under escort: 'My mother nearly died when I turned up between two military policemen, but they saluted her and handed me over like a parcel they'd been instructed to deliver.'[66]

He was medically discharged from the army, but it wasn't until a year later – 'the wheels of bureaucracy were turning slowly' – that he was instructed to report to the Jordan Hospital in Surrey. When he was shown his room, he was 'completely gob-smacked'. It suddenly struck him that this wasn't a hospital at all, but 'a leper colony'. He went around asking the other patients how long they'd been there and when they answered in years rather than months he thought, 'Oh my God . . .' He was given medication – DDS – but even after six months felt he was making no progress. When he looked at his fellow patients he realised that most of them had nowhere to go, whereas he had his 'mother and a lovely home'. With nothing to do all day, he began to court trouble. His doctor's notes tell their own story:

> 1/1/55. Has not got down to any studies yet – is kicking around aimlessly. To start gardening work on Monday.
> 12/1/55. Spoke to him about being out till 11.20 p.m. yesterday without permission . . . Missing gardening work as he is a hopeless slacker and backslider.
> 30/3/55. Began gardening last Monday . . .[67]

Patrick didn't mind the gardening because it was paid work – well, sort of: 'You didn't have to work that hard, you could skive and still get £1 at the end of the week.' And it was better than doing nothing. Boredom was the main enemy, which was why he visited the pub down the road where the attitude was 'We don't want you bloody lepers here' and got into an argument with the landlady.

Now a confirmed troublemaker, Patrick was ordered to leave the Jordan in July 1955 and attend the Hospital for Tropical Diseases in London as an outpatient. The medical officer of health for Hammersmith, who visited his home soon after, reported that he lived in 'a pleasant and sufficiently large flat with his mother and two sisters' and that he planned to go back to his old job as a mechanic in a firm in Chiswick High Road but had not yet done so because he would've had to explain why he'd failed to complete his two years of National Service. In October 1957 Patrick was readmitted to the Jordan Hospital 'owing to a severe reactional state', but warned about his conduct. His health may have improved as an inpatient, but his behaviour had not. He was discharged once again 'on disciplinary grounds' at the end of the following June. Dr Jopling provided a list of his shortcomings:

1) Refusal to get up in the mornings at a reasonable hour and to tidy his room.
2) Persistence in reporting to see me on Tuesday and Thursday mornings unshaven in spite of warnings that he should be washed and shaved before reporting for examination.
3) Rudeness to Mrs de M on one occasion when he shouted at her and abused her, resulting in Mrs de M feeling ill and very upset. On this occasion he was rude to Father J who tried to remonstrate with him.
4) Refusal to report at the Treatment Room at the proper times.[68]

Jopling added, 'As would be expected, this patient had to be taken off gardening work in view of his persistent slackness.' After his second discharge from the institution he loathed, Patrick managed to give the doctors the slip. Nearly four years later, the Hammersmith medical officer of health went to visit him but found that he was no longer living at the address he'd given. His sister told the MOH she had no idea where he was living or working: 'She thinks that he got a girl into trouble and got behind with his payments [of rent].' As far as she knew, Patrick was in good health.[69]

In his late sixties, and dying of cancer, Patrick could laugh with the doctors looking after him at the catalogue of his past misdemeanours. But at the time he had been – to use the psychological jargon – 'in denial'. About the time when he found work in a local engineering factory, where they had no inkling of his medical history, he said, 'I really did not care about Hansen's; at times I didn't think I even had it.' However, he did feel obliged to tell the woman he was to marry about it and was gratified by her response: 'Is that all?' she said, 'I thought you were going to give me the push!' They had children together and Patrick continued to avoid the doctors, though he kept taking dapsone (DDS) pills in the belief that they were all he needed to continue leading a normal life. But still his health deteriorated. What he hadn't realised was that he'd become dapsone-resistant; the magic pills were no longer working. In the end, even Patrick had to give in and seek medical advice; after years of missing appointments at the Hospital for Tropical Diseases despite repeated warnings of the serious consequences of a relapse, in 1987 he went to see the consultant leprologist there, Dr M.F.R. Walters, who said he'd never seen 'as gross a relapse of lepromatous leprosy'.[70]

Patrick's determined non-cooperation with the medical authorities was untypical of patients at the Jordan. Dr Jopling reckoned that the two most common psychiatric problems there were 'reactive depression and schizophrenia'. There were a few cases of suicide and attempted suicide due to one or other of these causes, or – in the case of a newly arrived Indian businessman who successfully did away with himself and left a note saying why – an inability to face the future. By contrast, in twenty-five years of work with Hansen's disease *outpatients* Jopling 'never encountered mental breakdown or attempted suicide'.[71] This observation tells its own story and strongly supports the notion that Patrick's otherwise unforgivably boorish behaviour was, in essence, a survival strategy. (The same applies to Peter Hall's occasional outbursts of rudeness in the face of persistent official questioning; in an uncomprehending, if not actively hostile, world he knew just how tenuous his freedom was.)

The Jordan Hospital closed in 1967, not through any shortage of patients but because a combination of new drugs – such as rifampicin, whose bactericidal properties minimised any public health risk associated with the disease – and outpatient clinics was proving more effective (and less expensive) than prolonged segregation in controlling leprosy. The remaining patients either went into sheltered accommodation or, in more chronic cases, to the Homes of St Giles. In nearly four decades between 1951, the year the disease became notifiable, and 1989 a total of 1,249 patients were treated for leprosy in England and none of them contracted it in this country; every single one – even the twenty who were English – was infected abroad.[72]

An American who was familiar with Carville visited the 'beautiful' Homes of St Giles in 1967 and was reminded of 'an exclusive country club'. Mavourneen Morriss and her husband were well received by the senior nun, who showed them round and introduced them to some of the patients. Morriss was just wondering if Peter Greave, whose *The Second Miracle* had made a deep impression on her, was still alive when Sister Gloria telepathically asked if she would like to meet him. She was delighted to make the acquaintance of this 'tall, angular man', who was interested in Carville and praised Stanley Stein and his editorial staff on the *Star* for doing such a 'wonderful job' in educating the public about Hansen's disease. Morriss found Greave's bungalow 'charming', like all the others at St Giles, but 'not quite as orderly' as some – though perhaps that was only 'to be expected of a sixty-year-old bachelor'.[73]

Leaving aside the fact that Greave wasn't a bachelor but a widower who'd been devastated by the early death of his much younger wife from cancer and, according to Les Parker, a friend at St Giles, 'never really recovered', this was something of an understatement. His rooms were a complete tip; he chain-smoked and dropped ash and cigarettes all over the floor.[74] He had never been tidy but following his wife's death, which forced him to return to St Giles after years of living in a Wiltshire village where she taught and he wrote and recorded unscripted talks for BBC radio, he ceased to care; he was finally losing his sight and all that remained for him was to complete his last – and greatest – book.

Les Parker recalls how Greave, before he went blind, would read him each chapter from whatever book he was writing as soon as he'd finished it. But lulled by the droning voice on one soporific summer's afternoon 'after a boozy lunch' Les fell asleep. Greave, who had 'a very short fuse', indignantly woke him up and dismissed him from his presence. Late that night there came a knock on Les's door and Les, who knew perfectly well who it was, called out, 'If it's anyone but Peter, come in.' Greave had come to apologise for his earlier petulance.[75]

Peter Greave died at St Giles in November 1977 at the age of sixty-seven. *The Seventh Gate* had received an enthusiastic reception when it had been published the previous year. But he would not have wished to live on, alone and sightless, into the 1980s when St Giles ceased to be a hospital and was taken over by a housing association catering for troubled youths, many of them with mental disabilities. Les Parker, one of a handful of Hansen's disease patients left, sympathised with the youngsters' predicament but questioned 'whether this population was best suited to join us at St Giles'. The remaining HD patients, who were used to '24-hour, 7-day-a-week specialized medical care', now had to make do with one part-time nurse. It was, of course, a matter for celebration that there was no longer any need for a leprosy hospital in Britain, but for survivors this progress had led to 'a feeling of abandonment'. They looked back nostalgically to the era when everyone at St Giles 'had the same problems and understood each other. In many ways' – as Parker told an audience at the fifteenth International Leprosy Congress in Beijing in 1998 – 'I feel more isolated and alone than ever.'[76]

Just down the road from St Giles is a small, overgrown graveyard with a lych-gate. A notice inside the gate draws attention to the number of rare plants and creatures that flourish in this tiny, chemical- and fertiliser-free nature reserve. Essex wildlife enthusiasts lovingly preserve its unkempt, wilderness state, but there is no mention of those who lie buried beneath the stone crosses on which the names are almost indecipherable even where the tangled undergrowth has not rendered them inaccessible, no mention of the cemetery's unique history as the final resting-place of leprosy patients and sisters who remain symbiotically linked even in death. What a contrast to the cemetery at Carville, where the grass is regularly mown and the graves tended with loving care. Yet in some ways the neglect of the graves is appropriate, a suitable memorial for those of whom Peter Greave, considering the centuries of vilification and abuse their kind had endured, writes:

> . . . when I think of this enormous span of time, a picture, vivid and compelling, forms in my mind. I see a great multitude of outcasts, a thousand ragged, lost battalions, stretching back through the ages, until they disappear below the curve of time. It seems impossible ever to calculate the hundreds of thousands of hearts this merciless disease has broken, the agonizing loneliness and misery left in its wake.[77]

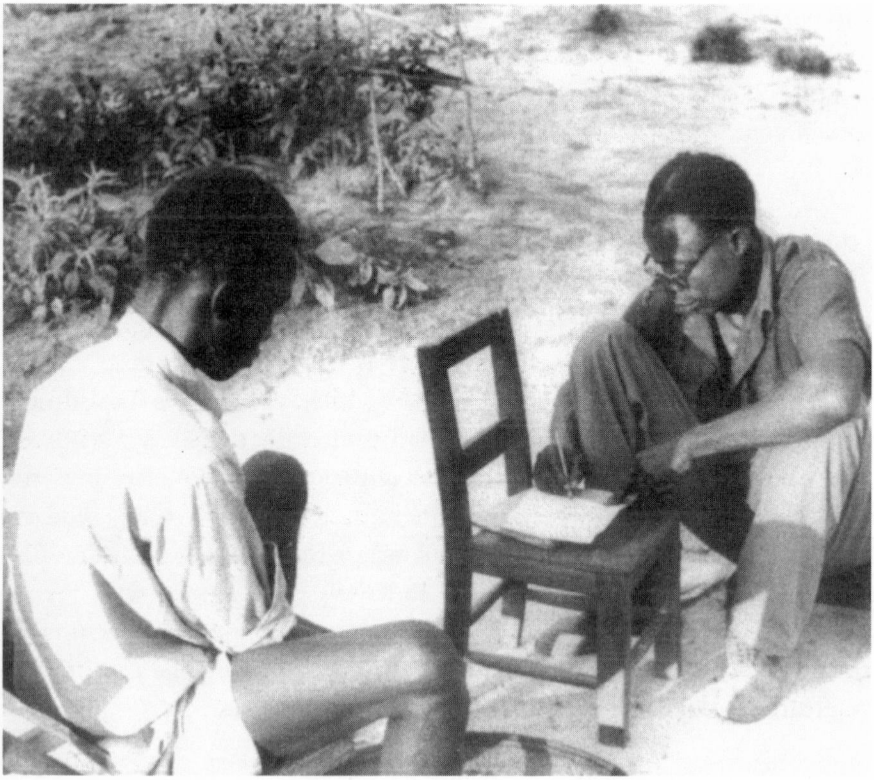

(Courtesy of Michel F. Lechat)

A leprosy patient and a medical auxiliary in the Belgian Congo in the 1950s

Chapter 12

'SAINT PAUL' BRAND AND 'MR LEPROSY' BROWNE

> . . . if I could choose one gift for my leprosy patients it would be the gift of pain . . .[1]
>
> Dr Paul Brand (1994)

When the 1968 International Leprosy Congress opened in London, the medical correspondent of *The Times* wrote that 'for generations [leprosy] has been trapped by various religious and charitable organisations with an almost proprietary interest in the disease' and welcomed its release from the shackles that had kept it 'out of the mainstream of medical progress and research'. A. Donald Miller, the long-serving general secretary of the Mission to Lepers (recently renamed The Leprosy Mission in deference to patients' sensitivity about the L-word), reacted with a mixture of bewilderment and indignation:

> This is not only a contortion; it is an absolute contradiction of the truth. We know that it was Christians, and particularly Christian missionaries, who were in the vanguard, not of trapping men with leprosy, but of bringing them liberty. It was where there was not the Christian spirit that leprosy victims were trapped, because of the ignorance and fear of men and women; trapped because of penal legislation, and trapped by the hopelessness of their disease.

Miller clinched the point with a roll-call of living British missionary doctors 'who have been liberating, not trapping, leprosy', including such honoured names as Ernest Muir, Robert Cochrane, John Lowe, T. Frank Davey, Paul Brand and Stanley G. Browne.[2]

The gospel may have been their inspiration but these men were certainly not unaware of the ambiguous historical relationship between missionaries and 'their' disease. Social prejudice against the disease, as Browne for one recognised, 'may even be engendered by Christian preachers who derive their ideas from Biblical references to "leprosy" and "lepers"'. On the other hand:

> Christian Missions have been the pioneers in showing Christ-like compassion and genuine sympathy for those afflicted with leprosy, and the emotional sentimentalism of a former generation is being replaced by practical help in curing the disease, in preventing the deformities it leads to, and in mitigating its psychological and social consequences.[3]

In their different ways, Brand and Browne did as much as any doctor – religious or secular – to advance the understanding and treatment of leprosy. Brand made his name in the field of reconstructive surgery, overturning the conventional wisdom about the relationship between the leprosy bacillus and disability in the process, and went on to cover all aspects of the physical and social rehabilitation of the patient. Browne's contribution was more in the field of public health; he conducted surveys and developed the concept of lay workers scattered over areas with high prevalence of the disease dispensing drugs aimed at both prevention and cure, and was himself crucially involved in experimentation with clofazimine, or B663, one of the three main anti-leprosy drugs used today. In their approach to leprosy in the sulphone era these two Christian doctors represented opposite ends of the spectrum: Brand always focused on care of the individual patient, while Browne's emphasis was more on the elimination of the disease.

Paul Wilson Brand was born in July 1914 in southern India. His parents were missionaries who eschewed the easy life of the plains for the challenge of the *Kolli Malai*, or 'mountains of death', so-called because they were the home of the malaria-carrying *Anopheles* mosquito. Jesse Brand, Paul's father, had trained as a builder, but both he and his wife Evelyn had done a short medical course as part of their preparation to be missionaries, and word of their medical skills soon got around among the hill tribes, who – for want of the real thing – took to calling them 'doctor' and lining up outside the door of their self-built bungalow for treatment. Despite recurrent bouts of malaria, Paul and his sister Connie had an idyllic childhood in the Kolli hills, which imbued Paul with a lifelong love of nature, of animals and, in particular, birds.[4]

His parents encouraged the children's interest in their work, so Paul was surprised to be sent into the house one day when three strange-looking men approached. He was so curious that he 'sneaked out and peered through the bushes'. He was amazed to see his father put on a pair of gloves to remove dirty bandages from hands and feet missing a number of digits before dressing the purulent sores he'd exposed. Was his father afraid? Jesse did not joke with these men in the way he did with other patients and when they'd gone, leaving a basket of fruit as a token of gratitude, Evelyn burned both basket and gloves – 'an unheard-of act of waste'. Paul and Connie were ordered to keep away from the spot where the men had been: 'Those men were *lepers*, we were told.'[5]

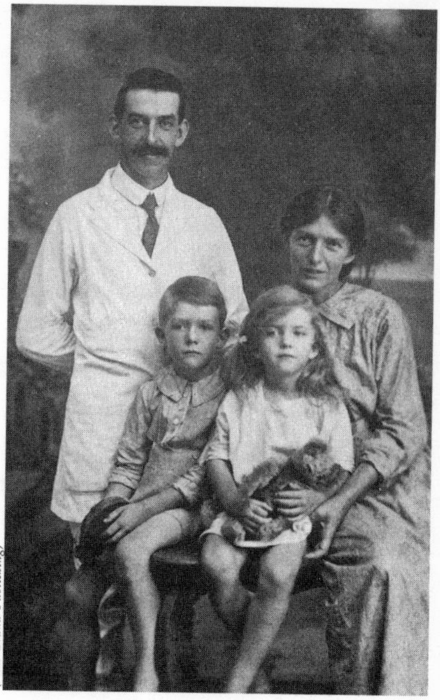
(Paul Brand Publishing)

Jesse and Evelyn Brand, with their children Paul and Connie

At the age of nine, Paul was sent home to England, along with Connie, for their formal education. Like so many other sons and daughters of the empire, he found the adjustment from the spacious, vibrant and mysterious life of the east to the cloistered, regimented existence of an English boarding school difficult, and he lived for his parents' long and detailed letters; his mother's were full of the doings of local people, his father's with drawings and notes of all he had observed on his walks in the forest. Paul had to wait six years before the news that he'd been longing for came: Jesse and Evelyn were taking a year's home leave – and just at the time when Paul was beginning to think about his own future career and wonder what he should do with his life. The joyous prospect of this parental visit was still fresh in his mind when a telegram arrived announcing his father's death. Jesse, just forty-four, had died of blackwater fever, a lethal complication of malaria. As Brand puts it, 'The mountains of death had claimed yet another victim.'[6]

Sea mail took such a long time to arrive that Paul continued to receive his father's lively and informative letters for months after he'd learned of his sudden death. So when these letters stopped coming it was as though his father had died a second time. Meanwhile, his mother's letters were becoming increasingly distracted and a member of the family was despatched to India to bring her home. When she arrived, a year or more later, Paul was shocked to see how greatly she'd aged. Of course he'd changed, too; he was no longer a young lad of nine, but an adolescent teetering on the brink of adulthood. Even so, he could not reconcile the 'hunched-over figure with hair prematurely gray and the posture of a woman in her eighties', who had to grasp the railing for support as she came down the gangplank, with the 'tall, beautiful woman overflowing with energy and laughter' of his memory. He could barely bring himself to call her Mother.[7]

Yet this same broken woman, who castigated herself over and over again for her husband's death and wondered how she would ever be able to carry on in the hills without him, returned there a year later and set about 'the work of medicine, education, agriculture, and teaching the Gospel' with renewed determination, riding tirelessly over the mountains on Jesse's old horse. The horse – and others – died, but she kept on; and when she grew too old to ride (or, as she preferred to put it, the horses too old to be ridden), she traversed the mountain ranges on foot, 'leaning heavily on tall bamboo poles which she grasped in each hand'. The fact that she was officially retired by the mission in her seventieth year made no difference; she went on just as before, earning herself the title of 'Mother of the Hills' among the tribes to whom she'd devoted her life. Her proudest achievement was to rid the hills of the guinea worm parasite that had plagued the people until she taught them to guard their wells from animals and children and to strain their water before drinking it. 'Granny Brand' had become a local legend well before she died in 1975 at the age of ninety-five.[8]

Fatherless, Paul Brand sought to follow in his father's footsteps. He left school at sixteen and served a five-year apprenticeship in the building trade, learning 'carpentry, architecture, roofing, plumbing, electricity, and stone-masonry'. The last-named was his favourite and, like a latter-day Jude the Obscure, he visited the great English cathedrals and ran his hands 'over the rippled texture of stone pillars and arches, awed by the realization that each tiny ridge marked the rise and fall of a medieval mason's wooden mallet'. Like his father, too, he signed up for a year's course at the Livingstone College Medical School, but more out of a sense of duty than from any great love of medicine. So he was pleasantly surprised to find 'that the science of medicine could tap into the sense of wonder I already felt towards nature' and that clinical work, such as tooth extractions, 'drew on the manual skills I had developed as a carpenter and mason, and had the excellent advantage of ending someone's toothache'. Nevertheless, he persisted in his plan of becoming a missionary builder in India and went to the Missionary Training Colony, which 'combined the rigors of Sparta, the ideals of Queen Victoria, and the jolly teamwork of the Boy Scouts'.[9]

It was no good. Medicine had become his passion. He resigned from the Colony and in 1937 went to University College Hospital medical school in London. His training was overtaken by the outbreak of the Second World War, which inevitably broadened his experience as he worked through nights of the blitz performing surgical operations while still a student. During the war he got married to a fellow medical student called Margaret Berry whose father was a doctor, too. The first of their several children was born in 1944 and by the time Brand, now a Fellow of the Royal College of Surgeons, received a telegram from Dr Robert Cochrane inviting him to teach surgery at the Christian Medical College at Vellore, in south India, Margaret was pregnant again. Paul turned down the offer, remarking that, among other things, he was awaiting his military call-up as well as a second child. But he'd reckoned without Cochrane's persistence. The 'irrepressible Scotsman' known as 'Uncle Bob' turned up in London and brushed aside all Brand's objections; he even persuaded the War Office to accept Paul's time in India as the equivalent of military service. As for family, Vellore was a 'wonderful place for women and children' and Margaret (who supported the idea) could join Paul as soon as she'd had the baby and was ready to follow him.[10]

Until his ship docked in Bombay, Brand had little idea of the imaginative hold the land of his childhood still had on him. Quoting Kipling – 'Smells are surer than sounds or sights to make your heart-strings crack' – he refers to India as 'a land of limitless redolence'. He pooh-poohs the notion that western doctors working in third world countries are 'self-sacrificing heroes' and asserts that they're 'having the time of their lives':

> I know too many physicians in the West who spend half their hours filling out insurance forms, wrangling with government health programs, choosing computerized record-keeping systems, shopping for malpractice insurance, listening to pharmacy sales reps. Give me India any day.[11]

Though he was employed as a lecturer in surgery at Vellore, Brand was soon drawn into Cochrane's speciality – leprosy. Uncle Bob saw it as his job to bring leprosy into the mainstream of medicine (*pace* the remarks of *The Times*' medical correspondent). He described himself as a gadfly: 'I like to tease the professors and researchers, and if they can't believe what I say, then I tell them to start finding out the truth.' He challenged Brand to 'find a solution to the problems of deformity in leprosy', taking him to the huge Lady Willingdon Leprosy Sanatorium at Chingleput, near Madras, where Brand, once he'd got over the shock of the 'gargoylish appearance of the advanced leprosy patients', turned his attention to their hands: 'Never in my life had I seen so many stumps and claw-hands . . . Some hands lacked thumbs and fingers altogether.' He couldn't believe what Cochrane was telling him, that no orthopaedic surgeon had worked in leprosy 'even though it has crippled more people than polio or any other disease'.

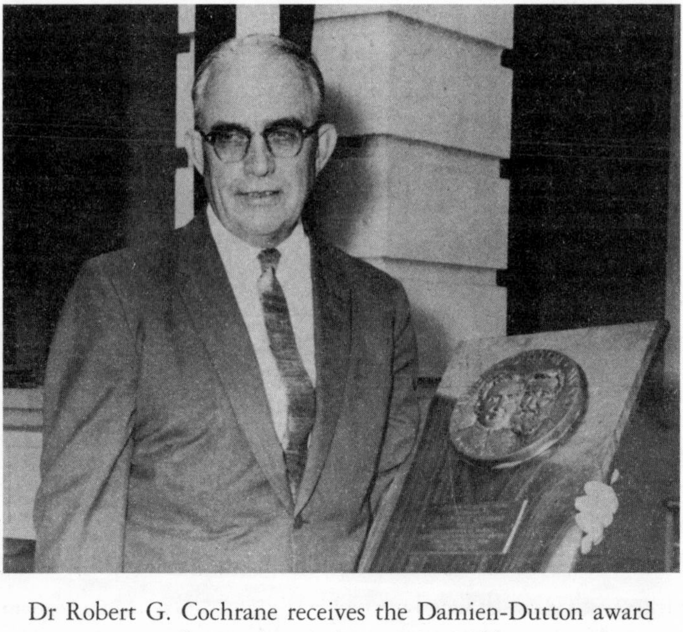

(*The Star*)

Dr Robert G. Cochrane receives the Damien-Dutton award for services to leprosy in 1964

> 'You're thinking of leprosy like other diseases, Paul,' [Cochrane] said. 'But doctors, like most people, put it in a separate category altogether. They view leprosy as a curse of the gods . . . You'll find priests, missionaries, and a few crackpots working in leprosy settlements, but rarely a good physician and never a specialist in orthopedics.'[12]

As a surgeon 'who loved hands', Brand was appalled at the extent of the damage he saw that day. He could only shake his head sadly at such 'waste'. These poor ruined creatures with their claw-hands . . . Or so he thought until one of them, responding to his invitation to squeeze his hand, held it in such a vice-like grip that he had to beg him to let go – 'in this one man's grip I had first-hand proof that a "useless" hand concealed live, powerful muscles. Paralysis? My own hand still ached from his grip.' He asked himself why it was that this man who could not separate his fingers to pick up a pencil had such a strong grasp. Now that Brand's mind as well as his sympathy was engaged, Cochrane knew he'd enlisted a powerful ally in his 'religious crusade', his war against leprosy.[13]

Brand set out to learn all he could about the disease. At the fourth International Congress of Leprology, which had been held in Cairo in 1938, much attention had been given to typology and 'tuberculoid leprosy was admitted to the classification'. At the other end of the scale, what had previously been known as the 'cutaneous' form of the disease 'became the lepromatous type'. These now came to be regarded as the 'polar forms' of leprosy, with lepromatous (and borderline) cases being seen as 'the main source of infection'.[14] In tuberculoid cases, as Brand now learned, many of the symptoms – 'patches of dead skin, loss of sensation, and a little nerve damage, but no extensive disfigurement' – resulted from 'the body's own furious autoimmune response to the foreign bacilli'. But one in every five patients lacked natural immunities and these were the ones who were classified as lepromatous and ended up in places like Chingleput, where one of the local names for leprosy was 'creeping death'.[15]

Brand admitted to a 'deep-seated prejudice and fear' of the disease:

> Patients presented the most horrible, purulent sores for treatment, and often the pungent odor of pus and gangrene filled the storeroom. Even though I had heard Bob Cochrane's assurances about the low contagion rate, I, like most people who worked with leprosy back then, worried constantly about infection.

He recalls that on one occasion when he flew back to England he was horrified to discover that he had no sensation in the heel of one foot:

> A dread fear worse than any nausea seized my stomach. Had it finally happened? Every leprosy worker recognizes insensitivity to pain as one of the disease's first symptoms. Had I just made the wretched leap from leprosy doctor to leprosy patient?

He knew only too well what to expect: 'Ordinary pleasures in life would slip away. Petting a dog, running a hand across fine silk, holding a child – soon all sensation would feel alike: dead.' Of course he didn't have leprosy; he was 'only a weary traveller made neurotic by illness and fatigue'. But constant exposure to chronic lepromatous cases of the disease induced a mortal dread of this affliction in even the most level-headed of leprosy workers in the days when the concept of a cure was still a radical departure.[16]

Once Brand's humane sympathy and scientific curiosity were aroused, however, his commitment to patients and research alike was absolute. He worked steadily, collecting data from 2,000 patients at Chingleput and elsewhere, and while he conducted his tests he listened to their stories. Both tests and stories revealed a pattern. The stories were invariably of rejection and despair, and they gave Brand an unforgettable sense of 'the human tragedy of leprosy'. The tests revealed what he had suspected at the beginning: 'frequent paralysis in areas controlled by the ulnar nerve, moderate paralysis in the median nerve, and very little in the radian nerve.'

Autopsies were almost impossible to arrange in India because of religious objections from both Hindus and Muslims, but when a chronic leprosy patient with no known relatives died Brand was given twenty-four hours to perform one before the corpse was cremated. He took full advantage of this unique opportunity, working with a colleague through the night. His findings confirmed that nerve swellings occurred 'only where the nerve lay close to the skin surface, and not in the deep tissues'. These swellings 'were in fact evidence of the body's own defensive response to an invasion' and though the implications of what the autopsy revealed – that 'to multiply, leprosy bacilli prefer the cooler temperatures that prevail close to the surface (this also explains why they seek refuge in testicles, earlobes, eyes and nasal passages)' – would not be fully appreciated for some years, Brand had learned enough to undertake reconstructive surgery on claw-hands.[17]

The difficulty was to find anywhere to perform the operations since leprosy patients were not welcome in ordinary hospitals such as the one at Vellore. But 'after much lobbying the [Vellore] hospital did grant permission for us to open a Hand Research Unit – we dared not use the word leprosy – in a mud-walled storeroom attached to the outer wall of the hospital compound'. For the surgeon, 'transferring tendons from one place to another' might be a relatively simple operation, but the patient had to make a mental adjustment to 'a brand new set of realities' and that could be a problem. At the heart of it was an issue that loomed ever larger in Brand's thinking, the issue of pain – pain as a necessary warning system:

> Pain, along with its cousin touch, is distributed universally on the body, providing a sort of boundary of *self*. Loss of sensation destroys that boundary, and now my leprosy patients no longer felt their hands and feet as part of self. Even after surgery, they tended to view their repaired hands and feet as tools or artificial appendages. They lacked the basic instinct of self-protection that pain normally provides.[18]

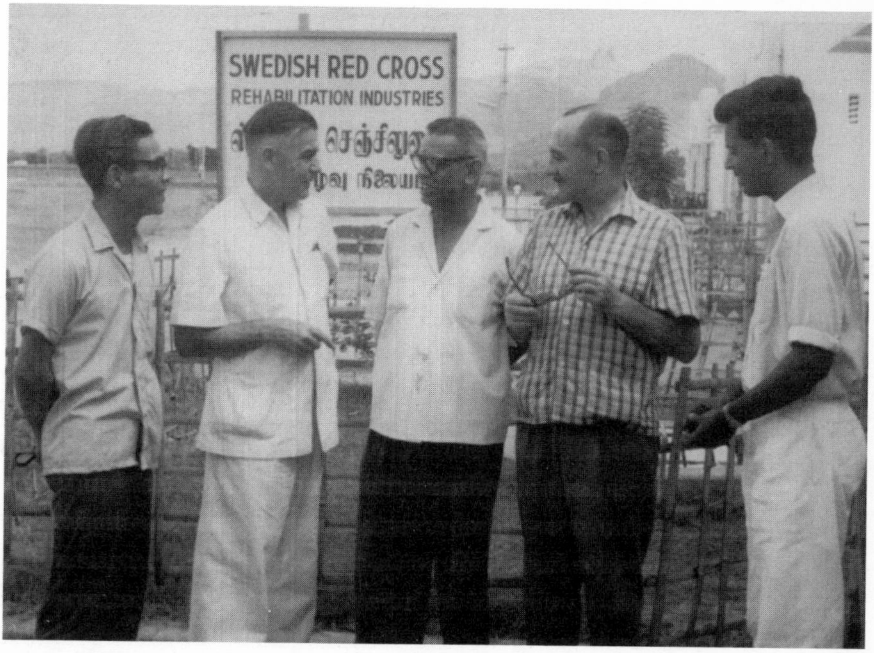

Dr Paul Brand (*second from left*) with colleagues in south India

(Paul Brand Publishing)

Even allowing for this, Brand was mystified when some of his post-operative patients, who had been lectured again and again on the importance of taking care of their reconstructed hands and feet, lost parts of their fingers or toes. It was almost as though the hoary old myths about body parts dropping off were true. The patients themselves were unable to explain what had happened; all they knew was that whatever it was, it happened at night. So one of the patients on the boys' ward undertook to stay awake and keep watch while the others slept. What he observed was 'a scene straight out of a horror movie': in the depths of the night a rat climbed on to the bed of a fellow patient and started to nibble the boy's finger. Deprived of sensation in his hand and therefore feeling no pain, the lad did not even stir, let alone attempt to shake off the rat. But the appalled watcher sounded the alarm and, as everyone woke with a start, the rat scurried off. The solution was simple: 'we went into the cat breeding business.'[19]

The more Brand thought about missing fingers and toes in advanced cases of leprosy, the more he questioned the conventional wisdom that attributed them to the inexorable progress of the disease. Clearly they did not 'simply drop off'; the presence of a nail bed at the end of a foreshortened finger meant, rather, that 'something was causing the body to consume its own finger from inside'. The culprit, he was convinced, was the malfunction of the pain warning system. Whereas normal healthy individuals adjusted their shoes if they were uncomfortable, or put on another pair to avoid getting blisters and running the risk of infection, leprosy patients without sensation in their extremities were incapable of making such adjustments and therefore developed infections. As x-rays revealed, 'tiny pieces of bone fragment break off and are extruded with the discharge from the wounds until eventually the infection leads to the loss of toes or even the entire foot'. Yet leprosy patients made no compensatory adjustment of gait to keep off the injured part, but continued to walk without a hint of a limp, seriously exacerbating their lesions. Brand writes:

> I was now ready to go public with the theory that painlessness was the only real enemy. Leprosy merely silenced pain, and further damage came about as a side effect of painlessness. In other words, all subsequent damage was preventable.[20]

Though Brand was a pioneer in the field of reconstructive surgery for leprosy patients, he wasn't the only surgeon to perform such operations; he would later discover that in the United States Dr Daniel C. Riordan had been operating on claw-hands on weekly visits to Carville since 1949. Riordan regarded reconstructive surgery as the 'second and still not adequately utilized weapon' in the fight against the 'red devil Hansen's bacillus' (the first being sulphone treatment).[21] But he was unlikely to come up against the kind of problem Brand faced when the first of his surgical volunteers, an educated man by the name of John Krishnamurthy, complained that his new hands were 'not good hands'. They looked fine to Brand; in fact, he thought they were beautiful and said so. 'Yes, yes,' Krishnamurthy replied, 'but they're bad *begging* hands' – by which he meant that in comparison with his old claw-hands they were ineffective in soliciting alms; and since for a person whose face still bore the marks of leprosy there was no other means of making money, he found himself worse off than before. This exchange brought home to Brand how he and his colleagues must lift their sights 'from the narrow field of surgery on hands and feet and bring the whole person into view'.[22]

Another of his patients became an important ally in achieving this aim. Professor T.N. Jagadisan was a Tamil brahmin from a family poor in material wealth but rich in Sanskrit culture. His father, a victim of the 1918 flu pandemic, had died when Jagadisan was only nine years old and he'd become head of the family 'with a little sister and a mother who was far from being equal to face any responsibility and totally lacked any initiative'. At fourteen he was married to a cousin, and though the marriage was a success, he writes of marriage 'before one reaches physical, mental and emotional growth' that it 'inflicts a psychological trauma and deprives the couple of the real joy of a wedding which is their due, and cripples from the start the growth of their matrimonial life'. But more crippling even than early marriage was Jagadisan's discovery, while still a schoolboy, that he had leprosy, something he had to keep secret for as long as he possibly could. He had known from the age of six that his paternal uncle, with whom he lived in some intimacy, had the dreaded *Kushtarogam*. This meant that he was able to diagnose his own condition without benefit of doctors. He didn't allow his secret to get in the way of his intellectual aspirations and he ignored the early inroads of the disease as he battled to earn a living for himself and his family during the Depression of the 1930s. He succeeded in becoming, first, a teacher and then a university lecturer in English and got to know many of the leaders of India's struggle for independence, including the Mahatma Gandhi.[23]

It wasn't until 1943, when he was refused a teaching post on account of his leprosy – despite the fact that he had a medical certificate from Dr Robert Cochrane to say that he was non-infectious – that he decided to 'come out as a leprosy worker':

> I was familiar with the wild fear and prejudice of people towards leprosy and the consequent social injustice to which the innocent sufferers are subject. But yet, it was as though I saw the figure of this prejudice staring me in the face for the first time and arresting my serious attention. A clear pronouncement of fitness from the highest medical authority did not help, even though the appointing authority displayed the greatest goodwill! What a strange and unjust position to be in! But it was there. I knocked against the granite wall of ignorance and prejudice. There was only one thing to do, to work for the removal of this wall . . .[24]

Later that year Jagadisan became publicity officer for the British Empire Leprosy Relief Association in Madras (which would be transformed into the Hind Kusht Nivaran Sangh, or Indian Anti-Leprosy Association, after independence). He was soon faced with an agonising personal decision. His mother, now over fifty, was showing signs of lepromatous leprosy which, unlike his tuberculoid strain, was infectious. Both he and his sister had young children in the house and, though his mother tried hard to keep her distance, home isolation was impracticable. Rather than put the children at risk, he decided to commit her to the leprosy sanatorium at Chingleput, though it made the whole family miserable and he himself 'could not have been more remorseful and grief-stricken if I had murdered my mother'. She took her separation from the family hard and did not become reconciled to her fate until 1947 when she moved to another refuge. And she died less than two years later.[25]

Jagadisan's work with BELRA brought him into close contact with Robert Cochrane, who became a 'very dear friend' as well as a mentor. On one occasion he took Cochrane to meet Gandhi, who listened to them intently and then – since he was observing silence at the time – wrote on a piece of paper:

> You have preached to the converted. My interest in the leper problem is as old as my residence in South Africa . . . I would like you to send a detailed

> plan with expenditure to go to the Board [of the Kasturba Gandhi National Memorial Trust]. No thanks needed.

In the December 1945 revised edition of his Constructive Programme, designed – in Gandhi's own words – 'to build the nation from the bottom upward', the Mahatma 'included the service of leprosy patients as an item'.[26]

Though they were both devout Hindus, Gandhi and Jagadisan deeply admired Christ and his teachings and approved of the spiritual dimension involved in missionary work with leprosy. Gandhi spelt out his own philosophy in a conversation with his follower Manohar Diwan – who'd earned his approbation by setting up a leprosy institution – and Jagadisan. He told them:

> Leprosy work is not merely medical relief; it is transforming the frustration in life into the joy of dedication, personal ambition into selfless service. If you can transform the life of a patient or change his values of life, you can change the villager and the country.

Gandhi's genius may have resided in his unique ability to invest politics with a spiritual dimension, but he was also quite capable of practical intervention: when Cochrane and Jagadisan informed him of a government proposal to introduce compulsory sterilisation of leprosy patients he used his influence to prevent such harsh and unnecessary legislation.[27]

Jagadisan, with his devotion to 'the twin causes of leprosy and literature', was himself an influential and gifted speaker and writer. As chairman of the Social Aspects Panel at the Seventh International Congress of Leprology held in Tokyo in November 1958, he insisted that 'real rehabilitation occurs only when the rehabilitated person lives and works in the environment of a normal society'. Japanese policy towards leprosy was still so segregationist that no doubt he had his hosts in mind when he insisted that any arrangement that 'perpetually keeps those recovered from leprosy in special colonies defeats the very purpose of rehabilitation which is restoration to normal life'. Even the 'outstanding work' of Eunice Weaver in organising *preventoria* all over Brazil for the uninfected children of leprosy patients came in for a measure of criticism; from the replies he'd received to a questionnaire he had sent out to leprosy workers in a number of countries, Jagadisan concluded that there

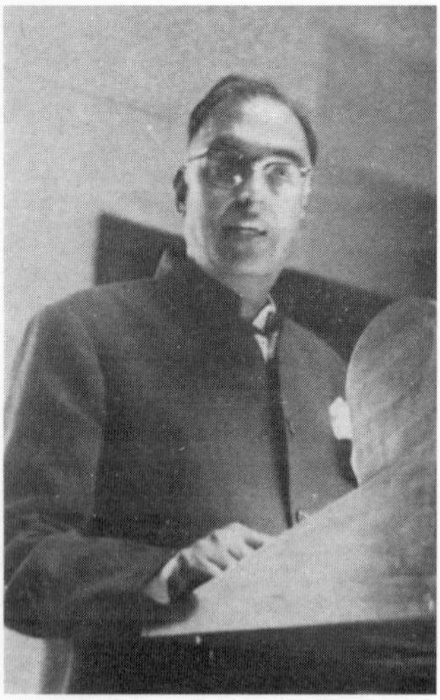
(The Star)

Professor T. N. Jagadisan

was 'a growing opinion against the organization of *preventoria*, even if the necessary resources could be found'. Mrs Weaver vehemently denied that *preventoria* stigmatised the children who grew up in them, but there was a feeling among other workers that these children, like leprosy patients themselves, sometimes found it hard to adjust to the outside world later in life: 'A Philippine authority says, "they have been saved from the disease but many of them become displaced persons all their lives." '[28]

At the Tokyo conference Jagadisan praised the 'pioneering efforts of Dr Paul Brand and others' in correcting deformities, particularly of the hands and feet, and he was at one with Brand in stressing that 'psychological rehabilitation should keep pace with physical rehabilitation'.[29]

Jagadisan himself had benefited from Brand's corrective surgery. In the past, when he'd travelled around India as secretary of the Hind Kusht Nivaran Sangh making speeches, he'd used his claw-hands to demonstrate that deformity was no cause for shame. But this hadn't prevented him from volunteering for reconstructive surgery once Brand had established its effectiveness. Afterwards, he continued to travel and make speeches, 'but now held up his hands, exclaiming, "Look at my Brand new hand!" to show that these deformities were reversible'.[30]

Professor Jagadisan died in 1991 and in his obituary Paul Brand noted that he entitled his autobiography *Fulfilment Through Leprosy*, not – as might be expected – 'Fulfilment *in Spite of* Leprosy'. Brand thought Jagadisan would have achieved greatness in the literary field regardless of any disease, but 'he became truly great through having the disease and then demonstrating that the human spirit can rise in triumph above it'.[31]

Brand's wife Margaret, in the intervals between having children (they had six in all), 'made one of the first systematic studies of the onset of blindness in leprosy patients' and husband and wife worked together as a team to try and prevent this 'most feared complication of leprosy' – made so much worse by the impossibility of developing a compensatory sense of touch in insensitive (or missing) fingers. Margaret observed that many patients were going blind as a result of not blinking, and Paul developed an operation whereby he connected functioning muscles at the corner of the mouth to paralysed eyelids, thus enabling the patient to blink without consciously having to think about it. Brand also found himself called upon to perform plastic surgery, rebuilding collapsed noses and replacing vanished eyebrows. Fortunately, he'd had some wartime experience in follow-up treatment for badly burned RAF pilots operated on by the pioneering plastic surgeon, Sir Archibald McIndoe, at his famous Burns Unit in the East Grinstead Hospital.[32]

Brand knew that paralysis and loss of sensation resulted from swollen nerves, but still he 'had no clue as to what was actually killing the nerves'. He sought the help of various neurologists, but most were as puzzled as he was. There was one exception. Dr Derek Denny-Brown was a 'brilliant' New Zealand neurologist working in Boston, and he explained to Brand that the pressure inside the nerve sheath became so great that it squeezed out the blood supply and the nerve died of inanition. For the first time, Brand felt he understood the process:

> As the leprosy bacilli invade nerves, the body reacts with a classic response of inflammation, causing the nerve to swell. Bacilli multiply, the body sends in reinforcements, and before long the expanding nerve is pressing against its sheath . . . A dead nerve will no longer carry the electric signals for sensation and movement.

(Years later another doctor discovered that the bacilli sometimes attacked the nerves directly, destroying the myelin coating of the fibres, but this was a 'less common' cause of paralysis.[33])

In the new leprosy hospital he was instrumental in having built at Karigiri, near Vellore, Brand and his colleagues pioneered a radically different approach to the 'cure' of leprosy than that adopted by the World Health Organization. The WHO had targeted the disease for eradication – a worthy aim, especially when backed by generous funding, but one that encouraged a statistical, rather than a caring, approach to patients: 'Once drugs had killed off the active bacilli in a patient, WHO pronounced that patient cured. Subsequent damage to eyes, hands, and feet was regrettable, but not really their concern.' The breakthrough for Brand came in 1957 when an Italian filmmaker made a documentary about a village boy with claw-hands whose life was transformed by reconstructive surgery; funded by The Leprosy Mission, the film was widely shown and Brand's approach to rehabilitation began to attract international recognition. The WHO employed him as a consultant, and Karigiri 'became a regular stopping place for international leprosy experts and for all new trainees sponsored by WHO'.[34]

The next decade was a period of great personal fulfilment for Brand. Leprosy work, far from proving a dead end, became, in his own words, a 'vocation' rather than a 'mere avocation', calling on the whole range of his abilities. What he felt was his chief contribution, though, was something they did not teach in medical school: 'to join with my patients as a partner in the task of restoring dignity to a broken spirit.' That, for him, was 'the true meaning of rehabilitation'. In all this, too, he had 'a sharp, numinous sense of the hand of God leading me forward'.[35] With his family growing all the time, his wife engaged in the same useful work as he, and his mother still active in the hills where he'd spent his early boyhood, he had a sense of achievement that was not to be measured in the worldly honours and awards that also began to come his way.

The mid-1960s would bring a new and unexpected challenge in the form of an invitation to join the medical team at Carville, a switch from the third to the first world with a vengeance. The Brands wanted to return to the west for the benefit of their children's education and had planned to settle in England, where Paul at least would have had no difficulty in getting a senior medical post. But it was a different matter for Margaret, who would've had to take more exams to qualify for ophthalmology, the area of medicine in which she had *de facto* become an expert. Part of the attraction of Carville was that she wouldn't have to requalify and could develop the work she'd been doing in India. Husband and wife would both benefit from the extra resources and unparalleled facilities of the best-endowed leprosy hospital in the world. So after some soul-searching they accepted Dr Edgar Johnwick's invitation to come to the United States and 'entered the alien world of Cajun cooking, Huey Long-style politics, and riverboat legends'.[36]

Sadly, Dr Johnwick died of a sudden heart attack before they arrived, but 'his humane reforms were well under way and the last discriminatory barriers [at Carville] soon fell'. The Brands went ahead with their American adventure despite the loss of their friend and sponsor. If Paul ever feared that working in America might not be challenging enough he had only to remind himself of the claim of a physiotherapist friend in India 'that, paradoxically, more educated societies are more likely to stigmatise disease'. This friend had cited New Guinea and central Africa as 'more accepting of leprosy patients than Japan, Korea, and the United States'. And if Brand doubted the extent of anti-leprosy prejudice in the States, a new friend, the celebrated Stanley Stein, then in the last year of his life, could put him right on that score. Stein was ailing fast; his drug resistance forced the doctors to use the powerful antibiotic streptomycin, which in his case had the side effect of causing deafness; so he was almost entirely cut off from human contact, as Brand memorably relates:

> A visit to Stanley during the last months of his life was nearly unbearable. Unable to see, unable to hear, unable to feel, he would wake up disoriented. He would stretch out his hand and not know what he was touching, and speak without knowing whether anyone heard or answered. Once I found him sitting in a chair muttering to himself in a monotone, 'I don't know where I am. Is someone in the room with me? I don't know who you are, and my thoughts go round and round. I cannot think new thoughts.'[37]

At Carville, Brand focused his research on the effects of insensitivity on the feet. His interest, as ever, was in leprosy but as the disease affected only a minuscule proportion of the US population – some 6,000 in all – it was virtually impossible to raise the necessary funding. It wasn't until he realised that his research would be equally valuable in countering the long-term effects of diabetes, another disease that can cause insensitivity (and is huge in the United States), that the big bucks rolled in. The measure of Brand's success at Carville was that whereas in the six years previous to his arrival there had been twenty-seven amputations performed, in the next few years there were none. Once again he succeeded in demonstrating that much of the damage traditionally attributed to leprosy (and, in this case, diabetes as well) was in reality the direct result of the absence of pain. 'Silencing pain, without considering its message', Brand writes, 'is like disconnecting a ringing fire alarm to avoid receiving bad news.' His version of Descartes' famous dictum was: 'I hurt, therefore I am'.[38]

The problem for leprosy (and diabetes) patients was that they didn't hurt, or not in the right way – since an absence of pain did not imply an absence of suffering. In the most advanced cases, like Stanley Stein at the end of his life, patients might feel no pain at all, but they suffered as greatly as anyone possibly could. As one of Brand's Indian patients put it, 'I'm suffering in my mind because I can't suffer in my body'. Apart from losing sensation and sometimes sight too, 'they lost their physical attractiveness, and because of the stigma of the disease they lost their feeling of acceptance by fellow human beings'.[39]

Brand had extraordinary empathy with his patients. When he eventually retired in 1986, one Carville patient said of him:

> I will always remember his special way of touching and holding my foot. It was as if he was touching and holding a delicate, precious though broken instrument. But I didn't only receive the benefit of his professional skill, but also the privilege of his sincere friendship, Christian love and compassion.[40]

It was at Carville that Brand acquired the sobriquet of 'Saint Paul'.

* * *

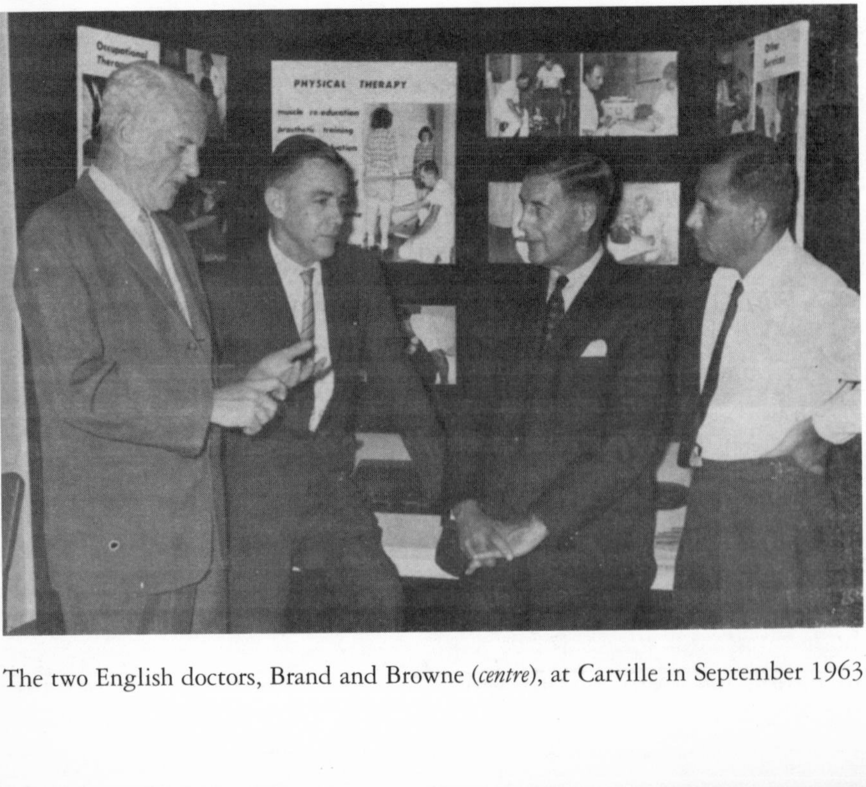

(The Star)

The two English doctors, Brand and Browne (*centre*), at Carville in September 1963

One of several projects for which the fertile Brand acted as midwife was the All-African training centre for leprosy rehabilitation at Addis Ababa in Ethiopia known as ALERT. In the early 1960s the International Society for the Rehabilitation of the Disabled (now Rehabilitation International) appointed Brand chairman of the World Committee on Leprosy Rehabilitation, and in 1963 a meeting was held at Carville to discover what was the world's most pressing requirement in this field. After a lively discussion it was decided that the 'greatest need was to train personnel to implement what was already known.'[41] And the continent that needed training most was Africa. But precisely where in that continent should a training centre be located?

This question brought Brand into a working relationship with his near contemporary and fellow medical missionary, Stanley Browne, who was asked to prepare a report for the committee on the most suitable sites, taking into consideration a number of conditions, including high incidence of leprosy, international accessibility, acceptance by a majority of the independent nations of Africa, a measure of political stability and the possibility of collaboration with an existing medical college. Browne had more than quarter of a century's experience of Africa, mostly in what was then the Belgian Congo, but latterly in Nigeria as well. So he was well qualified to answer this crucial question. 'I cast my mind back and forth over Africa, east, west and central, south and north', he recalled, 'and I came to the conclusion there were only two possibilities, one being Kampala, Uganda, the other Addis Ababa, Ethiopia. I could not foresee ten years of political stability in Uganda – how true that proved to be.'[42]

Brand and Browne's collaborative venture took shape. ALERT opened in Addis Ababa in 1966 and weathered social, political, funding and famine crises to grow – in Brand's words – as 'a living organism'.[43] It has survived into the twenty-first century, moving with the times as well as continuing to fulfil the need for which it was established.

Browne had in common with Brand practical Christianity and a passionate commitment to leprosy work, though he approached it in the more traditional way associated with Muir, Cochrane, Davey and other medical missionaries. Born in December 1907 in south-east London he was, as he put it, 'just a boy from an ordinary family in New Cross'. He was still under fifteen when he joined an organisation called Christian Endeavour and was baptised along with a dozen other youngsters, including his brother Frank. His eloquence earned him the nickname 'the boy preacher' in and around Bermondsey. His religious inspiration was matched by educational aspiration, but he came from a non-academic family without means, so he left school early and found a job as a clerk in the Town Hall at Deptford. This did not prevent him from continuing his studies in the evenings in order to get into university. His persistence paid off. Shortly after his mother's early death, he was interviewed for a Non-Vocational Scholarship at London University and won a place at King's College, where he studied medicine with a view to becoming a medical missionary. By the time he finished his clinical course in 1933, he had 'an impressive list of prizes and honours to his credit'.[44]

Browne knew exactly where he wanted to go. Like many of his generation, he'd been brought up on tales of African exploration, of 'Doctor Livingstone, I presume' and the opening up of the 'Dark Continent'. At Sunday school in south London at the age of nine or ten, he'd listened spellbound to a story of what had happened when the steamer in which the Baptist missionary W. Holman Bentley and his wife were travelling up the Congo stopped to pick up wood for fuel in an area occupied by a people notorious for their 'debauchery and cannibalism'. These people, the Bobangi, did a war dance on the banks of the river to prevent anyone from the steamer landing, but when Bentley got his wife to give their newborn baby – 'the first white baby to be born in the Congo' – a bath in full view of the hostile crowd on shore their anger turned to delight and the missionaries were welcomed ashore. The man who told the story thirty years later was the 'Bentley baby' himself, and when he asked which boys and girls would 'follow Jesus even to Congo' young Stanley was among those who eagerly raised their hands.[45]

Ten years later, in July 1927, Browne attended a missionary exhibition at Central Hall, Westminster, and shook the hand of a Baptist missionary called Crudgington, who'd accompanied Holman Bentley on the first ever journey made by white men along the north bank of the Congo up the rapids as far as Stanley Pool (as it became known) in 1881. Of course this was nothing compared to H.M. Stanley's epic 999-day crossing of the African continent from east to west of 1874–77, which opened up the Congo to colonial exploitation by the egregious Leopold II, King of the Belgians, whose factotum Stanley became. Stanley was not a party to the atrocities committed by the king's men in pursuit of ivory and rubber – the routine cutting off of hands exposed in a consular report by Roger Casement in 1904 – but he was certainly ruthless and, when he found it necessary, brutal, as many gentler (in both senses of the word) spirits who volunteered to accompany him on later expeditions were shocked to discover. The Congo natives, at any rate, had little to thank him for: from the east they became the prey of well-armed 'Arab' slave traders like Tippu Tib who penetrated the hinterland in his wake, decimating whole populations; and from the west they fell victim to the systematic greed of Leopold II. In the midst of this barbarism the English and American Baptist missionaries whose example inspired the youthful Stanley Browne did what little they could to alleviate the worst conditions and exemplify a more peaceful mode of existence.[46]

Another decade would pass before Browne reached his destination, the Baptist Missionary Society hospital at Yakusu on the upper reaches of the Congo, a decade in which he completed his medical studies, worked as a house physician and spent several months in Belgium improving his French and studying tropical diseases. Although the Congo he went to in 1936 had long since ceased to be the private fiefdom of Leopold II and had become the responsibility of the Belgian government, there were plenty of reminders of the earlier, lawless days. On his arrival at the BMS station in Yakusu, Browne was greeted by an elderly missionary and his senior pastor, Lititiyo, who had first met in 1897, when 'the latter – a young brave in direct line of the Yaokanja chieftainship – was running from a village raid carrying a human leg he had just hacked off and was about to roast and eat'. And Browne soon found himself attempting to quell an outbreak of sleeping sickness in an area where many of the older villagers remembered going out as boys in war canoes to intercept H.M. Stanley's flotilla when the explorer made his first journey down that stretch of the Congo.[47]

Like Brand, Browne came to specialise in leprosy largely by chance. Sleeping sickness was being successfully eliminated and after the 1938 International Congress of Leprology in Cairo the government of the Congo set about tackling leprosy. First, the prevalence of the disease had to be established and to that end the English doctors at Yakusu were called upon to make a survey of the 10,000 square miles of forest for which they were responsible, a task that devolved upon Browne. He soon supplemented what he'd learned from textbooks of tropical medicine in Belgium with a diagnostic ability acquired with the aid of the local witch doctor and village chief who accompanied him on his trek through the district. Together they discovered 4,000 cases of active leprosy in a population of 60,000 and in one area alone found that nearly 50 per cent of the people had it, a figure so high that the authorities found it impossible to believe until they checked it out for themselves. Having found the spot with the highest leprosy prevalence rate in the world in his own backyard, so to speak, Browne concentrated on the disease.[48]

On leave in England at the beginning of 1940, he became engaged to Marion – 'Mali' – Williamson, an Oxford graduate, schoolteacher and daughter of missionary parents. Six months later she sailed to the Congo, where they were married. Over the next twenty years their life was centred on the leprosy settlement at Yalisombo, across the river from Yakusu. At first the missionaries had great difficulty in persuading infectious cases to come to the settlement. There was no social stigma attached to the disease in the Congo; people with leprosy were not ostracised or abandoned until they were no longer able to perform their normal functions and became a burden on the community. Villagers were unimpressed with the argument that their children were at risk of infection. When the site was first cleared and neat little wattle-and-daub huts were built, each with its own patch of garden, a few leprosy-affected people agreed to come, but only on condition they could bring their families – which created a new problem: how were healthy family members to be separated from the infectious? It scarcely mattered: within three months of the official opening the place was deserted.[49] The missionaries would not accept defeat; they decided that the trouble was lack of food, or of the right food. There was a war on and there were shortages everywhere, but the local administration was ready to help out. Yalisombo was reopened and though it hardly flourished – patients quarrelled, grumbled about the food and took off whenever they felt like it – it just about kept going. For Stanley Browne, the saddest moment came when he had to admit the brightest of the medical auxiliaries they had ever trained at Yakusu, a Christian convert called Dickie Likoso, who'd contracted the disease. And even Dickie's presence could not prevent another mass exodus of disgruntled fellow patients from Yalisombo. When *Bonganga* (white doctor) Browne was asked by local church leaders to speak about leprosy at their annual conference, he expressed his frustration openly:

> We've tried twice and we've failed twice. You remember how all the people at Yalisombo went away because they weren't getting enough

> food, and how we got good food supplies for them. And now they're going away again because they don't like the medicine we're giving them. Well, we haven't got any other medicine, so what else can we do? We've done our best, and we've failed.[50]

But even as he was speaking a small package was on its way to him from America containing the sulphone drug that would transform life at Yalisombo just as it was doing elsewhere. Since Diasone could have unpleasant side effects, such as vomiting and diarrhoea, Browne and his colleagues needed volunteers who were prepared to endure these in the hope of being cured. So Browne crossed the river to Yalisombo the next day and told the patients about the new medicine, which just might be the long-awaited cure for leprosy, asking if anyone was willing to try it. Only one person raised his hand but that person was Dickie Likoso, whose intelligence and medical knowledge – as well as the rapid inroads the disease was making on his body – made him the ideal guinea pig.[51]

The doctors anxiously monitored Dickie's intake of the drug, varying the dosage according to its effects on his blood and kidneys in particular. They suffered with him when his face swelled and he underwent the agony of a lepra reaction. They asked him if he'd rather they stopped, but he gritted his teeth and told them to go on. They sensed the tension in the other patients, who were also observing Dickie's progress. When they saw under the microscope that the bacilli were breaking up they began to believe the drug might be working; and soon it became obvious to everyone. Dickie's skin patches were regaining their natural colour and his ears were reverting to their normal size . . . 'The white man's new medicine was actually curing Dickie's leprosy.'[52]

From that moment on, there was no problem in attracting leprosy sufferers to Yalisombo. In the two years following Dickie's lone, brave gesture the community grew from just over 100 to over 1,000 patients. The difficulty now was getting hold of enough drugs to satisfy the ever-increasing demand. Browne found himself in the position of 'a general with an army strategically deployed but unable to go into action for lack of ammunition'. Then the US cavalry – in the shape of the American Mission to Lepers – came to the rescue, granting enough supplies to cover the entire 10,000 square-mile area. Now it became a question of training a sufficient number of *infirmiers*, or medical auxiliaries, to 'embark on a campaign of war against leprosy throughout the whole district'.[53]

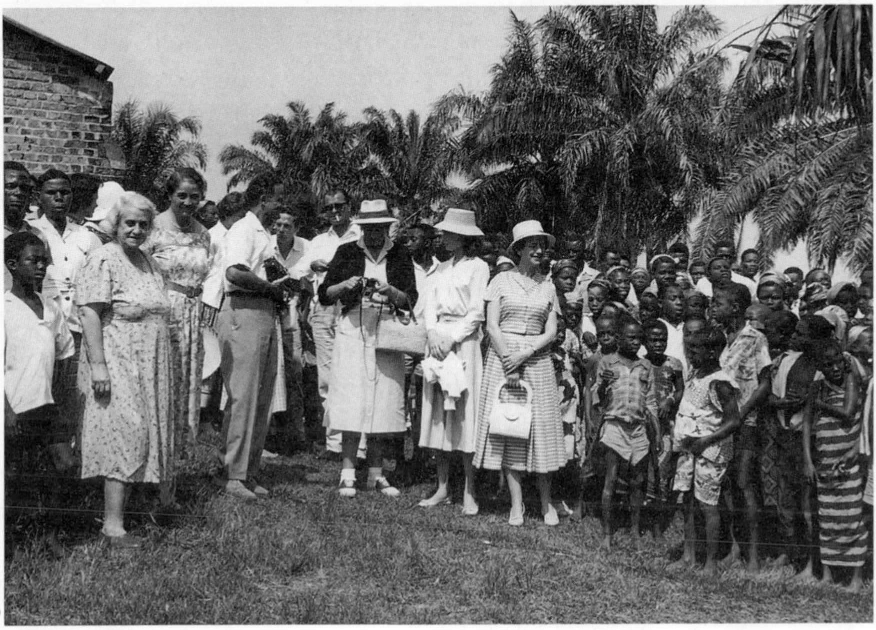
(©TLM)

The cast of *The Nun's Story* after filming at Yalisombo: (*left to right*) Peter Finch, Mrs Fred Zinnemann, Audrey Hepburn and Peggy Ashcroft

The ubiquitous Dr Robert Cochrane, in his new role as Technical Medical Adviser to the American Mission to Lepers, visited Yalisombo and reported enthusiastically about both the institution – whose laboratory and dispensary buildings were 'first class' – and the man behind it, who was 'really brilliant . . . and quite modest about it all'. Dr Browne's records were the best he'd ever seen and he was not just an 'unusually gifted and dedicated man' but 'first and foremost a missionary seeking by every means in his power to extend the Kingdom of God'.[54]

Encomiums of this sort helped to spread the fame of Yalisombo abroad. But it was still a surprise when two 'huge, gleaming American cars' rolled into the BMS compound at Yakusu and a party of filmmakers emerged whose spokesman greeted Browne with the words, 'Dr *Stanley* Browne, I presume.' The producer-director Fred Zinnemann told Browne, 'We are going to shoot some scenes for *The Nun's Story* in Stanleyville [Kinshasa], and are looking for a place where we can shoot some of the sequences at a bush hospital where lepers are treated.' Browne's wife Mali could see her husband wince at the casual use of the word 'leper' and the eminent visitor was left in no doubt that it had 'been banned by common consent by those who are trying to help the victims of this terrible disease'. So much so that when, some time later, the cast attended a 'Grateful Samaritan' service for forty-six patients who were receiving their certificates of discharge, Mali noted how well the lesson had been learned: ' "And some *patients*" – Peggy Ashcroft avoided, with a smile, the banned word "lepers" – "some patients will be going out, cured, soon?" '[55]

After that initial misunderstanding filming went ahead, with cast and crew becoming involved in sanatorium life – once Browne had reassured them on the remoteness of their chances of contracting leprosy – and patients eagerly entering into the spirit of the occasion, happy to recreate the 'sadness and hopelessness' of a leprosy dispensary twenty years earlier, before the advent of the wonder drugs. Even Stanley Browne had a role: Zinnemann gave him a megaphone and 'jokingly appointed him "assistant producer" for the day'. *Bonganga*'s knowledge of the people and their language enabled him to 'coax and persuade them to remain still and quiet when required'.[56]

Zinnemann and his stars were not the only famous visitors to a leprosy settlement in the Congo in the late 1950s. In 1959 at Yonda,

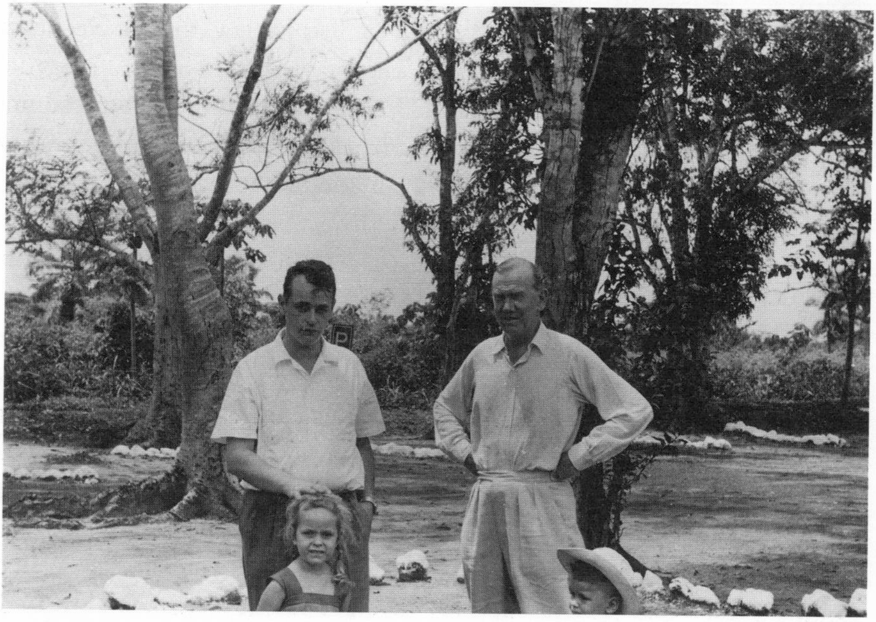

(Courtesy of Michel F. Lechat)

Dr Michel F. Lechat and his children with their distinguished guest, the novelist Graham Greene, at the Yonda leprosy settlement in the Equator Province, Stanley Browne's Belgian friend and colleague Dr Michel F. Lechat played host to the distinguished author of *The Power and the Glory* and *The Heart of the Matter*, who was researching the background for a new novel, which would be called *A Burnt-Out Case*. Graham Greene's visit was arranged through a mutual friend and initially at least was not entirely welcomed by Lechat, who feared that it might 'upset the delicate balance between myself and the mission'. How would the good fathers respond to a maverick Catholic writer like Greene? But he needn't have worried: Greene was 'the opposite of a journalist, and he inspired great confidence'. Despite being such a formidable observer, he 'never looked at people as though they were butterflies or cockroaches. He was part of daily life'. That was his strength, 'his perfect integration in whatever routine there might be, or however unusual the situation (and perhaps preferably when the situation *was* unusual)'.[57]

Though years later Greene confessed that his last, and worst, bout of depression coincided with the gestation of *A Burnt-Out Case* – 'very likely the result of his two-year cohabitation with the deeply depressive Querry, the central figure of the book' – he showed no sign of it at Yonda; he simply 'went his own way and got things organised'.[58] But his 'Congo Journal', like the novel that came out of this experience, does make rather glum reading; a Conradian gloom seems to pervade the 'heart of darkness' that is Yonda (Lechat says Greene was reading, or re-reading, *Heart of Darkness* at the time); and Greene, apart from recording facts and observations about leprosy, typically questions the nature of religious involvement. 'The vanity of being something special – even in disease', he notes at one point. 'Should one class Father Damien among the leprophils?' At another: 'The sisters who sometimes resent leprosy being cured. "It's a terrible thing – there are no lepers left here."'[59]

Not surprisingly, *A Burnt-Out Case* got a hostile reception from (Protestant) Christian leprosy workers when it came out. Reviewing the novel in the *Star*, Robert Cochrane accused the author of sensationalism, of misrepresentation of leprosy – 'the impression is given that the great majority of persons when they get leprosy are "cured" but the cure is through mutilation' – and of a medieval approach to the disease in that Greene used the word 'leper . . . no less than 51 times'. Cochrane wrote, 'Querry's God [and by implication Greene's] is not the God of the Christian.' And he concluded by saying, 'to those who suffer from leprosy, many of whom will read the book, this novel will bring pain and distress, and for this reason, it would have been better if it had never been written.'[60] But Lechat will have no truck with such special pleading. He defends Greene's right as a novelist to 'choose any topic he feels appropriate' – provided he treats it with respect, as he asserts Greene does. Leprosy is no more 'the exclusive domain of the leprologist' than love and war are the exclusive domains of the sex counsellor and the retired general.[61]

The entry in Greene's Congo Journal for 17 February 1959 reads: 'In the evening heard over the radio news of disturbances in Brazzaville: one feels that European Africa is rapidly disintegrating.'[62] The Belgian Congo certainly was and, following independence in 1960, the country descended into a civil war made all the dirtier by the behind-the-scenes involvement of western powers circling like vultures over a corpse ready to gorge on its easy pickings. The Brownes, who had three growing sons, had already left the Congo in 1958, well before the mass exodus of foreign doctors at the time of independence, but Stanley could take some satisfaction from the fact that leprosy work in the eastern half of the country, at least, was being carried on by the African medical auxiliaries he had so conscientiously trained over the years. In the 1970s, however, when he and Mali revisited Yakusu, in what was now Zaire, they found it in a state of neglect, and the 'efficient medical service, with its network of dispensaries spreading over thousands of square miles' that had been their pride and joy, had been 'almost completely disrupted'. As for the patients, they were told: 'The dispensaries were closed. No more medicine. Lists of patients' names destroyed . . . There are again many people with leprosy . . .'[63] The usual sickening aftermath of a civil war, in fact.

In 1959 Browne was offered the post of director of the Leprosy Research Unit at Uzuakoli in Nigeria. As this was a government rather than a missionary appointment it meant a great deal more money than he was used to getting and provided him with an ideal situation in which to pursue his research interests. His predecessor Frank Davey, along with John Lowe, had pioneered oral treatment with dapsone, using much smaller doses than had at first been thought necessary. Browne was the first to use the drug B663 – clofazimine – on patient volunteers. The trial was so successful that B663 became the drug of choice in cases of dapsone resistance and was also found to be effective in treating lepra reaction in cases of lepromatous leprosy.[64]

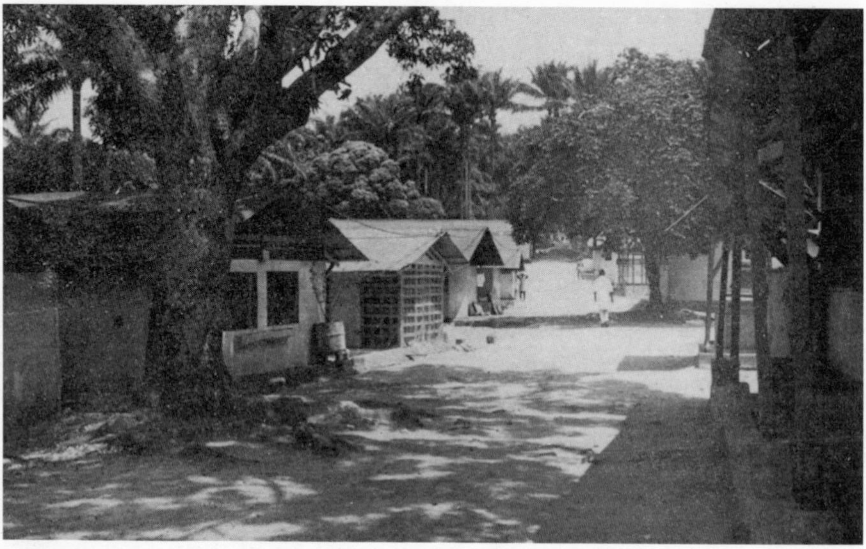

(The Star)

The 'village de lumière' at Lambarene

The Brownes returned to England in the mid-1960s, when Stanley took over a number of prestigious posts from Robert Cochrane. He became director of the Leprosy Study Centre Cochrane had set up, consultant adviser to the government and to the Leprosy Mission, and medical secretary of BELRA's successor, LEPRA. By this time he was indeed 'Mr Leprosy' (as his biographer entitled her book about him), travelling the world, giving lectures and writing innumerable articles and scientific papers.

One of the places he visited in his capacity of medical secretary of LEPRA was the Albert Schweitzer Hospital at Lambarene in Gabon, shortly after the great man's death in 1965. He pronounced it 'a disgrace'. But Schweitzer's biographer James Brabazon takes issue with him, arguing that Browne's judgement was clouded by his own bias towards preventive medicine over 'what he regarded as the more showy side of doctoring – surgery'. The fact that the Schweitzer hospital was not devoted solely to the 'fight against leprosy' was 'enough to damn it' in the eyes of a man who was as single-minded in his commitment to that fight as Browne was. According to Brabazon, this was unfair since the government had taken over campaigning in the villages for early treatment, and the leprosy village at Lambarene continued to exist 'for one reason only – the cured lepers refused to go home' (Schweitzer had given his word that they might stay as long as they lived).[65]

Though it was popularly supposed that the Schweitzer hospital had always concentrated on leprosy, that was by no means the case. It was really only in the ten or fifteen years following the Second World War and the discovery of an effective treatment for the disease, when nowhere else within hundreds of miles in what was then French Equatorial Africa could provide the sulphones, that leprosy took precedence at Lambarene. Even during that period there was considerable infighting among the medical staff, with a dynamic young nurse called Trudi Bochler frequently clashing with Schweitzer himself 'in her determination to see that "her" lepers got a fair share, or if possible more than their fair share, of the available facilities'.[66] In 1953 Schweitzer had undertaken to use his Nobel Peace prize money to build a leprosy village, and it was through Bochler's persistence that the village did eventually get built, but once the government took over the leprosy campaign it became little more than a refuge for chronic cases who did not want to go home or had no homes to go to.[67]

Browne's critical attitude towards the Schweitzer hospital probably had quite as much to do with its perceived shortcomings in hygiene and sanitation as with any preconceptions he may have had about priorities in the treatment of leprosy. But Brabazon's strictures are not without some force. On the one hand, Browne recognised the need for rehabilitation services for leprosy patients; on the other, he regarded them as 'low-priority projects' in comparison with prophylactic measures (such as BCG vaccination in areas where it had proved effective) and early treatment that would obviate the need for rehabilitation. '*Prevention*', he would insist, 'is the gospel we are trying to preach today to everybody concerned with leprosy – patients, doctors (including surgeons), physiotherapists, shoemakers – everybody.' Prevention of leprosy, and prevention of disability through recognising and treating the disease in its early stages, should be the aim, and indigenous medical auxiliaries the means of putting it into effect:

> The practical and practicable ideal in poor developing countries would be a leprosy service, rural and urban, completely integrated into a comprehensive medical scheme aiming at the control and eventual eradication of the major endemic diseases, coupled with the raising of the standards of nutrition and hygiene, and a determined and persistent campaign of education of all members of the community in the principles of positive health.[68]

Browne lived long enough (he died in 1987) to see the optimism of the post-war era fade as drug resistance made itself felt and the incidence level of leprosy throughout the world remained worryingly constant despite the WHO's eradication campaign. He became chairman of the medical commission of ELEP (the Federation of European Anti-Leprosy Associations) and moved more and more in the rarefied world of acronyms and international congresses and conferences, which is reflected in the kind of WHO-speak of the above extract. But he had worked long enough in the field to have a solid grasp of essentials and rightly warned against complacency, just as Paul Brand did.

Though he'd retired seven years earlier, Brand was invited to deliver the inaugural address at the Fourteenth International Leprosy Congress in Orlando, Florida in 1993. He applauded the success of multiple drug therapy (MDT), which had been introduced in the 1980s to combat dapsone resistance and hasten the elimination of leprosy, and praised the WHO for the progress of its programmes for reducing the prevalence of the disease throughout the world. But as a kind of elder statesman no longer at the centre of the struggle he took upon himself the role of Cassandra, using examples from his long experience to urge caution in proclaiming victory over an inadequately understood and still dangerous adversary. He recalled how, forty years earlier, in the midst of wildly over-optimistic forecasts of dapsone's ability to eradicate leprosy, he had visited a distinguished Harvard epidemiologist and WHO adviser to try and engage his interest in rehabilitation and the man had responded to his pitch with a kindly smile:

> 'Dr Brand, you are wasting your time,' he said. 'The time and money that you spend on one deformed leprosy patient; if it were spent on Dapsone treatment would result in the cure of fifty patients, who then would not become deformed. For the greatest good we have got to write off the present generation of deformed leprosy patients. If we put all our effort now into killing bacteria, the next generation will grow up without any leprosy at all.'[69]

The point of this anecdote, Brand said, was to demonstrate 'that PROPHESY IS A DANGEROUS GAME IN BIOLOGY'. To make it even clearer, he fantasised that the mycobacteria were holding a parallel congress while the Orlando congress was going on, taking stock of *their* situation and planning their future strategy:

> Perhaps their President, who this year may be the virus of AIDS, has just presented their Nobel prizes. One would have been given to *Mycobacterium tuberculosis*, for having emerged in some countries from the category 'No Public Health Problem' to that of MAJOR Public Health Problem, while most doctors were looking the other way. The other prize might be going to the Parasite of Malaria, which had succeeded in the clever strategy of remaining NEARLY ERADICATED for long enough to persuade most malariologists to move into other studies, then only to come roaring back, resistant to most anti-malarial drugs, and carried by mosquitoes that had become resistant to common insecticides. At the same congress a group of mycobacteria may be reading a paper in which they outline a plan by which *M. leprae* will become resistant, perhaps to clofazimine, by the year 2000. Such a congress of germs would probably welcome a statement from our congress here declaring them to be no longer a problem to public health.[70]

Brand concluded his characteristically trenchant and still pertinent address by restating his medical creed: 'The surest way to keep up pressure on *M. leprae* is to keep up our concern and our care for every individual patient who suffers from leprosy or from its late results.'[71]

This fine surgeon, who on his retirement had settled in Seattle, died on 8 July 2003, nine days short of entering his ninetieth year.

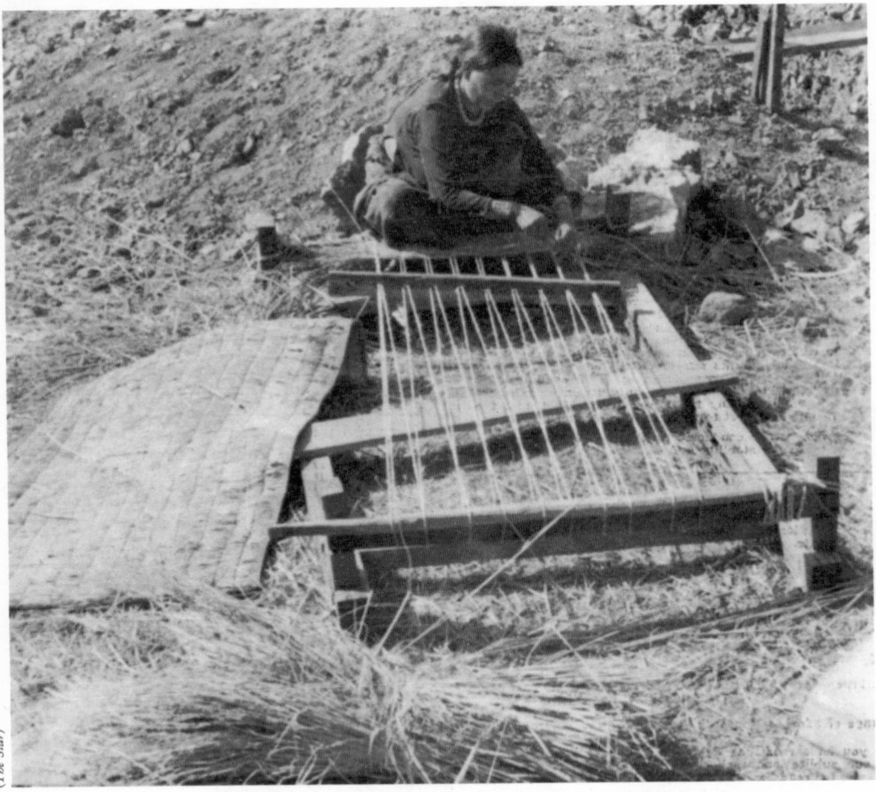

(The Star)

A Nepalese leprosy patient weaving a straw mat

Chapter 13

LEPROSY IN ONE COUNTRY . . . AND BEYOND

The seriousness of the leprosy problem in any country is, roughly speaking, directly proportionate to the state of economic backwardness. In other words, leprosy poses the greatest problems in those lands which, by reason of low *per capita* income, are least able to devote sufficient funds to its control.[1]

Dr Stanley G. Browne (1972)

To most people who can point to it on the globe, Nepal means mountains like Everest and Annapurna, trekking, Sherpas, Gurkhas, the pagoda-style architecture of the ancient monuments of the Kathmandu valley, and tourism – at least until recently, when the activities of the Maoist guerrillas frightened most of the tourists away. Yet as late as the beginning of the 1950s this Himalayan kingdom was a closed country, largely inaccessible to foreigners and right off the tourist map.

For over a hundred years it had been ruled by a Nepalese shogunate, the autocratic Rana dynasty that accorded the hereditary kings divine status even as it robbed them of temporal power and kept them in virtual imprisonment. But in 1951 King Tribhuvan, with the backing of the government of newly independent India, to which he had managed to escape, turned the tables on the Ranas and put an end to their regime.[2] Though democracy (or 'demo*crazy*' as sceptical foreigners are more inclined to call it) took a further forty years to come into being and is still a very fragile plant, the floodgates had been opened and first a trickle and then a torrent of foreign advisers, aid workers and tourists poured in, with their thick wallets and good intentions, transforming the face of the country without ever quite managing to alleviate the desperate poverty that still afflicts so many of its people.

Among the first to take advantage of this new opportunity were the Christian missionaries, who had been gathering on Nepal's Indian border. In 1950 they were granted permission to enter the country 'for educational and medical purposes only'. Nepal was – and is – a Hindu kingdom (though by no means all its inhabitants, even then, were Hindus) and there was to be no proselytism, no attempt to win converts to Christianity – though how you could hope to muzzle missionaries once you'd allowed them in was another matter.[3]

So from the beginning there was considerable tension between Nepal's Hindu hierarchy and the incoming westerners: however much the missionaries' medical and other skills might be in demand, their ideas were felt to be alien, even subversive. Both sides were wary of one another, and the early missionaries were careful not to provoke the authorities into taking away their visas. For foreign nationals, that was the only form of redress open to the government: expulsion from the country. For Nepali Christians it was a different matter: they could be – and were – imprisoned, abused and pressurised into denying their God. Some did renounce their faith, at least for the duration of their imprisonment, but the more determined among them set about converting the other inmates, thus earning still greater obloquy – or glory, depending on your point of view.

In 1955 a commission from the Mission to Lepers spent two weeks in Nepal, assessing the prospects for leprosy work there. Three of its five members were Indian Christian doctors and the other two were British laymen (who immediately ran into visa problems). They learned that in some government circles at least there was considerable unease at the number of different missionary organisations vying with one another to obtain permission to carry out medical work in Nepal.[4]

Early arrivals included the American doctors Robert and Bethel Fleming who struggled for five years to obtain official approval for the Shanta Bhawan Hospital they set up in Kathmandu. But that was nothing to 'Dr Bob', who, unlike his wife, was not a medical doctor but an educationalist; he was wont to say, 'We Christians waited two thousand years to get into Nepal. Then when the Lord was ready, he sent a bird to show us the way.' (Dr Bob was a keen ornithologist and himself resembled a bird, especially when seen beside his statuesque wife.)[5] In their wake the Presbyterians and several other Protestant groups from many different countries that had workers along the Indian border joined together to form the United Christian Medical Mission to Nepal. At Tansen, in west Nepal, the UCMM was already engaged in leprosy work, and further north the Nepal Evangelistic Band (soon to be renamed the International Nepal Fellowship, or INF) was pioneering similar work in Pokhara through the efforts of a couple of doughty British nurses called Eileen Lodge and Betty Bailey, who had arrived in 1953.[6]

The government of Nepal was unable to provide the Mission to Lepers commission with countrywide leprosy statistics; at that time most people, including officials, regarded Nepal as synonymous with the Kathmandu valley; neither the hills to the north, east and west, nor the long, thin strip of plains to the south known as the Terai counted for much in a land still largely devoid of roads and modern communications. Within the valley itself there was a government leprosy home at a place called Khokana, situated on the banks of the Baghmati River some six miles south of the city of Kathmandu. This was already a hundred years old and was little more than 'a living burial ground' for the afflicted. Originally the sexes had been segregated, but in 1934 a severe earthquake had demolished the women's quarters, and the women had moved in with the men. This resulted in a population explosion and, by the time of the commissioners' visit, a quarter of the 480 or so residents were children.[7]

The state leprosy officer who accompanied the commission to Khokana had not been there for more than two years because the only available vehicle had broken down and hadn't been repaired or replaced. This was typical of the neglect of the institution and its inhabitants. The visitors were appalled by the conditions: the buildings, though substantial, were in a state of disrepair; the rooms small, dark, airless and smoky, with four people crammed into each; and there was no sanitation. Basic food and clothing were provided and an auxiliary came in twice a week to give treatment in the outdated form of hydnocarpus (chaulmoogra) injections to those few patients who bothered about it (the state leprosy officer bemoaned the fact that he could not obtain dapsone, though workers at the UCMM clinic at Bhatgaon, one of the three historic cities of the Kathmandu valley, were giving it to their leprosy patients). The patients had no activity to occupy them and nowhere else to go, and the children, who might or might not have leprosy, ran wild. 'It was terrible', the commissioners reported, 'to see such neglected men, women and children amidst such majestic hills and luscious rice-fields.'[8] They compared the hopelessness and apathy of Khokana (and they heard that the other governmental institution at Malunga, near Tansen, was even worse) with the busy and devoted anti-leprosy work being done by missionaries at Tansen and Pokhara. At Tansen, despite the ban on proselytism, evangelistic work was being 'carried on within the hospital compound' by the Swedish minister there; and in Pokhara the Nepal Evangelistic Band had set up its own Nepali-run church, and the Shining Hospital – so called because it consisted of aluminium Nissen huts that reflected the sun – was winning over the local people in spite of considerable opposition from the Brahmins, or priestly caste. In Pokhara, too, Eileen Lodge and Betty Bailey, along with Dr Lillian O'Hanlan, were prospecting for a site for a dedicated leprosy home. So far they had only about fifteen leprosy patients, but they were convinced there were many more who remained hidden for 'fear of being incarcerated in Malunga'.[9]

The Mission to Lepers acted on its commissioners' advice and took up the challenge of tackling the problem of leprosy in Nepal, a country so poor that 'the total national income was not sufficient to pay even the salaries of Government officials and employees', according to what the commission had been told. The Mission invited Dr Cecil Pedley, an ophthalmologist and committed Christian who was working in northern India and was keen to go to Nepal, to work in Kathmandu on their behalf and help develop the site of the new Mission to Lepers Kathmandu Valley leprosy hospital at Anandaban. To avoid misunderstanding, the general secretary, Donald Miller, spelled out at length the conditions under which the government of Nepal was prepared to allow missionaries into the country; and Pedley sought clarification on the points that bothered him before agreeing to go. Miller approved of his reluctance to commit himself to a situation where his conscience might come into conflict with official policy, but gently reminded him that it was 'never justifiable simply to use other men's physical needs as a kind of strategic instrument for ulterior ends'.[10]

Although he was already over fifty, Dr Pedley spent the best part of the next sixteen years in Nepal. When the Medical Secretary of the Mission to Lepers, Dr N.D. Fraser, visited Kathmandu in the early spring of 1960, Pedley acted as his host. Fraser found him an engaging

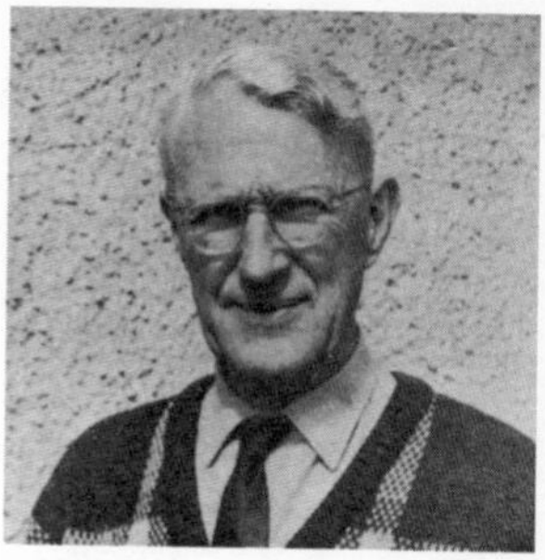
(The Star)

Dr Cecil Pedley

companion, who did all his own cooking and washing up and was happy to give up his room to his guest and sleep in a tent outside. But he doubted that Pedley was the right man to oversee the project of establishing a leprosy hospital at Anandaban, where a thorough grasp of accounting was essential, snap decisions had to be made and teamwork was paramount. Dr Pedley was self-reliant to a fault and found it difficult to delegate work and responsibility to others who might be more competent in their particular areas of expertise than he was, so Fraser concluded that he might be better employed as an eye specialist in a United Mission to Nepal (or UMN, as the UCMM had become) leprosy hospital.[11]

Which explains why, for most of his sixteen years in Nepal, Pedley was based in Tansen. In a series of letters and newsletters to fellow Christians in the United Kingdom, he described his work in this outpost and the trials and tribulations of a group of more or less staunch Nepali Christians who fell foul of the law and were sent to prison for periods of up to six years. He made regular monthly visits to the government leprosy settlement at Malunga, a day's trek over the mountains from Tansen, and found it a 'sad place' from which he would sometimes come away feeling 'very discouraged'. There were about 170 inmates, of whom some twenty-five were children, and had it not been for these monthly visits they would have had no medical attention whatsoever. But he did manage to get some people returned to their villages, armed with certificates confirming that their disease was no longer active.[12]

Pedley felt particularly sorry for the children who, like everyone else at Malunga, had nothing to do and got little or no education. Nubile girls were particularly at risk of exploitation. On one visit, he found that a healthy sixteen-year-old had been 'married' off to an elderly, deformed Brahmin despite the opposition of the girl's mother, a chronic sufferer whose own deformity – she had lost both feet and many of her fingers – rendered her powerless to intervene, especially after she had been walled into a corner of the vast barn-like room where, at the opposite end, her aged 'son-in-law' sat reading his holy books. Pedley rescued two other healthy girls of a similar age, who seemed to him susceptible to the Gospel, and found them work as nursing aids at Tansen – though a couple of years later one of them later ran

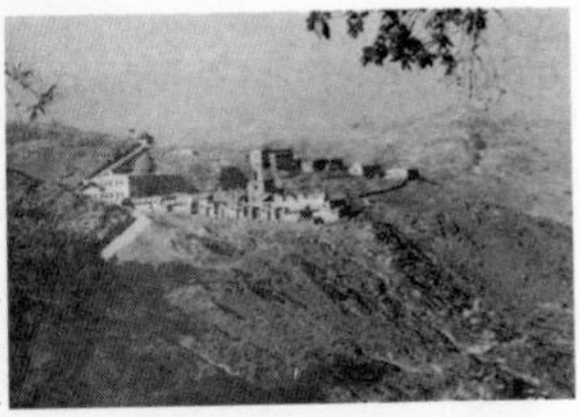
(The Star)

The General Mission Hospital at Tansen

off with a Hindu hospital worker who already had a wife and three children.[13]

In 1963, Dr Pedley felt the 'winds of change' blow through Nepal so far as leprosy work was concerned. About a hundred Khokana inmates who were discovered not to have leprosy (though born of leprosy-affected parents) were discharged; they staged a demonstration outside the palace of King Mahendra (Tribhuvan's successor) to publicise their plight as homeless, landless indigents – since leprosy law in Nepal obliged people with leprosy to give up their lands and spend the rest of their lives in a government leprosy settlement, and made no provision for children born there. The king responded by calling for an anti-leprosy campaign, and the World Health Organization undertook a pilot survey to discover the extent of leprosy in the country. At the same time, the medical director of the government hospital in Kathmandu, known as the Bir Hospital, Dr Giri Prasad, went on a tour of southern India under the auspices of the WHO and was inspired by a visit to Dr Paul Brand's surgical reconstruction unit at Vellore. On his return he argued for the admission of leprosy patients to the Bir Hospital for surgery.[14]

In April of that year the government's chief leprologist, Dr Indra Bahadur Mali, who had trained in Calcutta under Ernest Muir, took advantage of an audience with the king to press for the introduction of modern sulphone drug treatment in place of the outdated chaulmoogra oil – to which the king agreed. That same month Dr Mali arrived unexpectedly in Tansen and asked Pedley to accompany him on the first ever visit by a senior Ministry of Health official to the government settlement of Malunga. Dr Mali and others put pressure on the government to repeal the leprosy laws, but without effect: the antiquated laws were still in place when the new Statute Book was published in June. Sensing that the king, who had consented to open the new Mission to Lepers leprosy hospital at Anandaban later in the year, was on his side, Mali continued to campaign for a change in the law. He used the results of the WHO survey, which estimated that there were at least 100,000 leprosy sufferers in the country, or 1 per cent of the population of ten million, to argue against their compulsory confinement at Khokana and Malunga on the grounds of both expense and public health: it cost the government half a million rupees a year simply to feed and house the inmates, and it did not require great imagination to see that these settlements, given the number of children born in them, were 'factories for the manufacture of leprosy in the country'.[15]

Pedley himself was caught up in the process of change when Dr Mali invited him to Kathmandu to talk to the Director of Health Services about the leprosy work being done by the United Mission at Malunga and Tansen. He was then taken on a tour of government leprosy institutions in the Kathmandu valley, where he marvelled at the progress being made. Modern drugs were now being dispensed at clinics and at Khokana, where for the first time there were plans to build a workshop for the rehabilitation of healthy inmates at least. He helped make history by participating in an eye operation on a leprosy patient in the Bir Hospital – 'the first operation for the correction of a deformity caused by leprosy ever to be performed in a Government Hospital'. He gave an illustrated talk and displayed handicrafts made by leprosy patients at Tansen to Ministry of Health officials, who eagerly sought his views.[16]

Pedley reported that the intense lobbying had been successful: he'd heard that the king, shortly before his departure in September on a visit to Israel, had revoked the leprosy laws. But this seems to have been wishful thinking; the repressive legislation remained (and, as far as can be ascertained, still remains) on the Statute Book.

Equally, if not more, serious from Pedley's point of view was the introduction of stringent new laws against the spread of Christianity in Nepal: in addition to penalties for those who tried to convert Hindus, there were penalties even for those who 'converted themselves'. Since the wave of imprisonments of Nepali Christians in 1960 indigenous church leaders had been too afraid to baptise anyone, though there were converts clamouring for baptism. Now they would be even more afraid. So what was to be done? For Pedley the answer was simple: 'Prayer, more prayer, and yet more prayer.'[17]

In 1966, Dr I.B. Mali spent three weeks at Carville as part of his training for a master's degree in tropical medicine at Tulane University. Interviewed by the *Star*, he compared the facilities at the United States leprosarium with the lack of them at Khokana, where there was no electricity or heating, only a few cold-water taps and outside latrines, and soap was a luxury.

> But I have read about Carville as it was only thirty-five years ago [he went on] and in some ways, Carville seemed even worse off then than Khokana does now. For at Khokana, no barbed wire encloses the compound, no identifying cards are issued, and no patient assumes a pseudonym 'to protect his family'.[18]

Yet his hope that, just as Carville had emerged from its dark age through the efforts of its patients, the conscience of the country and occasional disbursements from a well-stocked treasury, Khokana might do likewise seemed unlikely to be realised. Nepal was too poor, the majority of its people too intent on survival to enjoy the luxury of a social conscience, and leprosy patients too cut off and cowed, not to say illiterate, to mount a campaign of protest at their treatment – no mute inglorious Stanley Steins at Khokana.

But the inmates of a government leprosy settlement were quite capable of making their feelings known, as Cecil Pedley discovered to his cost on a routine visit to Malunga in January 1967. His team from Tansen was confronted by a deputation of four men, who told them that the people of Malunga no longer wanted them to come and give out medicine. When asked why, the men said that they 'interfered with their way of life' – by which they meant that the Christians tried to discourage the amount of intermarrying that went on. The men cheerfully admitted that they came to the settlement in the hope of finding a partner and having children, regardless of whether they already had a wife and family in their village. According to Pedley, what they were really trying to say was: 'We don't come in here to get better; we want to stay here for life and we have no intention of returning to our villages where we are not welcome.' Pedley felt hurt at being rejected by the patients and perhaps he exaggerated their lack of desire to get better since they still wanted to get their medicine, but from a government doctor rather than the United Mission.[19]

There was a valid medical reason for his disapproval of intermarrying in these institutions, namely, anxiety over the fate of the children born in them; but there can be little doubt that the sexual licence also offended his Christian sense of the sanctity of marriage, or that a number of patients, in their turn, resented the attempts of the United Mission to reform them spiritually as well as treat them physically. At the same time his contention that Khokana and Malunga should be 'sealed off' and most of the inmates treated as outpatients in the community, and that the continued existence of the two settlements served only to perpetuate the belief that leprosy was incurable and its sufferers incapable of leading normal lives, was unexceptionable.

Pedley was hopeful that the first leprosy conference ever to be held in Nepal, which took place in Kathmandu in March 1969 with such eminent leprologists as T. Frank Davey and Stanley G. Browne in attendance, would give a new impetus to leprosy work and hasten the repeal of the anachronistic segregation laws.[20] And when Stanley Browne came to write his report of the conference for the Leprosy Mission, whose medical consultant he was, he too was sanguine, claiming it had done more to change official attitudes towards leprosy in a week than had been achieved in the previous twenty years.[21]

The conference was jointly sponsored by the government of Nepal and the WHO and was chaired by Dr I.B. Mali. It soon became clear to Browne that the missionaries had a great deal more practical experience of leprosy than the government doctors and that much of the pressure to change the laws came from them. But there were important contributions from government representatives, too. A dermatologist spoke out against the legal discrimination, pointing out that though regional governors and magistrates rarely invoked the law, those who stood to gain by it, such as moneylenders and grasping relatives, frequently did, with the result that the victim was segregated for life in one or other of the government institutions. Not only that, but leprosy was still legal grounds for divorce, and marriages could be dissolved if it was shown that one of the partners had been concealing the disease at the time they were wed.[22]

Browne went to Khokana to see the conditions there for himself. 'In all my travels', he wrote, 'I have never seen such a depressing, crowded, filthy, hopeless, useless, immoral, terrible place.' He described how nearly 600 people were crammed into a single three-storey building that was a veritable rabbit warren of tiny, low, dark, mud-floored rooms. Children, 'who had no need or indeed right to be there', gathered at the window apertures. Browne could scarcely contain his indignation:

> The listless and apathetic dehumanised inmates have nothing to do to occupy their minds or their hands, no contact with the outside world, and no hope for the future. They are the victims of society, and of the

discriminatory and coercive legislation. They cannot be released. Some have been there for fifty years or more.[23]

Despite the availability of dapsone, few bothered to take it. Two nursing sisters did what they could, 'ministering to these ungrateful, cantankerous, uncooperative people, dressing their wounds and trying to inspire some self-respect and hope'. So far as Browne was concerned, the only relief was provided by a cell of some thirty Christian patients – 'an oasis of hope and cheer amid the prevailing squalor and filth and stench'. It was imperative, he felt, that no new patients should be admitted, and that over the next few years the existing population be weeded out by a medical team and only those incapable of any kind of rehabilitation be allowed to remain. Those in need of surgery might be taken to one of the Kathmandu hospitals, or to the Leprosy Mission hospital at Anandaban – though Anandaban, which Browne also visited, was itself in need of reform, or at least strong leadership to provide a sense of direction.[24]

Six months after Browne's visit, Dr Pedley was back in Kathmandu for a meeting at the 'spacious' office of the Director of Health Services, where he was disappointed to learn that the iniquitous old law still stood: 'The local governor or the magistrate shall send the leprosy patient to the place meant for him by His Majesty's Government.' But a new interpretation was to be put on the words, 'the place meant for him'. Instead of admitting new patients to the already overcrowded settlements of Khokana and Malunga, which together now had well over 1,000 inmates, the government proposed to send them to the mission-run hospitals at Anandaban, Pokhara (where the INF leprosy hospital, Green Pastures, set up in the 1950s by Eileen Lodge and Betty Bailey, was now well established) and Tansen. The representatives of these institutions protested. Of course they were happy to think that Khokana and Malunga were to be sealed off, but they disapproved of the element of compulsion – not to say expulsion – conveyed by the words 'to the place meant for him' and pressed once again for abrogation of the law.[25]

One of the proposals of the conference of March 1969, the formation of a Nepalese Leprosy Relief Association under royal patronage (the presence of a princess throughout the proceedings had given them additional authority), had been immediately adopted. NELRA, as the association became known, still exists. It was set up as a non-governmental organisation with a threefold aim: of working towards reform of the medical and legal system so that leprosy patients might be diagnosed and treated scientifically and humanely; of improving conditions at Khokana and Malunga; and of contributing to plans for a national leprosy control campaign. The Nepalese committee asked for the loan of an adviser from a voluntary organisation to get the project started, and the Danish medical missionary, Dr Johannes G. Andersen, took up the challenge; he arrived in Kathmandu in January 1970.[26]

Andersen set about his task with a will. He examined the relevant legal texts and, while reluctantly accepting that some might remain on the Statute Book so long as they were not used to harass leprosy sufferers and their families, he was adamant that the segregation law should go, regardless of whether or not it was actually being implemented. As for Khokana and Malunga, which NELRA was committed to reforming, he strongly felt that they, too, should go; but that would have to be done in stages. The first priority was to stop all admissions; the next was to return to their homes all those who were socially and medically equipped to cope and had homes to go to. For those with no homes, the aim was to resettle them on land specially provided for the purpose, as a kind of staging post between involuntary segregation and normal village life.

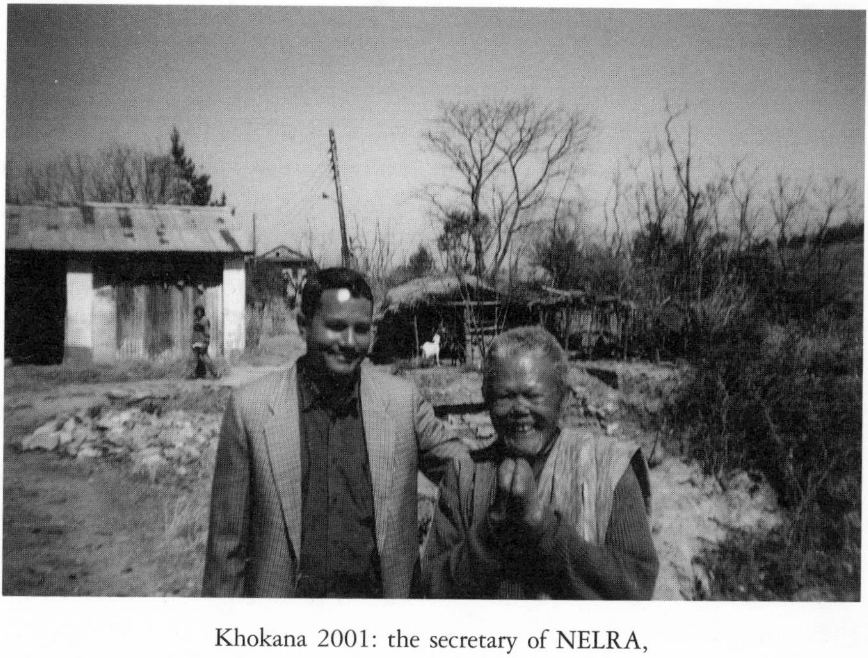

(author photo)

Khokana 2001: the secretary of NELRA, Bidur Basnet, with a long-standing leprosy patient

And finally, for those inmates who were physically or mentally too far gone to reintegrate into society, it was proposed 'as a purely temporary measure' that they be maintained at Khokana. The price of remaining in public care, however, would be compulsory vasectomy – since they could not take care of themselves, offspring should be out of the question. As it was, there were a number of children, many of them orphans, who would have to remain at Khokana, but they were to be looked after in a special rehabilitation home, funded by German money.[27]

When a survey was undertaken to assess the resettlement potential of the patients at Khokana, it almost resulted in a riot. The bemused inmates feared they were about to be thrown out of the only home they knew. On hearing of threats of violence a high-ranking government official who was also on the committee of NELRA had to go there to explain that the purpose of the survey was to see how best to improve their conditions. After that, most were happy to co-operate.[28]

Andersen had a problem of his own. At first he couldn't understand why, when he had the backing of two princesses and ready access to many of the most influential people in government, including a very supportive Director General of Health, all his initiatives were being blocked. For instance, no sooner had it been officially agreed that no more patients should be sent to Khokana than six new patients were admitted. The finger of suspicion pointed at Dr Mali, who combined the role of government chief leprologist with that of secretary of NELRA. Whether or not Mali felt that Andersen was usurping his authority, he did his utmost to sideline NELRA's adviser. Andersen was kept waiting outside the meeting at which he was supposed to present his report, supposedly just for quarter of an hour while internal business was being discussed, but in the event for four hours. By which time the meeting was over and most of the committee were puzzled as to why Mali, not Andersen, should have presented a report he clearly knew very little about and made comments on it. Everyone but Mali subsequently apologised to Andersen for this slight.[29]

Mali was in an invidious position. He was being asked to implement a new policy that was not backed by the law and, as he kept reminding Andersen, so long as the law was not changed he was powerless to do anything. Andersen suspected him of either playing for time, perhaps in the hope that once the adviser had gone he might get the credit for the reforms (to which the Danish adviser said he was welcome), or simply not wanting things to change – at least not to the extent proposed.[30] In the light of Mali's past record, the latter suspicion seems unjust. It is more likely that he was being cautious because his involvement in earlier efforts to change the law had made him justifiably sceptical of the success of this latest attempt and, unlike Andersen, who would be flying out of the country in a few months' time, he would have to live with the consequences.

The scheme for resettling those people from Khokana who were capable of returning to normal life but had no homes to go back to went ahead. An area of jungle in the western Terai was earmarked for this experimental settlement, which was not to become just another enclave like the leprosy settlements that were supposedly being phased out, but was to be a transitional stage in the process of reintegration into society. The person charged with the responsibility for making it work was Eileen Lodge, who had left Green Pastures in Pokhara after more than fifteen years of leprosy work. She spoke fluent Nepali and had already offered her services to the leprosy control project. The idea was that she should accompany the resettlement group to their destination and be on hand to advise and help them become normal citizens once again.[31]

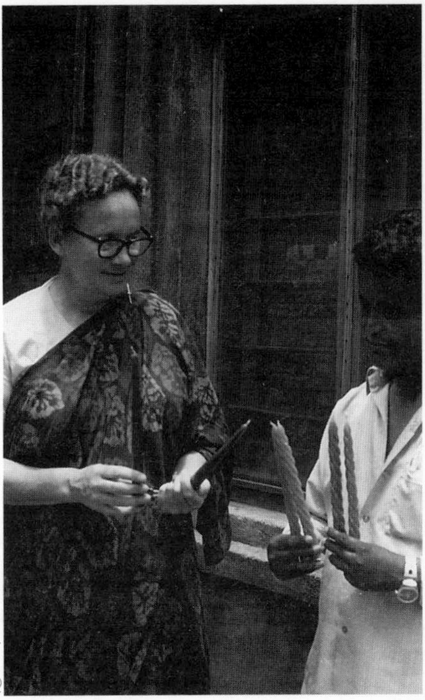

(©TLM)

Eileen Lodge, the doyenne of leprosy workers in Nepal, with a candle maker

Thirty years later, Eileen Lodge referred to this episode as 'the fiasco down in Khokana' and said she'd been 'driven to distraction' by the grim conditions and the impossibility of getting anything done at a government institution. Bureaucracy was anathema to her, and Nepalese bureaucracy was more labyrinthine than most. She was used, as she put it, to 'playing it by ear': two or three times during the 1960s she had driven a Land Rover from the UK overland to Nepal, bringing with her essential equipment for the Green Pastures hospital. She did get involved in the rehabilitation of patients from Khokana, but on her own terms. In 1972 she set up the Nepal Leprosy Trust and went to live in a house with three leprosy families, who made a living out of manufacturing candles; by doing all the marketing themselves they became a part of the community.[32]

Her next venture was to move into an old Rana palace south of Kathmandu on the road to Anandaban and turn it into a transit house for farming families, who had to get used to handling their own money – since they got no cash at Khokana, only rations. At first there was some local opposition to this farming project and people threw stones on to the palace roof. But the leprosy patients kept a low profile and did not retaliate, so eventually the locals left them alone. Eileen Lodge accompanied these farmers out to Bardia in the western Terai and stayed with them for the first ten days; the Nepal Leprosy Trust gave them rations while they were settling in, and provided them with animals, water pumps and tools to enable them to get started. These pioneers were followed by two or three other groups of leprosy settlers (or re-settlers) during the 1970s and 1980s, some of whom were quite seriously disabled. They even started a technical school, but that closed in 1990, though it was still desperately needed – not just for leprosy sufferers but for all the young school leavers without skills.[33]

The year 1990 saw the revolution that transformed Nepal into a constitutional monarchy and replaced the *panchayat* system of royally appointed central and local authorities with elected government. This has not proved an unmixed blessing, in that the corruption that brought down the *panchayat* system has been equally evident in the new democracy and, in addition, whichever political party has been elected has been more intent on holding on to the perquisites of power than on improving the lot of the people. Yet there have been gains, not least in religious tolerance. Foreigners are still forbidden to proselytise, but Nepali Christians and the increasing number of Muslims in the country are free to worship as they will.

In 1990 the Nepal Leprosy Trust was in the process of trying to set up a new leprosy hospital in the central Terai, and the coming of democracy complicated an already difficult task. But in other respects the founding of Lalgadh went so smoothly that Eileen Lodge saw it as a miracle. 'The hand of God was everywhere evident', she said. From a chance encounter with the commander-in-chief of the Nepalese army, which led to an immediate offer of help – it turned out that the general's grandfather had owned more than 20,000 acres of land in the area and he himself had been born there – to the discovery that the springs on the property yielded enough water to obviate the need to excavate a dry river-bed, everything fell into place.[34] Now Lalgadh is a busy hospital, catering for a large region north of the Indian border in which the dominant ethnic group is the Maithili people, who speak a language closer to Hindi than Nepali.

But Eileen Lodge has moved on and, despite suffering from diabetes and being well over the age at which most people retire and put their feet up, become active in the eastern region of the Terai, an area 'overflowing with leprosy' and, like Lalgadh, close to the Indian border, 'with all Bihar to the south of us'. Her latest organisation, the Nepal Leprosy Fellowship, has its headquarters in Dharan (for many years the British Gurkha HQ and main recruiting centre in Nepal, too) and once a month, on a day set aside for leprosy, sends mobile teams round all the health posts in the region to take skin smears.[35] Since 1987, the leprosy control programme has been integrated into the basic health services of Nepal, but the trouble is, in many parts of the country those health services are very basic indeed and the diagnosis and treatment of leprosy require special knowledge and skills.

One successful recent initiative has been a media campaign. This was conducted as part of a government-sponsored national leprosy elimination campaign, backed by the World Health Organization. The WHO had independently engaged the BBC (and a charitable trust set up by the BBC called the Marshall Plan of the Mind, or MPM) to look into the possibility of organising media-based leprosy awareness campaigns in five countries with a high rate of endemicity – the other four countries were India, Brazil, Ethiopia and Indonesia. (According to the WHO, just twelve countries provide over 90 per cent of leprosy cases in the world, and Nepal ranks sixth among them.) The BBC-MPM did a feasibility study and came up with a proposal to mount campaigns in each country with the aim of giving a 'new face to an old disease'. And in 1998–9 Nepal became the first country to conduct such a campaign.[36]

The object of the campaign was threefold: to make people aware of the symptoms of leprosy; to convey the message that it was curable, and that medicine was available free of charge; and to reduce the

Kun Junika Paap Ho

Some say it's the result of sins in a former life
Some say it's a curse from a former life
But more than my wounds it hurts me more
When some say my life is over

Friends turned away, friends left my side
I don't mind the attitude of others
But even my very own cut off ties from me
I became a speck of dust in the eye
I became a thorn in the flesh
I'm a person too
Although I'm human I became distanced from humanity

What's the difference between you and me?
I'm just like you too
I too have feelings
I'm a person just like you
I too have desires, let me weave my own sweet dreams
I'm a person, let me live like one

Sins, curses don't mean a thing
I'll write my own destiny
I'm a person, I'll put together my world

Voice Over

It's not a sin, it's not a curse
Leprosy is just a simple disease
If you recognize the signs and get treatment on time, you can be cured
Let's get treatment on time
Let's chase the disease, not the people out of our community
Let's make a leprosy free society
Let's increase mutual understanding

(*Leprosy Review*)

Translation of the Nepali media campaign theme song

stigma and fear associated with the disease. The state television and radio participated and a number of celebrities from film and TV gave their services either for free or at a fraction of their normal charge. The campaign theme song, posters, TV and radio documentaries, dramas and comedies, and – since television and radio are still luxuries and have yet to penetrate some parts of Nepal – street theatre all pressed home the message that leprosy was not a sin or a curse, but a disease like any other. A crucial aspect of the campaign was the involvement of a number of leprosy-affected people from different social classes and with different levels of impairment. All they had in common was that 'they had overcome leprosy, not only physically but also socially, emotionally and psychologically'. They were interviewed and told their stories on TV and radio; they were photographed hobnobbing with celebrities; and they appeared on a poster depicting nine people and asking the question, 'Which of these people has leprosy?' The answer: 'None, they have all been cured.'[37]

The effectiveness of the media campaign was put to an immediate test in the elimination campaign's 'search week', when hundreds of government health workers combed the country for new cases of leprosy. In six days they came up with nearly 12,000, and what amazed everyone involved was how readily people came forward for treatment. Almost overnight, it seemed, the fear of being stigmatised that for years had kept people with leprosy in hiding had been replaced by an eagerness to be cured. The example set by those who had risked scorn and derision by showing their scars in public not only encouraged more timid souls to seek treatment; it also proved cathartic to the participants themselves. As one of them remarked, referring to his early experience of leprosy:

> The villagers had several meetings and they tried to kick me out of the village. At that time I felt like committing suicide . . . Now all the villagers call me *Hakim* [leader]. A leader! 'Oh, Ram Nandan is an important man – a leader'.[38]

The media campaign was a one-off event, involving outsiders who would depart or return to their normal activities, and the difficulty has been to sustain the impetus it created. Leprosy workers have tried in various ways. At Lalgadh, for instance, they resorted to street theatre and put on popular shows in the district – 'the people who get leprosy don't get to see television or listen to the radio'. But when they conducted research into the extent of public prejudice against leprosy-affected people they found little difference in the attitudes of those who had seen their shows and those who hadn't: both displayed a greater tolerance than the stories

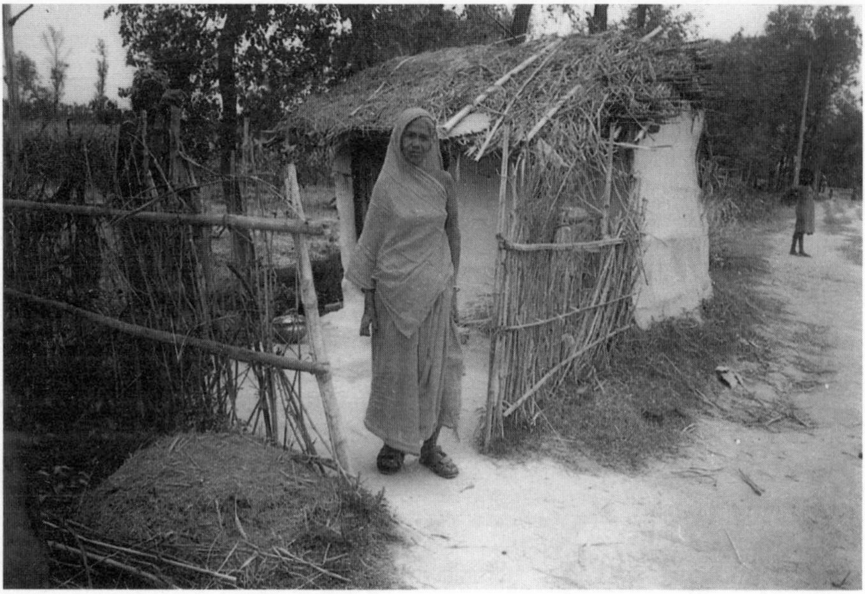
(author collection)

Deuna Devi, in front of her wattle-and-daub hovel

of their patients had led them to expect. This suggested either that patients had internalised the stigma of leprosy and imagined disapproval or rejection where none was intended, or that the public said one thing and did another. Perhaps there was an element of both.[39]

Deuna Devi was a Maithili woman whose husband had left her for another woman when she developed leprosy and whose only child had died in infancy – an unremarkable event in that part of the world, where appalling sanitation and the lack of potable water make dysentery commonplace. She had been ostracised and driven out of the community, not even allowed access to the village water supply until a deputation from Lalgadh succeeded in convincing the village development committee (VDC) that she was entirely non-infectious, a 'burnt-out case' who represented no health risk whatsoever despite the deformities of her hands and feet. But by then the damage was done and though the villagers relented to the extent of allowing Deuna Devi to use the communal water supply nothing could alter her conviction that they all hated her.[40]

She lived in a tiny, crudely thatched wattle-and-daub hovel; its nearest European equivalent would be a moderately spacious dog kennel. There was scarcely room for even so small a woman as she was to stretch out on the mud floor to sleep. The whole hut and yard would have fitted into an average-

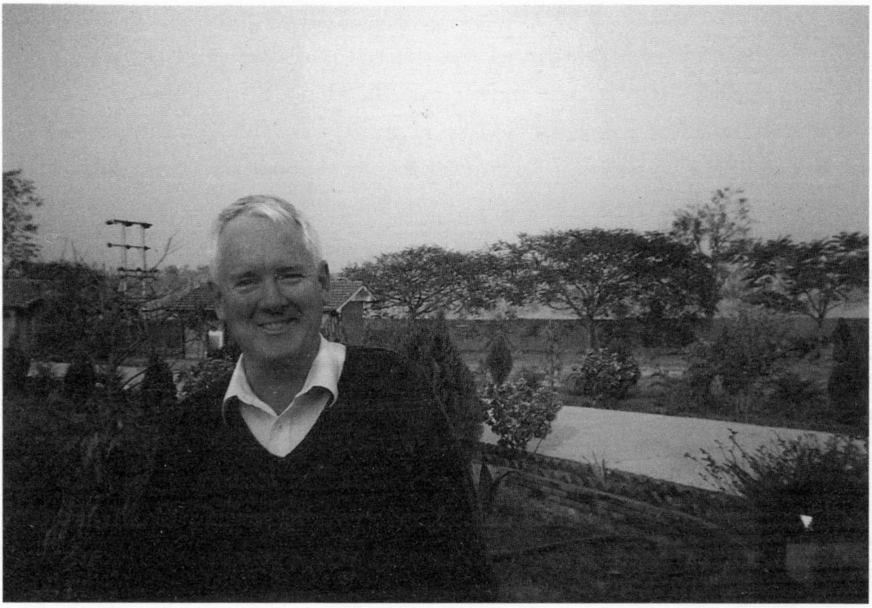

(author photo)

Dr Hugh Cross at Lalgadh in 2001

sized western living room. Yet, disabled as she was, she kept the place spotlessly clean. It was a long walk to the village and the nearest bus stop and, since Deuna Devi's dwelling was right next to a dirt road, every bullock-cart, tractor and 100 cc motorbike that came past either spattered her with mud or choked her with dust, according to the season.

The Nepal Leprosy Trust had undertaken to build her a new house (at a cost of about £150). It would be bigger and better, and on a more accommodating site within the boundaries of the village. Her ex-husband was dead now, like her child, but his second wife, whose attitude the Lalgadh social worker who often visited the village described as 'very bad', remained implacably opposed to her predecessor. Without the support of the Trust, Deuna Devi could have done nothing; even with it, she felt isolated and vulnerable. In 2001 the Trust was seeking funds to initiate a scheme whereby people affected with leprosy, like Deuna Devi, would attend VDC meetings, find out what was most needed in their village and report back to the Trust, which would then try and get something done about it. The idea was that if a person who'd had leprosy could become a kind of liaison officer, both the individual and the community would benefit.[41]

The programme director at Lalgadh in 2001 was Hugh Cross. He was originally from Zimbabwe, though he'd worked for many years in the UK as a shepherd before training as a podiatrist and taking up leprosy work. He was particularly struck by the harshness of life for women in rural Nepal, with or without leprosy. In one of the wards at Lalgadh there was a listless girl who at the first sign of leprosy had been sold into prostitution – from which she'd been rescued by the Nepal Leprosy Trust – *by her own mother*. This was shocking, yes, but not illogical when every aspect of the situation was taken into consideration. Poor women in rural areas were little more than beasts of burden at the best of times, their only other function in life being to produce children. A young girl with leprosy had no prospect of marriage and so became an economic liability; in a world in which survival was the priority and sentiment a luxury, selling her into prostitution was no more than realising a failing asset. Married women with leprosy were scarcely better off since, like Deuna Devi, they were almost invariably deserted by their husbands – and *vice versa*. In Hugh Cross's experience, women who had leprosy became apathetic, many of the younger ones openly talking of suicide as the only alternative to a life without purpose, and some doing more than talk of it.[42]

Their realism could be breathtaking. Cross took to noting down some of the stories he heard: Thamini Majhini's, for instance. Thamini was an

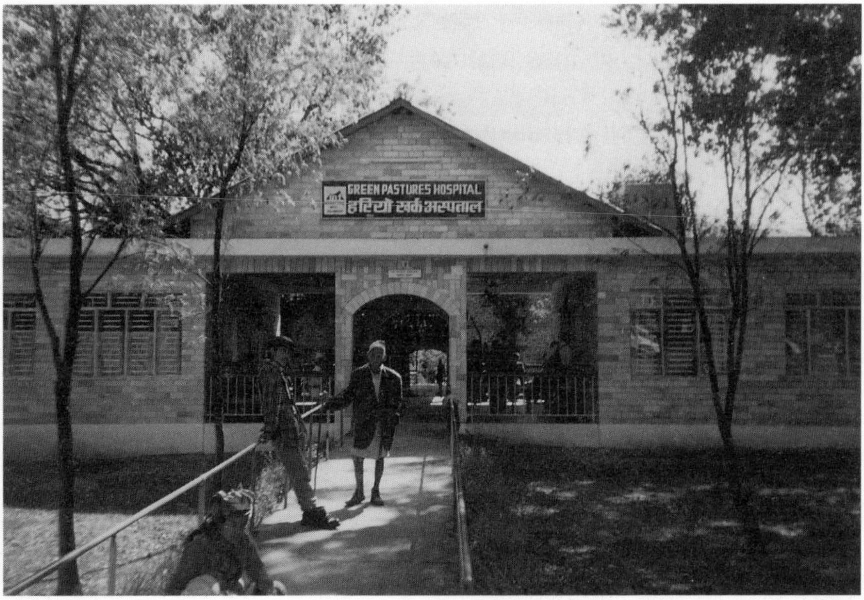

(author photo)

Green Pastures, 2001

illiterate hill woman, 'so shrivelled by hardship that she looks like a seedless raisin'. She had lived in her village for years with untreated leprosy. It wasn't until she developed an ulcer on her anaesthetic foot that the villagers drove her out, obliging her to catch fish in the river and range through the jungle for food. Such hardships as hunger and pain she could endure, just as she put up with the fact that every year when the rains came her shack would fall down. What she could not endure was the isolation, the exclusion from the quarrels and intimacies of family life – in a Hindu culture, where the concept of self is weak, those of family and community are proportionately strong. For Thamini, the cause of her exclusion was not leprosy *per se* but the ulcer on her foot. So she inveigled a couple of men who were cutting bamboo into lending her a *kukri* (the heavy, curved, all-purpose knife made famous as a weapon by the Gurkhas) to cut a branch, and 'walked over to a fallen tree trunk, put up her foot and hacked it off with the borrowed blade'.[43]

Better to be an amputee than a *kori*, a Nepali word that is quite as derogatory as the English word *leper*. Several studies have pointed out that negative and hostile attitudes to leprosy sufferers are a response to deformity rather than to the danger of infection, which is far higher in the early stages of the disease before any outward and visible signs are manifest. According to one such study, it's a Catch-22 situation: 'Even nowadays persons affected by leprosy have to leave their village or are socially isolated. Therefore, it is understandable that persons affected by leprosy try to hide their disease out of fear of negative community actions.' They put off seeking help or, having sought it, stop going to the clinic and taking their course of multiple drug therapy (MDT) in the hope of concealing their disease (a pattern of behaviour known to professionals as 'defaulting' or 'non-compliance'); but in so doing they precipitate the very eventuality they dread most: the onset of deformity and the social segregation that brings.[44]

These findings, however, are challenged in another study, where only five out of 166 new patients who registered for treatment between October 1993 and March 1995 at the leprosy outpatient clinic that the staff of Anandaban Leprosy Hospital hold weekly in Patan, the city adjacent to Kathmandu in the centre of Nepal, 'volunteered that social stigma delayed their presentation for treatment'. The most common cause of delay was 'failure to recognize the possibility of leprosy (87 cases, 52%)'. The authors of this study conclude that ignorance of the disease was a far more potent factor in holding patients back than fear of social consequences, 'though there is anecdotal evidence to suggest that some individuals were successful in concealing the disease from close relatives'.[45]

Green Pastures Hospital in Pokhara is no longer exclusively concerned with leprosy; it is now a general rehabilitation hospital and treats those who are disabled as a result of spinal injury or diseases like polio as well. The fact that it has opened its doors to these other patients – and they mix freely with the leprosy patients – is an indication of the changing perspective on leprosy in Nepal. And not just in Nepal. Throughout the world, 'integration' has been the watchword for the last thirty years or more, meaning the integration of leprosy into the general health services. In Nepal, as we have seen, the process was formally initiated in 1987.

In a paper presented at the Congress of the All-India Association of Leprologists at Bhopal in 1971, Stanley Browne had argued that, given leprosy had 'at long last' entered the mainstream of medicine – even if most medical schools continued largely to ignore it – there was no reason why it should 'maintain its splendid isolation from the rest of medicine'. Effective treatment was available, and with the growing understanding of the distinction between 'active leprosy infection and the late secondary sequelae of peripheral neuropathy', the infectious aspect could be seen to have a great deal in common with other mycobacterial diseases. As a result:

> On grounds of infectivity, curability, absence of an intermediate host, leprosy does not require a separate service. From the standpoint of risk to public health, and the risk of serious, sudden and widespread epidemics, leprosy cannot demand special medical consideration, or special legislative measures. Any special pleading must be on socio-psychological grounds and not on medical grounds.[46]

Separate services were expensive and it did not 'seem morally right to spend thousands of rupees on a single leprosy patient and do nothing for those who happen to be suffering from some other disease or disability'. The same applied to rehabilitation: 'Reconstructive surgery, physiotherapy, prostheses, vocational training, sheltered workshops, job placement, all should be organised for the total need, and not for leprosy victims alone.' Far from being a reviled and neglected outcast the 'ex-leprosy patient' in some communities was in danger of becoming 'an over-privileged and expensive non-productive citizen, making inordinate demands on the budget'.

If Browne overstated his case, it was because he had a particular axe to grind: where money was limited and a choice had to be made, he thought it better to spend it on the discovery and treatment of leprosy in its early active and curable phase rather than on damage limitation in chronic cases. Better still to prevent it, if that were possible. His clinching argument in favour of integration was that 'the very existence of a separate and distinct leprosy control programme, be it ever so successful, serves indirectly to reinforce and perpetuate the myth of the uniqueness of leprosy'.[47]

A decade later, his old colleague from the Belgian Congo, Michel Lechat, sounded a warning note. Yes, of course leprosy management should be part and parcel of the general health services, but there was still considerable resistance to integration, not least in the ranks of the medical profession itself. Admission of leprosy patients into general hospitals was by no means universally welcomed. There was also the danger that the authorities would use integration as an excuse for reducing funding for leprosy control. So though integration was desirable as an ideal, it should be pursued only where it was practicable and did not jeopardise prospects of success: 'Patients come first; doctrine after.'[48]

Another worry is that since modern treatment, as defined by the WHO, has equated 'cure' with bacterial negativity rather than the absence of after-effects, the long-term care of leprosy patients is being overlooked. Leprosy remains a complex and troubling disease requiring specialised medical training and understanding not often found in a country's general health services. In the 'horizontal' (as opposed to 'vertical') model of health care favoured by the WHO, one in which all diseases are treated together and equally, so to speak, leprosy patients are likely to end up at the back of the queue, since their disease is not life-threatening and their needs are neither immediately obvious nor obviously immediate. By 1982, Stanley Browne himself had come round to this view and admitted that 'some ill-considered and premature attempts at integration have left the HD sufferer worse off than before'.[49] The late editor of the *Star*, Emanuel Faria, speaking at the 1993 International

Leprosy Congress in Orlando, Florida, gave the patient's perspective. He said that 'unless we are able to do something for the deformed patients or prevent disabilities, there's no HD control'. He didn't think it was right to be 'talking about curing the disease when there are so many people suffering from the effects of the disease'.[50]

Among leprosy workers in Nepal, as elsewhere, there is considerable anger and disillusion, not over the WHO goal of eradicating the disease (as who would not wish to see an end to this scourge?), but over the way the WHO measures and presents statistics in order to give the impression that 'elimination' – defined as a rate of prevalence of less than one case per 10,000 population – is imminent. The definition of a leprosy case, so far as the WHO is concerned, is someone undergoing multidrug therapy; leprosy-affected persons who have not registered for treatment, or have completed their course of MDT, do not count, no matter what they may require in the way of drugs, clinical care, or rehabilitation. They may have lasting nerve damage, but they don't have 'statistical leprosy'.

Furthermore, in 1998 the WHO changed the rules regarding MDT – halving the length of treatment from twenty-four to twelve months in cases of 'multibacillary' or lepromatous leprosy at the more infectious end of the scale, and from twelve to six months for 'paucibacillary' or tuberculoid leprosy at the less or non-infectious end. While any reduction in medication is to be welcomed provided the treatment remains effective, the jury is still out on the efficacy of the reduced MDT. But what it has unquestionably achieved is a further reduction in statistical leprosy.

Then there is the matter of how statistical leprosy is determined. At Green Pastures, Alison Anderson of the International Nepal Fellowship charted both the 'prevalence' and the 'incidence' of leprosy in the Western Region of Nepal over the last decade of the twentieth century. While prevalence – i.e., the number of people who registered for treatment during that ten-year period – showed a satisfactory drop from 8.5 to 5 per 10,000, incidence – defined as the number of newly detected cases starting treatment in the same period – recorded a worrying rise from 3 to 5 per 10,000.[51] The intensification of the leprosy elimination campaign in the late 1990s may account for the rise in newly discovered cases, but if there was no real increase there was absolutely no decline either. The best that could be said was that incidence was probably stable. No prizes for guessing which yardstick the WHO uses.

For the WHO, which has been predicting the eradication of leprosy for years ('the eradication of leprosy research, more like', one disillusioned researcher suggested) and is responsible for disbursing huge sums of international money to achieve that aim, the elimination campaign *has* to be a success. And to some extent it has been a success – not least in providing the impetus (and funds) to tackle this enduring problem in the poorest countries in the world, like Nepal, which have nearly all the cases. In the sense that it flourishes in conditions of poverty and malnutrition, leprosy is a political disease, and the WHO has done its part in highlighting this and working with national governments to eliminate it.

But the pressure to succeed does not justify the sleight of hand involved in using prevalence rather than incidence as the measure for achieving 'elimination'; in Alison Anderson's words, this is 'just a technical hoax'. All diseases are ultimately tragedies at a *personal* level, as she says. 'Elimination may solve our political, financial, public health and statistical problems, but only eradication will end the human tragedy.' And eradication 'requires a reduction in incidence, so that each year fewer people get the disease'. In Nepal, as in other endemic countries, this is not happening.[52]

When the elimination of leprosy (as a public health problem) failed to be realised in the year 2000, the WHO intensified its campaign and created the Global Alliance for the Elimination of Leprosy (GAEL) along with the Nippon Foundation, the drug company Novartis and the governments of the endemic countries to achieve what it called the 'final push'. But sceptics now claim that the elimination campaign is based on a fundamental misconception. They question the WHO assumption that 'the chain of transmission will be broken when the prevalence rate drops below the target rate' and the disease phased out. As the director of Netherlands Leprosy Relief, Kommer L. Braber, wrote in a letter to the editor of the *Leprosy Review*, 'To my mind it is highly speculative, if only because most infectious leprosy patients have already transferred the bacteria to the people around them before they are diagnosed and placed on MDT.' In Braber's opinion, transmission of leprosy might not decrease for years to come: 'We should not be surprised if six, ten or even thirty years from now, the number of new cases will still be in the region of 500,000 per year world-wide.'[53]

If leprosy had been 'just another communicable disease' it might have been a suitable candidate for a 'final push', but it was not and a leprosy patient was 'not just someone in need of MDT'. The major problem with leprosy was nerve damage leading to disability, and the major cause of this damage was the time lag between the first appearance of the disease and the start of MDT. So anti-leprosy programmes should forget about prevalence and focus on shortening this time lag – 'once the nerves are impaired, the major battle is lost'. Braber was not so much pessimistic as realistic: 'We may never rid the world of leprosy as a bacterial disease, but we do have the means to eliminate leprosy as a disabling disease. Prevention of nerve damage and disability in every patient should become the core of leprosy control.' What he feared might happen after 2005, the deadline for the 'final push', was that the WHO and its sponsors would look for fresh challenges outside the field of leprosy, whether or not they'd reached their prevalence target, and national governments and health authorities would follow suit in declaring leprosy no longer a public health problem – and where would that leave 'the "ex"-leprosy patient and the millions who will need MDT after 2005'?[54]

The British government leprologist and senior lecturer at the London School of Hygiene and Tropical Medicine, Dr Diana Lockwood, concurs with this view. 'The purpose of controlling leprosy', she writes in the *British Medical Journal*, 'is to reduce the rate and severity of disability. The key to effective management of leprosy is early diagnosis and treatment and early recognition and management of nerve damage, combined with effective health education.' Leprosy is not an easy disease to diagnose and the integration of specialised leprosy programmes into primary health care will mean that many patients go undiagnosed, thereby adding to the misleading impression that the incidence of leprosy is on the wane. Both the WHO and a group of experts brought together by the International Leprosy Association (ILA) considered how to simplify diagnosis, and while the WHO line is that 'in 70% of patients, diagnosis can be made by a single sign: an anaesthetic skin patch', the ILA group 'found that the other 30% are multibacillary patients, who are more likely to be infectious and to develop nerve damage'.[55] In other words, the patients in greatest need of treatment (both from their own and from a public health point of view) are the ones most likely to be missed or misdiagnosed in the WHO-sponsored Brave New World.

Another cause for concern is that the WHO technical advisory group have now recommended that all leprosy patients, 'regardless of type', should be given a six-month triple drug regimen – a sort of one-size-fits-all treatment: 'This would simplify leprosy treatment but give 60% of patients a third drug that they do not need, and it would undertreat patients with a high bacterial load.' What is more, it is proposed to implement this treatment without a formal trial.[56]

Part of the difficulty, as Dr Lockwood points out, is that in the world of leprosy there are different perspectives: 'WHO has a global public health view, treating populations, whereas the leprosy non-governmental organisations have a stronger focus on treating individuals.' The International Federation of Anti-Leprosy Associations (ILEP) was to have been part of the Global Alliance when it was formed in 1999, but when some of its members questioned GAEL policies it was excluded from the partnership. Such high-handed behaviour does not inspire confidence in the integrity of the WHO and its private partners.

Lockwood describes the elimination of leprosy as a 'virtual phenomenon'. It will be the 'elimination of registered cases through very short treatment regimens'. There is 'no evidence [the] predefined prevalence will reduce transmission, incidence, or the annual number of new cases'. Like Braber, she worries over what will happen to leprosy control programmes in endemic countries like Nepal once the WHO has (or hasn't, as the case may be) achieved its increasingly meaningless goal. Questions abound:

> Who will provide drug treatment after 2005? Who will train the primary health care workers once the vertical programmes have been disbanded? What plans are being made for the long-term care of patients with nerve damage, who will continue to present for many years to come?[57]

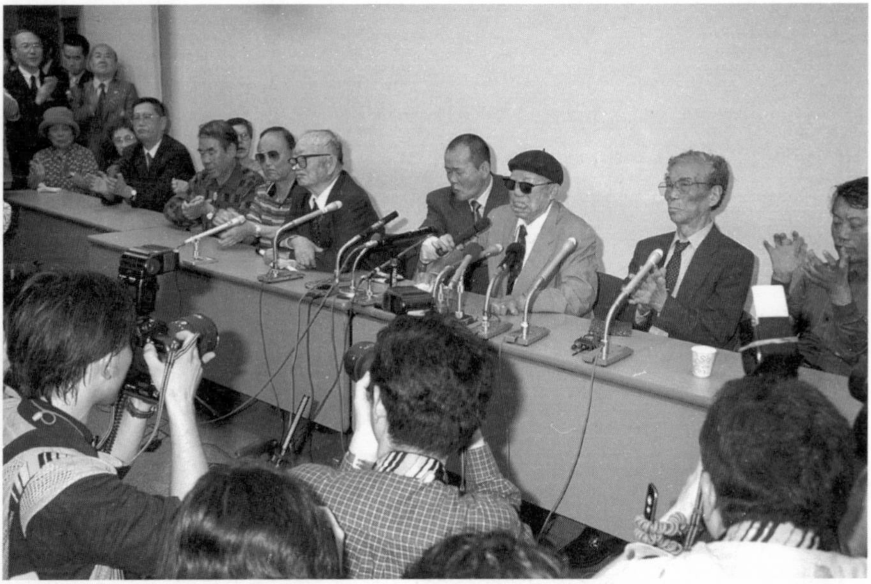

(*Photograph by Nobuyuki Yaegashi*)

Ex-patients applaud the decision of the Japanese government on 23 May 2001 not to appeal against the Kumamoto district court ruling that the Leprosy Prevention Law was unconstitutional

Chapter 14

A KIND OF CLOSURE

If Nepal proved reluctant to repeal the leprosy segregation law – and India as recently as in the 2002 National Public Health Act included 'Special provisions regarding leprosy' reminiscent of legislation enacted by the British authorities over a hundred years earlier[1] – Japan was unique in continuing to use isolation as the main means of leprosy control long after other countries had abandoned it as unnecessary. The Leprosy Prevention Law of 1907 that Hannah Riddell had been instrumental in framing as a relief measure was revised in 1931 to make it harsher and again, more controversially, in 1953, and was not finally abrogated till 1996![2] As an economically developed country in Asia, Japan might have been expected to take the lead in treating its leprosy patients in a humane way. But instead of getting the best of both worlds, they got the worst. They were incarcerated, deprived of human rights and if they married subjected to sterilisation and forced abortion; at the same time, like their US equivalents, they had to change their names to obviate stigmatisation of their families.

During the Second World War they suffered quite as much in their homeland as did their counterparts in occupied countries like Malaya and the Philippines. The influential Dr Kensuke Mitsuda, the 'Father of Leprosy Relief Work' in Japan, was so infected by the fascistic mood of the time that in 1941 he called for the round-up of all leprosy sufferers and their confinement in state-run institutions. In one leprosarium, so it was said, 'dozens of patients committed suicide' and hundreds, if not thousands, more ran away, never to be heard of again; yet to remain (and this applied to all the over-crowded sanatoria) was 'to be sentenced to what amounted to death by malnutrition'. And the post-war political reconstruction hardly touched them: 'the principle of absolute isolation of leprosy patients remained unchanged for several decades that followed as if there had been no change in the country and the world.'[3]

Mitsuda was still playing a prominent role in dictating policy in 1951. He and two other directors of state-run leprosaria testified before a government public health committee.

> It is necessary to have laws which make it possible to force leprosy patients to be contained in sanatoria even if it is against their will [they claimed]. Sterilization is a good way to ensure that the disease will not be transmitted among family members. To escape from a sanatorium should be made a crime . . . and as such be punished.[4]

Fifty years later the elderly Kaoru Matsumoto, a dignified, blind Japanese Christian and former head of the patients' association at the Tama Zenshoen leprosarium, recalled how, though women patients were fenced off from the men, young men and women would meet at the fence and talk and fall in love, and how the men would climb over the fence after dark to consummate these so-called 'commuter marriages'. The authorities knew all about them, of course, and allowed them to happen on condition that the men had a vasectomy – 'an abominable system', Matsumoto said, 'which took advantage of a patient's vulnerability and forced patients in sanatoria to submit to what otherwise would have been unimaginable'.

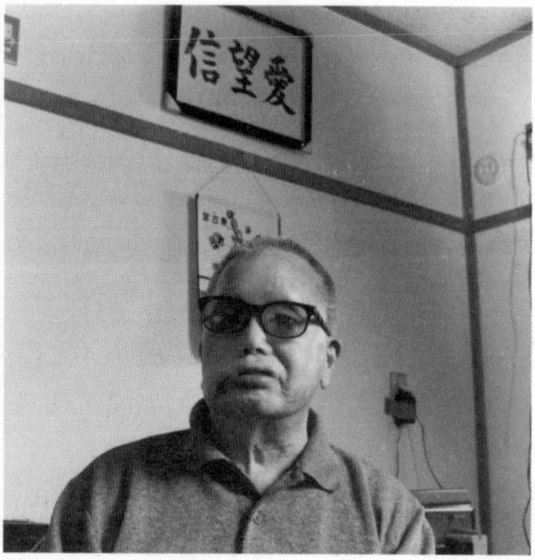

(Photograph by Nobuyuki Yaegashi)

Kaoru Matsumoto

> In the October of 1945, very soon after the end of the Second World War, I too had a vasectomy performed in order to marry. I agonized over whether to submit to the procedure but, in the end, love prevailed and it was performed.
>
> But when I found myself on the operating table, lying on my back and legs spread, panic set in and I was overcome with an urge to flee. This was a proce-

> dure to be performed on animals, not on a human being. When the procedure was over, I felt that I was a failure as a human being. As I slowly made my way back to my dormitory room, bent forward and gingerly walking with my legs spread out, I cried at how pitiful I was.[5]

As if that were not humiliating enough, there were no private rooms for married couples, so the husband still had to go to the women's quarters and spend the night with his wife in a room shared with seven other women, all sleeping almost on top of one another. Sometimes, if he had to get up during the night to answer a call of nature, he might find himself stumbling back into someone else's bed by mistake. Such 'tragicomedies' were not uncommon.[6]

Kaoru Matsumoto was one of the leprosy patients who, in the aftermath of the war and in the face of continuing indignities such as he described, formed an All-Japan patients' association, known as Zen Kan Kyo. The association petitioned the government to make the law less restrictive and punitive and demonstrated outside the Ministry of Health and Welfare building. But when the new law was passed in August 1953, it was found to be unchanged.[7]

During the 1950s a few 'mild cases' were discharged and in 1956 the Ministry of Health and Welfare initiated a rehabilitation project aimed at promoting this scheme; it peaked in 1960, when 216 patients were discharged. After that the number decreased. In 1964 the government offered a grant to help discharged patients find employment, but it was a case of 'too little, too late'.[8] The scheme was bound to fail, given the government's half-hearted approach. Leprosy was reckoned to be 'on the threshold of extinction' in Japan in 1964, and since virtually all patients were confined in institutions – the only places where sulphone treatment was available – the control of leprosy was seen simply as 'a matter of steering patients into the leprosaria'.[9] The same arguments that had raged over the decline of leprosy in late nineteenth-century Norway were rehearsed in late twentieth-century Japan: for every 'expert' who attributed it to the policy of isolation there were several others who regarded it as already underway before the policy took effect and ascribed it to a rise in the general standard of living.

When the Seventh International Congress of Leprology took place in Tokyo in October 1958, the subcommittee on social aspects, chaired by Professor T.N. Jagadisan, passed a resolution stating that 'where governments still enforce a policy of compulsory segregation, this should be totally abandoned'. As Dr T. Ozawa of the Ministry of Health and Welfare was a member of this subcommittee that overtly criticised his government's policy, the Japanese delegates faced a dilemma. They found a simple solution: the document containing this resolution was not translated into Japanese. Had Jagadisan been Japanese rather than Indian, he himself, as an ex-leprosy patient marked by the after-effects of the disease, would have been incarcerated in one of the sanatoria that he was visiting as a VIP. This could have been an embarrassing situation, but both hosts and guest behaved with impeccable politeness; when asked to comment on Japanese policy, all Jagadisan would say was, 'It may be all right at this stage, but you'll most likely eventually be treating on an out-patient basis like we're doing.'[10]

This still wasn't happening in 1972, when Dr Fujio Ohtani was appointed director of the national sanatoria division of the Ministry of Health and Welfare. Indeed, the number of patients treated on an outpatient basis had been declining since 1965. Far from any attempt to reintegrate patients into society, the 'only real effort expended was to improve the conditions in the sanatoria'. Ohtani threw himself into this business of improving conditions. He invited representatives of the Zen Kan Kyo into his office, where he served them tea; his aim was to get staff and patients to sit down together as equals and after about a year he was pleased to see that the divisions were breaking down. But the more involved he became, the more clearly he saw that he was caught on the horns of a dilemma. On the one hand, Japan's rigidly segregationist approach was isolating the country from the rest of the world and depriving patients of their human rights, no matter what was done to improve conditions in the sanatoria; on the other, these patients had been isolated for so many years that they had inevitably become institutionalised:

> They felt there was nowhere they could go without being subjected to discrimination other than the sanatoria, which had been established mostly in remote regions since they were first set up over half a century earlier. Some had friends and some had gotten married inside the sanatoria. For some, a unique culture and, in certain cases, religious organizations had evolved within the sanatoria. The sanatorium was really their home. The sanatoria had become a second home to many.[11]

The question Dr Ohtani had to ask himself was: if he espoused the repeal of the Leprosy Prevention Law, wouldn't that mean that he'd 'lose the basis necessary to work towards improving the terrible conditions'? What seemed to be needed – and was advocated by both Zen Kan Kyo and the Association of National Sanatoria Directors – was a partial revision of the law. What everyone, including the patients who in 1953 had fought for the abrogation of the law, feared was that if the law were repealed, the government would wash its hands of the ageing patient population, allowing conditions to deteriorate still further in the sanatoria, or worse, discharge patients who had no livelihood and nowhere to go. Yet when he considered how society regarded the disease and its victims, several of whom he counted among his friends, Ohtani remained uneasy, wondering if he wasn't guilty of settling for the easy option in concentrating on ameliorating conditions rather than going for the legal jugular.[12]

Through a series of promotions within the Ministry of Health and Welfare, Ohtani's 'real agenda remained the same – to liberate the Hansen's disease patients'. He was proud of his achievements: a bigger budget for medical treatment, increased allowances and pensions, more private rooms in place of open wards and, in 1979, an official change of name from 'leprosy' to 'Hansen's disease'. But looking back after his retirement from the ministry in 1983, he castigated himself for complacency:

> I now realize that I managed to delude myself into thinking that I was doing good things for the patients. In reality, I now know that I was merely a petty bureaucrat filled with a sense of self-importance for the token gestures I was involved in implementing. The truth was, I was a spineless coward and lacked ability.[13]

No Japanese HD patient would agree with Dr Ohtani's critical self-assessment. His involvement with leprosy did not cease with his retirement. Even when he was diagnosed with cancer in 1989 and had to undergo major surgery, from which it took him some years to recover, he worked on the task of creating a museum in the grounds of the Tama Zenshoen sanatorium. The HIH Prince Takamatsu Memorial Hansen's Disease Museum opened in 1993:

> The completion of the Hansen's Disease Museum has had far greater results than I had ever hoped for. It has truly served well as a vehicle to get across the message of the struggle of the Hansen's disease patients to fight the discrimination against them. It also served to give us the confidence we needed to go on to the next stage – namely to get the (New) Leprosy Prevention Law repealed.[14]

No sooner had Ohtani recovered his own health, however, than his wife fell ill, also with cancer. She had taken care of him for the previous four years; now it was his turn to look after her. But she died the following year, in 1994, and he was bereft. He lost all desire to live and work. In the space of just a few years he'd attended four family funerals, losing not only his wife, but both parents and another close relative as well. It was only through the support of leprosy patient activists such as Kaoru Matsumoto and other campaigners that he was able to pull out of his depression and resume the fight for the abrogation of the pernicious law. When it was finally repealed (along with those parts of the Eugenic Law that allowed for the sterilisation of HD sufferers) with effect from 1 April 1996, Ohtani gave all the credit to the Zen Kan Kyo, which had

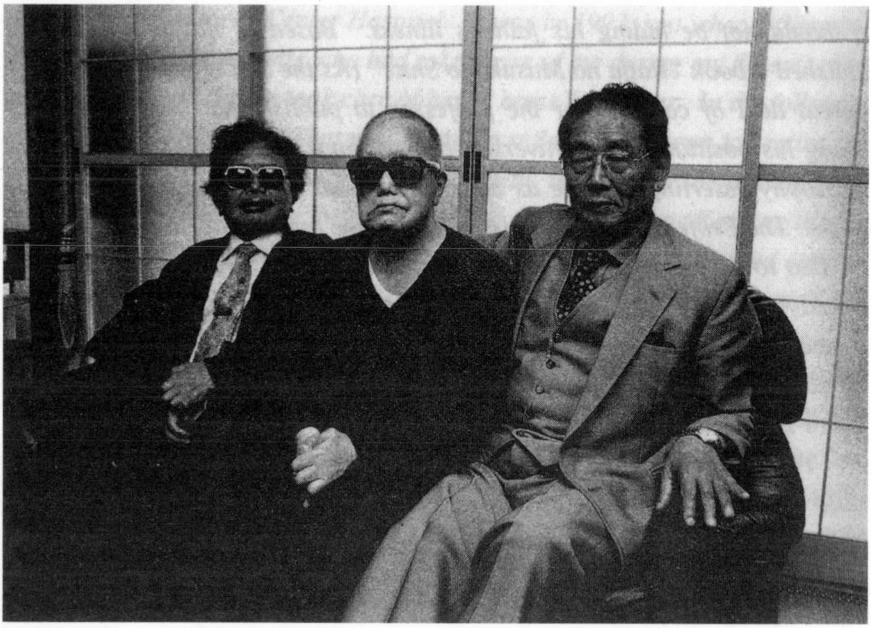

(Tofu Kyokai Foundation)

Dr Fujio Ohtani (*right*) with patient leaders Yasuji Hirasawa and Kaoru Matsumoto (*centre*)

struggled for over forty years to achieve this. Of his own part, he wrote characteristically: 'As one who once was an official within the Ministry of Health and Welfare, I reflect upon my responsibility for not making as much effort as I should have for which I deeply apologize.'[15]

At that time there were about 5,700 leprosy survivors living in fifteen sanatoria throughout Japan.[16] As Anwei Skinsnes Law, project co-ordinator of IDEA (the International Association for Integration, Dignity and Economic Advancement), whose aim is 'to decrease the social isolation felt by so many individuals affected by Hansen's disease and ensure that they are treated justly as citizens equal to all others', reported in the *Star*, 'Although their average age is seventy, they are determined to BEGIN new lives.'[17] The Zen Kan Kyo was renamed the Zen Ryo Kyo (National Association of Sanatoria Residents) and several of the erstwhile outcasts resumed their original identities and attempted to re-establish family ties that had been so cruelly severed.

This was not always possible. Tokie Nishi's story, recounted in the *Washington Post*, is not untypical. Aged seventy-one in 2001, she had been living an institutional life for fifty years, though she'd been cured of the disease soon after entering a sanatorium. When she'd been diagnosed with leprosy in 1949, aged nineteen, her mother had pleaded with the doctors to let Tokie stay at home, but this had not been permitted. There'd been a two-year standoff during which Tokie's parents held out against the authorities, but then the neighbours found out and the social pressure became so intense that her parents had had to give in. Her father had taken her to the station and there they'd parted – in silence and misery.

> For a few years, she was allowed to visit her home once a year, but her mother eventually told her to stop coming. 'The pressure of discrimination was so harsh on her,' Nishi said. 'I was the only daughter she had, and I think she paid the highest price. She was so sad. I do not know if she is alive or dead.'[18]

Tokie Nishi was in no doubt as to why the authorities had segregated people like her: 'The government kept people inside not to prevent the spread of leprosy, but because we were "the shamed".'[19]

The final act in the legal battle over the Leprosy Prevention Law took place on 11 May 2001 in the district court of Kumamoto (the city in which Hannah Riddell had begun her leprosy work 120 years earlier), when Judge Masashi Sugiyama ruled that the law was unconstitutional 'because it excessively restricted the rights of patients through a quarantine that was no longer needed after 1960'. The government was ordered to pay 1.82 billion yen (£10.4 million) in compensation to 127 mostly elderly former leprosy patients, and there were other lawsuits filed by former leprosy patients pending in Tokyo and Okayama.[20]

One of the leaders of the 127 plaintiffs was an eighty-two-year-old man who for sixty-one of those years had lived under the pseudonym Shigeo Arata. When the verdict was announced, he celebrated by reclaiming his real name, Tamiichi Tanaka. He'd run away from home when he contracted leprosy at the age of twenty-one and, after a failed attempt at suicide in a mountain crater, had voluntarily entered a state leprosarium under his assumed name. There he'd met his wife Mie, who was two years older. She became pregnant and, though she'd repeatedly begged to be allowed to have the baby, had been forced to have an abortion in the *sixth* month of her pregnancy. In 1998 Tanaka and (at that stage) twelve other former patients filed the damages suit, but got no support from the sanatorium's patient counsellor who did not even allow them to hold meetings with their lawyers on the premises. Eventually, with his wife in hospital suffering from senile dementia, Tanaka had been obliged to hand over the leadership of the ever-expanding group of plaintiffs in order to spend more time with Mie. But nothing could spoil the ultimate victory. A tearful but jubilant Tanaka exclaimed, 'We finally made it!'[21]

The success of the Kumamoto court case was in no small measure due to the testimony of Dr Fujio Ohtani, who had been called as a witness by both the plaintiffs and the defendants. Characteristically, he refused to meet and discuss his testimony with either side in advance but shut himself up for months to study all the available documentation before coming to court and giving his evidence. He spoke of his own part – 'as an administrator and a pragmatist' – in getting a 'bad law' repealed and argued that the real question now was, who had been responsible for maintaining such a law so long after there had ceased to be any justification for it? Dr Ohtani indicted not just the government and those individuals in the medical and legal professions and the media who had power and influence (including himself), but society in general for colluding in denying patients their basic human rights and dignity.

The only time Dr Ohtani lost his composure was when he was questioned about the reluctance of some ex-patients to leave the sanatoria now that they were free to do so. He angrily pointed out that, having been isolated for most of their lives and deprived of their freedom and dignity – their homes, families, their right to procreate, even their names – they could hardly be expected to accept society's change of attitude towards them at face value. No one who heard his contention that society had made them what they were, and it was only right that society should make amends, had any doubt that he was castigating himself for his own past actions as a high official in ameliorating conditions for patients rather than challenging the law head on from the very beginning.

Such was the effect of his testimony that when he finished speaking, everyone in the court stood up and applauded him. The eloquence and transparent honesty of the elderly Dr Ohtani had made the case unanswerable.[22]

In the United States, the final act at Carville – renamed the Gillis W. Long Hansen's Disease Center in 1985 – revolved around the 'stipend' or, to give it its official name, assisted living allowance.[23] This was an annual payment for life that the dwindling number of inpatients was offered by the government in 1998 as an inducement to move out, so that the facility might be closed down.

What had once been a swampy hell-hole in the back of beyond had long since been transformed into a fine estate comprising handsome buildings, a lake, a golf course and spacious grounds dotted with magnificent old oak trees – now sadly shorn of their decorative Spanish moss by pollution from the ubiquitous petrochemical works that the State of Louisiana has encouraged to spring up in the vicinity. But it was expensive to maintain. Given the history of Carville, it's a nice irony that in 1990 the government leased half of the place to the Federal Bureau of Prisons. There was not much fraternising between patients and prisoners, but during the period that the prisoners shared their quarters the patients noticed a marked improvement in the quality of the food served in the cafeteria.[24]

After that not entirely congenial arrangement had come to an end the question of what to do with Carville took on renewed urgency. One suggestion was to turn it into a National Park, as had happened in 1980 with Kalaupapa in Hawaii, where those patients who'd not wanted to leave the only home many of them had ever known were allowed to remain after it had ceased to be a leprosy settlement. But that came to nothing. The government eventually handed Carville back to the State of Louisiana and it was turned into a quasi-military camp for young people at risk run by the National Guard as part of its Youth Challenge Program.[25]

As in Japan where, by 2001, the average age of the surviving 4,500 or so former patients in sanatoria (or centres, as they'd become) was seventy-four, most of the hundred-odd remaining residents at Carville were old, some having been there for sixty years or more. Opinion was divided over whether or not to take the stipend: younger folk and those with families were keen to pocket the money and take their chance in the outside world, while many of the older single or widowed people were too institutionalised, too tired or too frightened to leave. The worry was that once those who'd chosen to take the stipend were out of the way the government might pull out of Carville entirely.[26]

On 11 March 1999, an 'International Day of Dignity and Respect', sponsored jointly by IDEA and the Carville Patients Federation, was observed at the Gillis W. Long HD Center as a way of drawing public attention to federal legislation that provided 'for removal of patients to

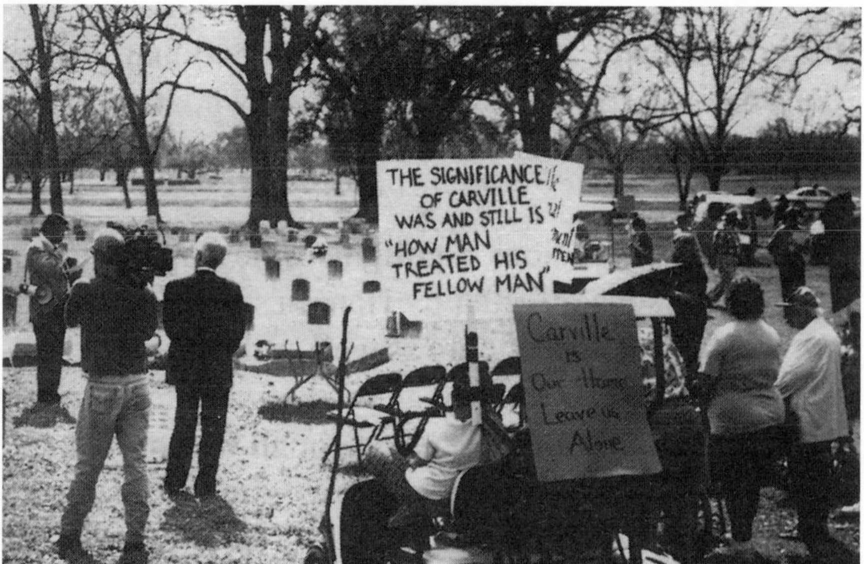
THE SIGNIFICANCE OF CARVILLE WAS AND STILL IS "HOW MAN TREATED HIS FELLOW MAN"
Carville is Our Home Leave us Alone

(©Pamela Parlapiano)

Carville cemetery on the first
'International Day of Dignity and Respect', 11 March 1999

another residence away from Carville'. Patients' representatives were seeking reassurance from the government that those patients who opted to stay should 'be allowed to remain at their Carville home for the rest of their lives'. Eleven days later, that reassurance was provided: patients were given the choice of staying at Carville 'as long as they want', or moving into 'a new assisted living facility in Baton Rouge' (this was the Summit Hospital, where Betty Martin ended her days), or living independently 'with a lifetime, annual, tax-free stipend of $33,000 and free medical care relating to Hansen's disease on an outpatient or short-term basis'.[27]

The last medical director of the GWLHD Center, Dr Robert R. Jacobson, felt that in the end the US Public Health Service handled the changeover from isolation at Carville to referral to outpatient clinics all over the country in the right way. The PHS's earlier attempt to drive the patients out of Carville back in the 1950s when Dr Gordon had been in charge had foundered because it had been premature; at that time there'd been virtually no facilities for Hansen's disease patients outside Carville.[28]

In 1999 fifty-eight patients chose to remain. Death took its toll and by 2001 their number had been reduced to a mere thirty-eight. Mary Ruth Daigle was one of them, a survivor from the heyday of Stanley Stein's *Star*, for which she'd worked as managing editor in the late 1950s and 1960s. Her elder sister Kitty had been married to Stein's successor as editor, Louis Boudreaux, but had died at the relatively young age of fifty-four. When her sister had left the family home in Texas in the 1930s, her mother had told Mary Ruth that she'd gone to college in New Orleans. It wasn't until five weeks before Mary Ruth joined Kitty at Carville that she'd learned the truth. Of course it had helped that she had a sister there: for instance, she didn't have to think up another name for herself since Kitty had already chosen an alias. Changing her name hadn't bothered her, though in 1990 when she and her late husband Wasey, another patient, had been travelling outside Carville and were worried about Medicare and Medicaid, they'd reverted to their real names.[29]

Small and apple-cheeked, Mary Ruth at eighty-two was unmarked by the disease that had kept her at Carville for the best part of sixty years. She worked as a volunteer in both the museum and the post office there. It amused her to think that at the outset of her working life, before she'd been diagnosed as having Hansen's disease, she had been working at her local

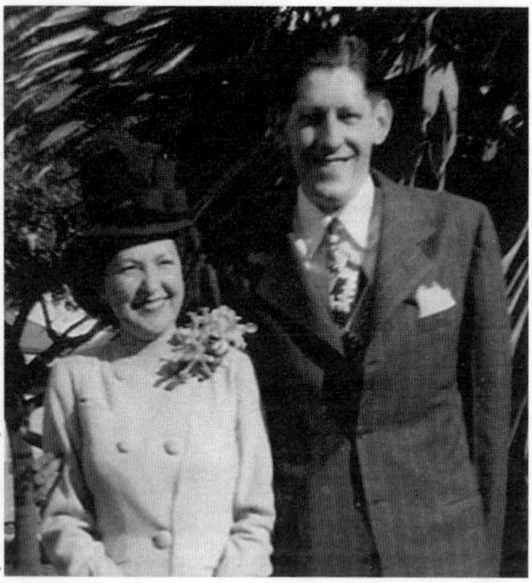

(from 'The texture of our souls')

Mary Ruth and Wasey Daigle on their wedding day at Carville

post office in Texas and now once again at the end of her days she was doing the same in Carville! Far from being afraid to die, she was almost impatient to be gone. In Carville's well-kept cemetery, three graves in a row contained the earthly remains of her brother-in-law, sister and husband and next to the last was an empty plot – waiting for Mary Ruth. That above all was what had kept her at Carville: her desire to be close to the beloved husband who had gone before her.[30] Now at last she has joined him.

Some Sisters of Charity remained, too, true to the pledge their predecessors had made to the patients more than a hundred years earlier never to desert them. Their number, like that of the patients, had dwindled. They had grown old along with their charges and some, at least, were saddened by the thought that their chosen way of life held so little attraction for the young. Like Carville itself, it seemed, they were part of a vanishing world.

The closure of Carville doesn't mean the end of Hansen's disease even in America, where between 300 and 500 cases still occur annually; the majority of these are from immigrant groups from Asia and South America but there are a few indigenous cases from the southern states as well.[31] Hence the continuing importance of scientific research. Since the 1970s the hopes of Carville's research department have centred on the nine-banded armadillo, whose low body temperature makes it the ideal experimental animal for HD research, given *M. leprae*'s predilection for peripheral nerves rather than the warmer central nervous system. This research department has now been relocated to the University of Louisiana at Baton Rouge.

The armadillo has proved to be an invaluable source of *M. leprae* bacilli, but researchers have yet to find a way of cultivating the bacillus *in vitro* (the third of 'Koch's postulates'). This is their Holy Grail, the achievement of which would make it possible to develop a vaccine as well as to solve the enduring mystery of how the bacillus is transmitted from person to person. It could be by any one of three routes: inoculation, or entry through broken skin; respiratory, breathing in the welter of germs known to be discharged from the noses of HD sufferers; or ingestive, through the gastrointestinal tract. This situation reminded the Indian Dr C.K. Job, who worked at Carville for many years, of the story of the blind men confronted by an elephant:

> One felt the trunk and said, 'Elephant is like a snake'; another felt its legs and exclaimed, 'Elephant is like a pillar'; yet another felt the tusk and thought, 'Elephant is like a spear'; and so on. Unfortunately, none of them saw the elephant. This may summarize our present position with regard to the mode of transmission of *M. leprae*.[32]

Back in the mid-1970s the leprologist Dr Olaf Skinsnes – the father of IDEA's Anwei Skinsnes Law – claimed that he and his team at the University of Hawaii School of Medicine had succeeded in growing the bacillus in a test tube. Unfortunately, when other scientists analysed Professor Skinsnes's supposedly 'pure' culture, they discovered that it contained at least two organisms, neither of which was *M. leprae*.[33] Respected leprosy worker though he was, Skinsnes came in for further criticism for failing to follow the 'accepted procedures for the positive identification of *M. leprae*' and for announcing his discovery through the medium of the popular press rather than reporting it in a reputable journal with supporting scientific documentation.[34]

The peculiarities of leprosy – for instance, the fact that for reasons unknown 'reactions' can happen before, during and after multiple drug therapy and that the symptoms of reactions and relapses are so alike that there's no way to distinguish between them except by monitoring the response to treatment – have led some clinicians and researchers to question the fundamental premises of orthodox leprology. The Argentine researcher Dr Meny Bergel called leprosy a 'metabolic disease' and attempted to rehabilitate Jonathan Hutchinson's 'fish hypothesis', and both he and the English clinician Dr Michael Corcos went so far as to deny that the disease was caused by *M. leprae*.[35] Bergel called *M. leprae* an 'opportunist' germ, likening its role to that of the staphylococcus in the diabetic, and saw its relation to the disease in chicken-and-egg terms, arguing that it was a case of 'because one is leprous one has Hansen's bacillus', rather than the other way round. 'Killing the Hansen bacillus in order to cure leprosy,' he maintained, 'is equivalent to kill[ing] the garbage collectors so that there won't be any more garbage.'[36]

Corcos, who was for many years a medical officer in the British colonial service in Nigeria and Trinidad, focused on the central paradox of the immune response to Hansen's bacillus – that at the 'tuberculoid' end of the spectrum damage is said to be caused by the *strength* of the response of the individual's immune system, while at the other, 'lepromatous' end it is the *absence* of response that supposedly causes the damage: 'Is a tuberculoid macule a form of "leprosy", or is it "resistance to the disease"? It is difficult to understand how it can be both.' To Corcos, who enthusiastically supported the *Star* in its campaign to do away with the stigmatising 'lepr-' prefix, orthodox definitions of 'leprosy' and its 'cure' seemed suspiciously circular: 'Thus "leprosy" may be loosely defined as the disease caused by the bacterium known as "*Mycobacterium leprae*". "*Mycobacterium leprae*", on the other hand, is the specific cause of the disease known as "leprosy".'[37]

Whatever the rights and wrongs of the case, the lack of certain knowledge over crucial aspects of Hansen's disease – such as, in Bergel's words, 'contagion, [the] penetration process of the causal germ and incubation period' – renders such speculation inevitable.[38] Unless or until a medical scientist makes the breakthrough that Skinsnes was so keen to achieve that he managed to delude himself, if not others, into believing he'd actually done it, doubts will remain. As another researcher wrote at that time: '. . . without culturing Hansen's bacillus in artificial media, hope of eradicating leprosy from the earth remains remote.'[39]

That may no longer be the case, however. Microbiologists have always talked in terms of *in vivo* and *in vitro*, but now there is a third way: *in silico*. The recently completed sequencing of the *M. leprae* genome has opened up the study of the biology of this organism and will enable researchers to get round some of the problems of not being able to cultivate it. The surprising thing is that in comparison with *M. tuberculosis* it has shed about two-thirds of its genes: where *M. tuberculosis* will have sixteen enzymes for metabolising fat, say, *M. leprae* will have just two, which doesn't leave much margin for error. The British leprologist Dr Diana Lockwood says: 'For me what's remarkable is that this incredible slimmed down organism with a minimal gene bank remains very successful and is clearly very well adapted for the particular niches that it lives in.'[40] Practically, scientists will now be able to investigate drug resistance. They will also be able to see precisely which genes enable *M. leprae* to bind to nerve cells and work out how to counteract this. Whether this is a breakthrough comparable to the cultivation of the bacillus remains to be seen but it certainly has great and exciting possibilities.

The persistence of HD, despite intensive elimination campaigns, has caused even orthodox leprologists to question the prevailing wisdom that the disease is transmitted exclusively from one human being to another. Both the nine-banded armadillo and the New World sooty mangabey monkey can be infected naturally in the wild as well as artificially when injected with human bacilli, but neither animal is considered likely to be a source of the human disease.[41] Though it was once thought that the bacteria could not survive for any length of time outside the human body, it is now known that they can survive for several months without a human host.[42] There is also the possibility of an extra-human reservoir of *M. leprae* not just in animals like the armadillo and mangabey monkey but in vegetation, or in the soil itself.

The Norwegian epidemiologist Lorentz M. Irgens and the German microbiologist Jindrich Kazda studied the voluminous patient register kept in the National Leprosy Registry of Norway from its establishment in 1856 to the registration of the very last patients in the 1950s. They fed detailed information on every patient's place of residence, age, gender, profession and family relationships into a computer and analysed the results. What they discovered was that the overwhelming majority of patients came from a limited number of more or less identical sites: 'isolated farms or hamlets near a fjord situated below a mountain range with a Southern orientation, and high atmospheric humidity.'[43] The inhabitants piped their water from mountain pools containing various kinds of moss, including sphagnum moss (which, curiously in this context, was dried out and used as a surgical dressing during the First World War). Kazda found that the combination of high atmospheric humidity and the intense heat generated by the sun made sphagnum moss the ideal incubator for a variety of mycobacteria, including one that was indistinguishable from *M. leprae*. When injected into the footpads of nude mice – the first animal model for leprosy developed by Dr Charles C. Shepard of the Public Health Service Communicable Diseases Center in Atlanta, Georgia, in 1960 – it produced identical lepromas to those found in leprosy patients. If Kazda is right, and leprosy bacteria do occur naturally in the environment, then contaminated drinking water would provide a simple explanation both for the occurrence of leprosy in particular, highly localised sites in nineteenth-century Norway and for its precipitate decline in the twentieth century, when poor farmers and fishermen were no longer dependent on mossy mountain sources for their drinking water.[44]

Hansen himself was alert to the possible climatic and environmental influences on the disease. As early as 1895 he wrote:

> Here in Norway where the people often go barefoot, wading in streams, marshes and rivers, the backs of the feet and the under part of the calves are frequently the seat of the first leprous eruption, not so often in the form of nodules, as of a dense, regular infiltration.[45]

Though there are still many unanswered questions concerning this most mysterious of diseases, in the western world at least Hansen's disease is now a rarity and can easily be treated in the community. The closure of Carville in the United States, and of St Giles in England, may lull us into complacency, so that we're all too ready to believe WHO propaganda about the imminent 'elimination' of leprosy throughout the world. But in great swathes of the third world, right across India and Nepal, Indonesia, Myanmar, sub-Saharan Africa, Mozambique, Madagascar, Brazil and Venezuela, the incidence of the disease remains constant and the problems relating to it manifold. And so long as that remains the case – and our understanding of the disease remains so inadequate – no amount of wishful thinking will consign it to history.

NOTES

Introduction

1 Ernest Muir, *Manual of Leprosy* (E. & S. Livingstone, Edinburgh 1948), p. 109
2 Patrick Feeny, *The Fight Against Leprosy* (Elek Books, London 1964), p. 105 – see also Donald Culross Peattie, *Cargoes and Harvests* (New York 1926), pp. 267–8, and J.F. Rock, 'Hunting the Chaulmoogra Tree', *National Geographic Magazine*, Vol. 41, 1922, pp. 242–76 (Rock attributes the legend to pre-Buddhist Burma)
3 Dharmendra, 'Leprosy in Ancient Indian Medicine', *International Journal of Leprosy*, Vol. 15, No. 4, Oct–Dec 1947, pp. 424–30
4 *Holy Bible* (King James authorised version), *Leviticus*, Ch. 13, verse 45; *Numbers*, Ch. 5, verse 2
5 John Updike, *Problems and Other Stories* (Knopf, New York, 1979), p. 181
6 Marlowe's *The Contentions* and *II Henry VI* and Shakespeare's *II Henry IV* – see Olaf K. Skinsnes and Robert M. Elvove. ' "Leprosy" in Occidental Literature', *International Journal of Leprosy*, Vol. 38, No. 3, 1970, pp. 294–307
7 Charles Creighton, *A History of Epidemics in Britain, Vol. 1* (London 1894; reprinted by Frank Cass 1965), p. 84
8 See, for example, Carole Rawcliffe, 'Learning to Love the Leper: Aspects of Institutional Charity in Anglo Norman England', *Anglo-Norman Studies XXIII*, 2000, pp. 231–50
9 James Y. Simpson, 'Antiquarian Notes of Leprosy and Leper Hospitals in Scotland and England', *Edinburgh Medical and Surgical Journal*, Vols 56 and 57, 1841–2, pp. 301–30 and 394–429
10 Michel F. Lechat, 'The Paleoepidemiology of Leprosy: An Overview', *International Journal of Leprosy*, Vol. 67, No. 4, Dec 1999, pp. 460–70
11 Creighton, *History of Epidemics*, pp. 107–8
12 Geoffrey Chaucer, *The Canterbury Tales: General Prologue*, lines 240–5:

He knew the taverns wel in every toun
And everich hostiler and tappestere
Bet than a lazar or a beggestere;
For unto swich a worthy man as he
Acorded nat, as by his facultee,
To have with sike lazars aqueyntaunce.

13 George Newman, *On the History of the Decline and Final Extinction of Leprosy as an Endemic Disease in the British Isles* (London 1895), pp. 32–3, 67
14 Charles A. Mercier, *Leper Houses and Mediaeval Hospitals* (London 1915), p. 21
15 Keith Manchester, 'Leprosy: The Origin and Development of the Disease in Antiquity' (from Danielle Gourevitch, ed., *Maladie et Maladies*, Libraire Droz, Geneva 1992), p. 46

16 Arno Karlen, *Plague's Progress: A Social History of Man and Disease* (Gollancz, London 1995), p. 85
17 Feeny, *Fight Against Leprosy*, p. 170
18 Anthony Weymouth, *Through the Leper-Squint: A Study of Leprosy from Pre-Christian Times to the Present Day* (London 1938), p. 147
19 A. Donald Miller, *An Inn Called Welcome: The Story of the Mission to Lepers 1874–1917* (Mission to Lepers, London 1964), p. 197
20 The Leprosy Mission International archives, newspaper cutting and letter from Betty Herring, dated Easter Morning 1937
21 Stanley Stein, *Alone No Longer* (The *Star*, Carville, La., 1974; first publ. 1963), p. 163
22 Stanley G. Browne, *Leprosy in the Bible* (Rushden, Northants, 1970; third edn 1979), pp. 7, 26
23 G.A. Ryrie, 'The Psychology of Leprosy', *Leprosy Review*, Vol. 22, Nos. 1 and 2, 1951, pp. 13–24
24 *The Lancet*, Vol. II (1823–4), pp. 149–50
25 Ryrie, 'Psychology of Leprosy'
26 Muir, *Manual of Leprosy*, p. 163
27 Definition of leprosy in www.tesarta.com
28 Muir, *Manual of Leprosy*, p. 3
29 Jonathan Hutchinson, *On Leprosy and Fish-Eating* (London 1906), p. 1
30 Author interview with Dr Diana Lockwood, London, 30 July 2003
31 R.H. Thangaraj and S.J. Yawalkar, *Leprosy for Medical Practitioners and Paramedical Workers* (Ciba-Geigy Ltd, Basle, Switzerland, 4th edn 1989), p. 27
32 Ibid., pp. 27, 24
33 Ibid., pp. 27, 59
34 Ibid., p. 64
35 Author interview with Dr Diana Lockwood
36 Thangaraj and Yawalkar, *Leprosy for Medical Practitioners*, p. 66
37 Author interview with Dr Diana Lockwood
38 Ibid.
39 Thangaraj and Yawalkar, *Leprosy for Medical Practitioners*, p. 76
40 Hutchinson, *On Leprosy and Fish-Eating*, p. 4

1 A New Disease in New Brunswick

1 Philip A. Kalisch, 'Tracadie and Penikese Leprosaria: A Comparative Analysis of Societal Response to Leprosy in New Brunswick, 1844–1880, and Massachusetts, 1904–1921', *Bulletin of the History of Medicine*, Vol. XLVII, 1973, pp. 480–512
2 *Report on Leprosy by the Royal College of Physicians* (London 1867), p. 3
3 Laurie C.C. Stanley, *Unclean! Unclean! Leprosy in New Brunswick 1844–1880* (Les Editions d'Acadie, New Brunswick 1982), p. 14
4 Cited in Kalisch, 'Tracadie and Penikese Leprosaria'
5 Ibid.
6 Ibid. – the words are taken from the 2 March 1844 resolution of the House of Assembly, New Brunswick, to send a commission of investigation to Tracadie
7 Ibid.
8 Stanley, *Unclean! Unclean!*, p. 18
9 M.J. Losier, *Children of Lazarus: The Story of the Lazaretto at Tracadie* (n.p., New Brunswick 1984), p. 19
10 Cited in Kalisch, 'Tracadie and Penikese Leprosaria'
11 Losier, *Children of Lazarus*, pp. 19–20
12 Kalisch, 'Tracadie and Penikese Leprosaria'
13 Losier, *Children of Lazarus*, pp. 19–20
14 Ibid.
15 Ibid., p. 21

16 See Stanley, *Unclean! Unclean!*, pp. 35–7, and Losier, *Children of Lazarus*, pp. 27–30
17 Losier, *Children of Lazarus*, p. 36
18 Cited in Stanley, *Unclean! Unclean!*, p. 34
19 Ibid., pp. 40–1
20 Ibid., p. 33
21 Kalisch, 'Tracadie and Penikese Leprosaria'
22 Losier, *Children of Lazarus*, pp. 53–4
23 *Report on Leprosy by the RCP*, p. xlvii
24 Ibid., p. lviii
25 Ibid., p. 4
26 Laurie C.C. Stanley-Blackwell, 'A Singular Obsession: New Brunswick's Leprosy Doctor', *International Journal of Leprosy*, Vol. 61, No. 4, Dec 1993, pp. 619–27
27 Ibid.
28 Letter of 28 Apr 1869, cited in Kalisch, 'Tracadie and Penikese Leprosaria'
29 Losier, *Children of Lazarus*, p. 81
30 Ibid., pp. 75, 80, 83
31 Stanley, *Unclean! Unclean!*, p. 47
32 Stanley-Blackwell, 'A Singular Obsession'
33 Ibid.
34 Losier, *Children of Lazarus*, pp. 109, 125
35 Cited in ibid., p. xi

2 The Father of Leprology

1 Frederick B. Watt, 'Foreword' to first English edition of G. Armauer Hansen, *Memories & Reflections* (German Leprosy Relief Association, Würzburg, Germany 1976), p. 10
2 Jonathan Hutchinson, *On Leprosy and Fish-Eating* (London 1906), p. 65
3 Cited in Zachary Gussow, *Leprosy, Racism, and Public Health: Social Policy in Chronic Disease Control* (Westview Press, Boulder, Col. 1989), p. 69
4 Peter Richards, 'Leprosy in Scandinavia', *Centaurus*, Vol. 7, No. 1, 1960, pp. 101–33.
5 H.P. Lie, 'Report of the Leper Hospital . . . in Bergen for the 3 Years 1899–1901', *Lepra*, Vol. IV, Fasc. 1
6 Lorentz M. Irgens, 'Hansen, 150 Years After His Birth, the Context of a Medical Discovery', *International Journal of Leprosy*, Vol. 60, No. 3, Sept 1992, pp. 466–9.
7 Gussow, *Leprosy, Racism, and Public Health*, p. 69
8 Th. M. Vogelsang, 'The Old Leprosy Hospitals in Bergen', *International Journal of Leprosy*, Vol. 32, No. 3, July–Sept 1964, pp. 306–9
9 Lorentz M. Irgens, 'Leprosy in Norway: An Interplay of Research and Public Health Work', *International Journal of Leprosy*, Vol. 41, No. 2, April–June 1973, pp. 189–98
10 Th. M. Vogelsang, 'Gerhard Henrik Armauer Hansen 1841–1912', *International Journal of Leprosy*, Vol. 46, No. 3, July–Sept 1978, pp. 257–323
11 Gussow, *Leprosy, Racism, and Public Health*, p. 71
12 Ibid., p. 72
13 Th. M. Vogelsang, 'Leprosy in Norway', *Medical History*, Vol. 9, Jan 1965, pp. 29–35
14 Henry Vandyke Carter, *Report on Leprosy and Leper-Asylums in Norway: With References to India* (London 1874), pp. 13–14
15 Ibid., p. 14
16 Gussow, *Leprosy, Racism, and Public Health*, p. 74.
17 Vogelsang, 'G.H.A. Hansen'
18 Ibid.
19 Hansen, *Memories & Reflections*, p. 70
20 Vogelsang, 'G.H.A. Hansen'; see also Ingvald Rokstad, 'Gerhard Henrich Armauer Hansen', *International Journal of Leprosy*, Vol. 32, No. 1, Jan–March 1964, pp. 64–70

21 Hansen, *Memories & Reflections*, p. 96
22 Vogelsang, 'G.H.A. Hansen'
23 Vogelsang, 'Leprosy in Norway'
24 Vogelsang, 'G.H.A. Hansen'
25 Morton Harboe, 'Armauer Hansen – The Man and His Work', *International Journal of Leprosy*, Vol. 41, No. 4, Oct–Dec 1973, pp. 417–24
26 Vogelsang, 'G.H.A. Hansen'
27 Hansen, *Memories & Reflections*, p. 98
28 Vogelsang, 'G.H.A. Hansen'; see also Knut Blom, 'Armauer Hansen and Human Leprosy Transmission: Medical Ethics and Legal Rights', *International Journal of Leprosy*, Vol. 41, No. 2, April–June 1973, pp. 199–203
29 Cited in Blom, 'Armauer Hansen'
30 Ibid.
31 Richards, 'Leprosy in Scandinavia'
32 Hansen, *Memories & Reflections*, p. 99
33 Ibid., p. 100
34 Irgens, 'Leprosy in Norway'
35 Vogelsang, 'Leprosy in Norway'
36 Cited in Gussow, *Leprosy, Racism, and Public Health*, p. 78
37 Hutchinson, *On Leprosy and Fish-Eating*, p. xv
38 H.P. Lie, 'Why Is Leprosy Decreasing in Norway?', *International Journal of Leprosy*, Vol. 1, No. 2, April 1933, pp. 205–16
39 Lorentz M. Irgens, *Leprosy in Norway: An Epidemiological Study Based on a National Patient Register*, *Leprosy Review*, Vol. 51, Supp. 1, March 1980, p. 113
40 Ibid., p. 125
41 Gussow, *Leprosy, Racism, and Public Health*, p. 81
42 S.R. Wood, 'A Contribution to the History of Tuberculosis and Leprosy in 19th Century Norway', *Journal of the Royal Society of Medicine*, Vol. 84, No. 7, July 1991, pp. 428–30
43 Vogelsang, 'G.H.A. Hansen'
44 Hansen, *Memories & Reflections*, p. 103
45 Ibid., p. 109
46 Ibid., p. 103
47 Ibid., p. 100
48 Cited in Vogelsang, 'G.H.A. Hansen'
49 Vogelsang, 'G.H.A. Hansen'
50 Hansen, *Memories & Reflections*, p. 84
51 Vogelsang, 'G.H.A. Hansen'

3 The Martyr of Molokai

1 Father Pamphile (ed.), *Life and Letters of Father Damien* (London 1889), pp. 93–4. As early as November 1873, Damien was writing to his brother, 'As for me, I make myself a leper with the lepers, to gain all to Jesus Christ. That is why in preaching, I say, *We lepers*, not, *My brethren*, as in Europe . . .' See also Gavan Daws, *Holy Man: Father Damien of Molokai* (Univ. of Hawaii Press, Honolulu 1973), p. 97
2 Zachary Gussow, *Leprosy, Racism, and Public Health* (Westview Press, Boulder, Col. 1989), p. 90
3 A.A. St M. Mouritz, *'The Path of the Destroyer': A History of Leprosy in the Hawaiian Islands* (Honolulu 1916), pp. 58–9
4 *Leprosy in Hawaii: Extracts from Reports* (Honolulu 1886), pp. 4–5, 8–10, 11
5 Ibid., p. 21
6 Ibid., p. 5
7 Ibid., pp. 40–1
8 Ibid., p. 44

9 Ibid., pp. 47–8
10 Ibid., p. 184
11 Ibid., pp. 51–3
12 Mouritz, '*The Path of the Destroyer*' p. 166
13 *Leprosy in Foreign Countries* (Honolulu 1886), p. 211
14 Mouritz, '*The Path of the Destroyer*', pp. 212–28; Report by Joseph Damien, Catholic Priest, to His Excellency Walter M. Gibson, President of the Board of Health on 'Thirteen Years' Residence and Labor among the Lepers at Kalauwao', 11 March 1886
15 Ibid.
16 Ibid.
17 A. Mouritz, *A Brief World History of Leprosy* (Honolulu, rev. edn 1943), p. 60
18 Hilde Eynikel, *Molokai: The Story of Father Damien* (Hodder & Stoughton, London 1999), p. 1
19 Ibid., p. 21
20 Pamphile, *Life and Letters of Father Damien*, pp. 76–7
21 Eynikel, *Molokai*, p. 69
22 John Farrow, *Damien the Leper* (New York 1937), p. 75
23 Eynikel, *Molokai*, p. 71
24 Pamphile, *Life and Letters of Father Damien*, p. 93
25 Eynikel, *Molokai*, pp. 77–8
26 Cited in Mouritz, '*The Path of the Destroyer*', p. 227
27 Ibid., p. 225
28 Ibid., pp. 225–6
29 Farrow, *Damien the Leper*, pp. 105–7; Daws, *Holy Man*, pp. 111–12; Eynikel, *Molokai*, pp. 99–100
30 Daws, *Holy Man*, p. 73
31 Ibid., p. 113
32 Pamphile, *Life and Letters of Father Damien*, p. 106
33 Charles J. Dutton, *The Samaritans of Molokai: The Lives of Father Damien and Brother Dutton Among the Lepers* (London 1934), p. 201
34 Ibid., pp. 67–9
35 *Leprosy in Hawaii*, p. 87
36 Ibid., pp. 115–16
37 Cited in Mouritz, '*The Path of the Destroyer*', pp. 221–3
38 *Leprosy in Hawaii*, p. 77
39 Daws, *Holy Man*, p. 126
40 Paul Bailey, *Hawaii's Royal Prime Minister: The Life and Times of Walter Murray Gibson* (Hastings House, New York 1980), pp. 235–6
41 Sister Mary Laurence Hanley OSF and O.A. Bushnell, *A Song of Pilgrimage and Exile: The Life and Spirit of Mother Marianne of Molokai* (Franciscan Herald Press, Chicago 1980), p. 142
42 *Leprosy in Hawaii*, pp. 113–14
43 Ibid., pp. 124–5
44 Ibid., p. 120
45 Ibid., p. 117
46 Mouritz, '*The Path of the Destroyer*', p. 54
47 Cited in Gussow, *Leprosy, Racism, and Public Health*, pp. 100–1
48 *Leprosy in Hawaii*, p. 138
49 Mouritz, '*The Path of the Destroyer*', pp. 54–5
50 Ibid., p. 55
51 *Leprosy in Hawaii*, p. 120
52 Ibid., pp. 147–8
53 Ibid., p. 151
54 Ibid., pp. 153–4
55 A.A. St M. Mouritz, 'Human Inoculation Experiments in Hawaii Including Notes on Those of Arning and Fitch' (condensed, arranged and annotated by H.W. Wade), *International Journal of Leprosy*, Vol. 19, No. 2, April–June 1951, pp. 203–15

56 Ibid.
57 'The Contagious Nature of Leprosy', *British Medical Journal*, 19 April 1890, pp. 917–18
58 Ibid.
59 Mouritz, 'Human Inoculation Experiments'
60 Eynikel, *Molokai*, p. 195
61 Charles Warren Stoddart, *The Lepers of Molokai* (Ave Maria Press, Notre Dame, Ind. 1893 edn), pp. 36–7
62 Ibid., pp. 38–9
63 The view that St Francis actually contracted leprosy, and that his stigmata and other symptoms were, in fact, caused by the disease is now widely accepted by members of the order. A paper on this topic was presented in Session 11 of the 30th International Congress on Medieval Studies at the University of Western Michigan, Kalamazoo, in May 1995, by Joanne Schaltzein OSF and Daniel Sulmasy OFM, of the Franciscan Institute. For a discussion of some of his symptoms see C. Rawcliffe, *Medicine and Society in Later Medieval England* (Sutton Publishing, Stroud 1995), p. 70
64 Cited in Stoddart, *The Lepers of Molokai*, p. 112
65 Mouritz, *A Brief World History of Leprosy*, p. 61
66 Ibid., pp. 59–60
67 Ibid., p. 61
68 Linda W. Greene, *Exile in Paradise: The Isolation of Hawaii's Leprosy Victims and Development of Kalaupapa Settlement, 1865 to the Present* (National Park Service, Denver, Col. Sept 1985), p. 164
69 Mouritz, *'The Path of the Destroyer'*, p. 76
70 Farrow, *Damien the Leper*, pp. 166–7
71 Hanley and Bushnell, *A Song of Pilgrimage and Exile*, pp. 223–4
72 Mouritz, *'The Path of the Destroyer'*, pp. 76–80
73 Bailey, *Hawaii's Royal Prime Minister*, pp. 218–32
74 Ibid., pp. 237–40
75 Ibid., pp. 259–62
76 Hanley and Bushnell, *A Song of Pilgrimage and Exile*, pp. 263–7
77 Daws, *Holy Man*, pp. 169–72
78 Ibid., pp. 180–1
79 Mouritz, *A Brief World History of Leprosy*, pp. 62–3
80 Edward Clifford, *Father Damien: A Journey from Cashmere to His Home in Hawaii* (London 1889), pp. 27, 57
81 Dutton, *The Samaritans of Molokai*, pp. 103, 105
82 Greene, *Exile in Paradise*, pp. 188–90

4 Mr Stevenson and Dr Hyde

1 RLS to Fanny Stevenson, Molokai, May 1889, cited in Alanna Knight (ed.), *Robert Louis Stevenson in the South Seas* (Mainstream Publishing, Edinburgh 1986), pp. 120–2
2 Cited in Nicholas Rankin, *Dead Man's Chest: Travels After Robert Louis Stevenson* (Faber, London 1987), p. 283
3 Ibid., p. 284
4 RLS to James Payn, Honolulu, 13 June 1889, cited in Knight, *Robert Louis Stevenson*, pp. 126–7
5 Dated Kalawao, 22 May 1889
6 RLS to Sidney Colvin, Honolulu, June 1889, cited in Knight, *Robert Louis Stevenson*, pp. 123–4
7 Ibid.
8 A.A. St M. Mouritz, *'The Path of the Destroyer': A History of Leprosy in the Hawaiian Islands* (Honolulu 1916), p. 288
9 Cited in Robert Louis Stevenson, *An Open Letter to the Rev. Dr Hyde of Honolulu* (Ave Maria Press, Notre Dame, Ind., 1927 edn), pp. 1–3
10 Ibid., pp. 8, 10, 16

11 Gavan Daws, *Holy Man: Father Damien of Molokai* (Univ. of Hawaii Press, Honolulu 1973), p. 137
12 Hilde Eynikel, *Molokai: The Story of Father Damien* (Hodder & Stoughton, London 1999), p. 315
13 Charles J. Dutton: *The Samaritans of Molokai: The Lives of Father Damien and Brother Dutton Among the Lepers* (London 1934), pp. 121–2
14 Ibid., p. 107
15 Daws, *Holy Man*, p. 228
16 Ibid., pp. 228–32
17 Mouritz, '*The Path of the Destroyer*', pp. 72–3
18 Ibid., pp. 73–4
19 Ibid., pp. 74–5
20 Jack London, *Tales of Hawaii* (Press Pacifica, Hawaii 1984), pp. 1–16
21 W.S. Merwin, *The Folding Cliffs: A Narrative of 19th-century Hawaii* (Knopf, New York 1998)
22 Dutton, *The Samaritans of Molokai*, p. 267
23 Ernie Pyle, *Home Country* (William Sloane Associates, New York 1947), p. 238
24 Sister Mary Hanley OSF and O.A. Bushnell, *A Song of Pilgrimage and Exile: The Life and Spirit of Mother Marianne of Molokai* (Franciscan Herald Press, Chicago 1980), pp. 383–5
25 Ibid., pp. 385–6
26 Katharine Fullerton Gerould, 'Kalaupapa: The Leper Settlement on Molokai', *Scribner's Magazine*, Vol. LX, No. 1, July 1916, pp. 1–18

5 An Imperial Danger

1 'The Father Damien Memorial Fund', *British Medical Journal*, 22 June 1889, p. 1424
2 H.P. Wright, *Leprosy: An Imperial Danger* (London 1889), pp. vii–viii
3 'Leprosy', *BMJ*, 15 June 1889, pp. 1364–5
4 *BMJ*, 22 June 1889 (and 20 July 1889)
5 W. Munro, *Leprosy* (Manchester 1879, reprinted from the *Edinburgh Medical Journal*, Sept 1876–Nov 1879), pp. 46–7
6 Wright, *Leprosy*, p. viii
7 *BMJ*, 15 June 1889
8 H. Vandyke Carter, *On Leprosy and Elephantiasis* (London 1874), pp. 210–11
9 Cited in Agnes Lambert, 'Leprosy: Present and Past. 1. Present', *The Nineteenth Century*, Aug 1884, pp. 210–27
10 Edward Clifford, 'The First-Born Son of Death', *The Nineteenth Century*, Oct 1888, pp. 576–8
11 Private information from Dr Shubhada S. Pandya
12 T.R. Lewis and D.D. Cunningham, *Leprosy in India: A Report* (Calcutta 1887), p. 67
13 Ibid., p. 68
14 Morell Mackenzie, 'The Dreadful Revival of Leprosy', *The Nineteenth Century*, Dec 1889, pp. 925–41
15 Ibid.
16 Ibid.
17 Shubhada S. Pandya, 'Anti-contagionism in Leprosy, 1844–1897', *International Journal of Leprosy*, Vol. 66, No. 3, Sept 1998, pp. 374–84
18 Mackenzie, 'The Dreadful Revival of Leprosy'
19 Pandya, 'Anti-contagionism in Leprosy'
20 Mackenzie, 'The Dreadful Revival of Leprosy'
21 Cited in S.S. Pandya, '"Very Savage Rites": Suicide and the Leprosy Sufferer in Nineteenth Century India', *Indian Journal of Leprosy*, Vol. 73, No. 1, 2001, pp. 27–36
22 Ibid.
23 Robert Needham Cust, *Memoirs of Past Years of a Septuagenarian* (Privately printed 1899), pp. 28–9
24 Edward Clifford, *Father Damien: A Journey from Cashmere to His Home in Hawaii* (London 1889), pp. 161–4

25 Govt of India, Home Dept, No. 39 of 1890, to the Rt Hon. Viscount Cross, GCB, HM Sec. of State for India, Simla, 22 July 1890
26 Pandya, 'Anti-contagionism in Leprosy'
27 Ibid.
28 *Leprosy in India: Report of the Leprosy Commission in India 1890–91* (Calcutta 1892), pp. 289–90 and 420–1
29 G. Armauer Hansen, 'On the Report of the Leprosy Commission in India, 1890–91: A Criticism', *The Lancet*, 30 Dec 1893, pp. 1053–4
30 British Library, Oriental and India Office Collections, India Office Records, V/8/62 India Acts, Act No. III of 1898
31 J. Lowe, 'A Curious Chapter of the History of Leprosy in India, the Indian Leprosy Commission of 1890', *Leprosy in India*, July 1939, pp. 82–6
32 Cust, *Memoirs*, p. 73
33 Robert Needham Cust, *Linguistic and Oriental Essays: Third Series* (London 1891), p. 579
34 Stephen Neill, *A History of Christian Missions* (Penguin London 2nd, 1986, reprinted 1990), p. 220
35 Cust, *Linguistic and Oriental Essays*, p. 576
36 A. Donald Miller, *An Inn Called Welcome: The Story of the Mission to Lepers 1874–1917* (Mission to Lepers, London 1964), p. 9
37 Cited in Cyril Davey, *Caring Comes First: The Leprosy Mission Story* (Marshall Pickering, London, 1987), pp. 58–9
38 Miller, *An Inn Called Welcome*, pp. 12–14
39 Davey, *Caring Comes First*, p. 116
40 Miller, *An Inn Called Welcome*, pp. 19–22
41 Ibid., pp. 25–7
42 S.G. Browne, 'The Leprosy Mission: A Century of Service', *Leprosy Review*, Vol. 45, 1974, pp. 166–9
43 The Leprosy Mission International, Minutes of Committee Meetings, 27 June 1901
44 Ibid., 12 Feb 1903 (from the first of three resolutions passed at the Conference of Superintendents of Leper Asylums held at Asansol on 30 Nov 1902)
45 Miller, *An Inn Called Welcome*, pp. 35–6
46 Davey, *Caring Comes First*, p. 51
47 The Leprosy Mission International, Wellesley Bailey to his wife, Purulia, 23 Dec 1890
48 The Leprosy Mission International, Dayamony to Miss Gurney, Purulia, 27 Oct 1897
49 Frank Oldrieve, *India's Lepers: How to Rid India of Leprosy* (London 1924), pp. 64–5
50 John Jackson, *In Leper-Land* (London 1901), p. 198
51 The Leprosy Mission International, Rev. F. Hahn, 'Purulia Leper Asylum Report', Lohardugga, 18 July 1899
52 The Leprosy Mission International, Rev. F. Hahn to Wellesley Bailey, 21 Sept 1897
53 The Leprosy Mission International, Extract of letter from Mary Reed, Chandag, 16 June 1898
54 The Leprosy Mission International, Mary Reed to Mrs Bailey, 8 July 1899
55 Miller, *An Inn Called Welcome*, pp. 119–20
56 Mission to Lepers in India and the East, '13th Annual Report for the Year 1904', *Lepra*, Vol. VI, Fasc. 1, p. 23

6 Two Women with a Mission

1 The Leprosy Mission International, Minutes of Committee Meetings, 9 March 1893 and 12 July 1895
2 Julia Boyd, *Hannah Riddell: An Englishwoman in Japan* (Charles E. Tuttle, Rutland 1996), pp. 11–12, 25
3 Ibid., p. 57
4 Ibid., pp. 74, 64, 98

5 'Leprosy in Japan', *BMJ*, 9 Jan 1892, p. 100
6 Cited in Boyd, *Hannah Riddell*, pp. 101–2
7 Cited in ibid., p. 54
8 Ibid., p. 123
9 Ibid., p. 140
10 Ibid., p. 143
11 Ibid., pp. 144, 150
12 Ibid., p. 149
13 Fujio Ohtani, *The Walls Crumble: The Emancipation of Persons Affected by Hansen's Disease in Japan* (n.p., Tokyo 1998), pp. 48–50
14 Boyd, *Hannah Riddell*, pp. 149, 152
15 Ohtani, *The Walls Crumble*, pp. 55–7
16 Boyd, *Hannah Riddell*, p. 151
17 Ibid., p. 193
18 Ibid., p. 171
19 Henry Johnson, *The Life of Kate Marsden* (London 1895, 2nd edn), p. 2
20 Ibid., pp. 2–7
21 Ibid., p. 9
22 Dorothy Middleton, *Victorian Lady Travellers* (Routledge & Kegan Paul, London 1965), pp. 128–9
23 Ibid., p. 130
24 Johnson, *The Life of Kate Marsden*, p. 11
25 Middleton, *Victorian Lady Travellers*, p. 132
26 Johnson, *The Life of Kate Marsden*, pp. 15–16
27 Ibid., p. 16
28 Middleton, *Victorian Lady Travellers*, p. 132
29 Johnson, *The Life of Kate Marsden*, p. 17
30 Kate Marsden, *On Sledge and Horseback to Outcast Siberian Lepers* (London 1883), p. 3
31 Middleton, *Victorian Lady Travellers*, p. 133
32 Johnson, *The Life of Kate Marsden*, p. 26
33 Ibid., pp. 31–4
34 Ibid., p. 36
35 Ibid., pp. 37–9
36 Middleton, *Victorian Lady Travellers*, pp. 133–4
37 Kate Marsden, *My Mission in Siberia: A Vindication* (London 1921), p. 12
38 Marsden, *On Sledge and Horseback . . .*, pp. 95–6
39 [W.T. Stead], 'The Quest for the Holy Grail: An English Lady among the Lepers of Siberia', *The Review of Reviews*, Vol. 6, July–Dec 1892, pp. 185–8
40 Marsden, *On Sledge and Horseback . . .*, pp. 82–4
41 Ibid., pp. 130–1
42 [Stead], 'The Quest for the Holy Grail'
43 Marsden, *On Sledge and Horseback . . .*, p. 143
44 Ibid., pp. 113–14
45 T.R. Lewis and D.D. Cunningham, *Leprosy in India: A Report* (Calcutta 1887), p. 30
46 [Stead], 'The Quest for the Holy Grail'
47 Ibid.
48 'Leprosy in Russia', *BMJ*, 18 June 1892, p. 1318
49 '"The Lepers of Siberia"', *BMJ*, 3 Dec 1892, p. 1247
50 'Help for Lepers', *BMJ*, 24 Dec 1892, p. 1402
51 *BMJ*, 21 Jan 1893, p. 135
52 '"Siberian Leper Fund"', *BMJ*, 15 July 1893, p. 141
53 Johnson, *The Life of Kate Marsden*, p. 55
54 'British Help for Siberian Lepers', *BMJ*, 20 Jan 1894, p. 152
55 The Leprosy Mission International, Charity Organisation Society Report, Case No. 16,929, 'The Kate Marsden Leper Fund', 27 July 1893

56 *The Times*, 16 and 18 Aug 1894
57 Ibid., 18 Aug 1894
58 Ibid.
59 Johnson, *The Life of Kate Marsden*, p. 57
60 St Francis Leprosy Guild leaflet, 'Kate Marsden – Founder of the Guild', n.d.
61 Middleton, *Victorian Lady Travellers*, pp. 144–5
62 National Archives and Records Administration (Record Group 90) – Records of the Public Health Service, Central File 1897–1923, Boxes 526 and 527, 4712/6. Kate Marsden to the Marquess of Lansdowne KG, dated 26 Kildare Terrace, Bayswater [London], 25 Nov 1901
63 Ibid.
64 Ibid., KM to the Rt Hon. Lord Pauncefote, dated Hotel Normandie, Broadway, New York City, 20 Dec 1901
65 Ibid., Sec. of the Treasury to Sec. of State, Washington DC, 8 Jan 1902
66 RGS Archives: from *The Hippodrome* Magazine, London, Xmas No., 1918
67 Ibid., letters from KM to the RGS of 20 June 1912 and 8 May 1916, and the President of the RGS's reply of 9 May 1916
68 Ibid., letter from Major Leonard Darwin to RGS of 2 July 1924 and Sec. of RGS's reply of 3 July 1924
69 Ibid., letter from Miss E. LL. Norris to Mr Hinks, RGS, of 31 Dec 1924 and Hinks's reply of 1 Jan 1925
70 Middleton, *Victorian Lady Travellers*, p. 145
71 William Millinship, 'Heroine of Russia cast out into the cold', *The Times*, 15 Aug 1994, p. 10
72 Ibid.

7 Veterans of the Spanish–American War, 1

1 Carville Museum (CM), Sisters of Charity Records (SCR): the Sisters' Diary entry for 27 Nov 1940 mentions a talk by Perry Burgess at Carville and gives Ned Langford's real name as Newsbaumer: 'It is understood that a part of this story was written by himself, this manuscript having been found among his possessions.' All quotes in this chapter not otherwise identified come from Perry Burgess, *Who Walk Alone* (Holt, New York 1940)
2 Cited in James Hamilton-Paterson, *America's Boy* (Granta Books, London 1998), p. 33
3 Ibid., p. 35
4 Ibid., pp. 37–8
5 Ibid., p. 38
6 Ronald Fettes Chapman, *Leonard Wood and Leprosy in the Philippines: The Culion Leper Colony, 1921–1927* (University Press of America 1982), p. 2
7 Victor Heiser, *A Doctor's Odyssey* (London 1936), pp. 234–5.
8 Ibid., pp. 239–40
9 Ibid., pp. 241, 243–4
10 Chapman, *Leonard Wood*, p. 11
11 Heiser, *A Doctor's Odyssey*, p. 228
12 Ibid., p. 244
13 Ibid., pp. 247–8
14 Ibid., p. 249
15 Ibid., pp. 260–1
16 Ibid., pp. 250–1
17 Ibid.
18 Katherine Mayo, *The Isles of Fear: The Truth about the Philippines* (London 1925), p. 161
19 Ibid., p. 162
20 Chapman, *Leonard Wood*, pp. 83–5, 89
21 Ibid., pp. 82–3, 89–90
22 Mayo, *The Isles of Fear*, p. 163

23 Chapman, *Leonard Wood*, pp. 90, 130
24 Ibid., pp. 90–1
25 Ibid., p. 92
26 Mayo, *The Isles of Fear*, p. 169
27 Chapman, *Leonard Wood*, p. 94
28 Ibid.
29 Mayo, *The Isles of Fear*, p. 169
30 *International Journal of Leprosy*, Vol. 13, 1945, pp. 126–7
31 Ibid., p. 70
32 Chapman, *Leonard Wood*, p. 129
33 *Leprosy Review*, Vol. VII, No. 3, July 1936, pp. 134–8
34 Ibid.
35 Cited in Burgess, *Who Walk Alone*
36 Perry Burgess, *Born of Those Years: An Autobiography* (Dent, London 1952), p. 63
37 Chapman, *Leonard Wood*, pp. 161–2
38 Thomas M. Johnson, 'Joey's Quiet War', *Reader's Digest*, 1964
39 Father Forbes Monaghan, 'The Story of Billy', *The Star*, Feb 1948
40 Ibid.
41 H. Windsor Wade, 'High Lights of Wartime Culion', *The Star*, Oct 1946, pp. 1–3
42 Burgess, *Born of Those Years*, p. 245
43 Chapman, *Leonard Wood*, pp. 162, 164
44 Ibid., p. 164
45 *The Star*, Oct 1946, p. 4

8 Veterans of the Spanish–American War, 2

1 Stanley Stein, *Alone No Longer* (*The Star*, Carville, La 1974), pp. 180–1
2 National Archives and Records Administration (Record Group 90), 'Historical Summary', 25 Sept 1908
3 Philip A. Kalisch, 'The Strange Case of John Early: A Study of the Stigma of Leprosy', *International Journal of Leprosy*, Vol. 40, No. 3, July–Sept 1972, pp. 291–305
4 Ibid.
5 Stein, *Alone No Longer*, p. 181
6 Kalisch, 'The Strange Case of John Early'
7 National Archives and Records Administration (Record Group 90), M.D. O'Connell, Dept of Justice, to Sec. of the Treasury, Washington DC, 28 Sept 1908
8 Ibid., L. Duncan Bulkley, 'Medico-Legal Aspects of the Case of John Early, Suspected Leper, Long Quarantined in Washington', read before the Society of Medical Jurisprudence, 13 Dec 1909
9 Ibid.
10 Ibid., Treasury Dept, Washington DC, to Captain Seaver, Salvation Army, 3 July 1909
11 Ibid., Bulkley, 'Medico-Legal Aspects . . .'
12 Ibid., Felix S.S. Johnson, American Consul, Bergen, Norway, to Asst Sec. of State, Washington DC, 20 Aug 1909
13 Ibid., Bulkley, 'Medico-Legal Aspects . . .'
14 Ibid., Egbert C. Everest, Counsel for John Early, Plattsburgh, NY, to Walter Wyman, Surgeon General, Washington DC, 8 Feb 1911
15 Kalisch, 'The Strange Case of John Early'
16 National Archives and Records Administration (Record Group 90), Rupert Blue, Surgeon General, Washington DC, to Asst Sec. Bailey, 4 May 1912
17 Ibid., Baylis H. Earle, Port Townsend, Washington, to Surgeon General, Washington DC, 20 May 1912
18 Ibid.

19 Ibid., Earle to Surgeon General, 22 July 1913
20 Ibid., Earle to Surgeon General, 30 May 1914
21 Kalisch, 'The Strange Case of John Early'
22 Ibid.
23 National Archives and Records Administration (Record Group 90), William H. Ford, Philadelphia Board of Health, to John B. Hamilton, Surgeon General, Washington DC, 31 Oct 1890
24 Ibid., 'National Control of Leprosy' discussion paper; see also Zachary Gussow, *Leprosy, Racism and Public Health* (Westview Press, Boulder, Col. 1989), p. 136
25 National Archives and Records Administration (Record Group 90), Walter R. Brinckerhoff, 'Leprosy in the United States of America in 1909'
26 H.M. Bracken, 'Report of the Committee of National Leper Homes', New Orleans 8 Dec 1902, *Lepra*, Vol. III, Fasc. 4 (1903)
27 Gussow, *Leprosy* . . ., p. 138
28 Cited in Kalisch, 'The Strange Case of John Early'
29 National Archives and Records Administration (Record Group 90), Office of the Surgeon General, Washington DC, 'Memorandum Relative to John Early', n.d. (but on internal evidence 1916)
30 Gussow, *Leprosy* . . ., p. 140
31 Stein, *Alone No Longer*, pp. 96–7
32 Fay F. Schamberg, 'The Unwanted Stigma of Leprosy', *The Survey*, 15 Apr 1929 (reprinted in the Chinese Mission to Lepers' *The Leper Quarterly*, n.d., no page ref.)
33 Isadore Dyer, 'The Sociological Aspects of Leprosy and the Question of Segregation', *Journal of Cutaneous Diseases, Including Syphilis*, May 1911 (no page ref.)
34 Stein, *Alone No Longer*, p. 98
35 Cited in Kalisch, 'The Strange Case of John Early' and Gussow, *Leprosy* . . ., pp. 145–6
36 Gussow, *Leprosy* . . ., pp. 140–1
37 National Archives and Records Administration (Record Group 90), Dr Oscar Dowling, President of the Louisiana State Board of Health, to Dr Rupert Blue, Surgeon General, Washington DC, 15 Nov 1918; and Rupert Blue to Oscar Dowling, 19 Nov 1918
38 Ibid., Brinckerhoff, 'Leprosy . . .'
39 Gussow, *Leprosy* . . ., pp. 49–55
40 Ibid., pp. 58–9
41 Dyer, 'The Sociological Aspects . . .'
42 National Archives and Records Administration (Record Group 90), Dr I. Dyer, Tulane Univ. of Louisiana, New Orleans, to Dr W.C. Rucker, Asst Surgeon General, Washington DC, 17 Nov 1915
43 Gussow, *Leprosy* . . ., p. 60
44 Prof. John Smith Kendall, 'Little Known Chapter in the History of Carville', *The Star*, Nov 1952, pp. 1–2
45 Gussow, *Leprosy* . . ., pp. 60–1
46 Carville Museum (CM), Sisters of Charity Records (SCR): Sister Ursula Bertschy, *The History of the United States Leper Colony* (thesis 1945), p. 100; 'Out of Darkness', *The Star*, Jan–Feb 1969, p. 4
47 'L.A. Carville from Carville, La', *The Star*, Nov–Dec 1954, p. 11
48 Gussow, *Leprosy* . . ., pp. 62–3
49 Cited in ibid., p. 64
50 CM, SCR, Sister Ursula, *The History* . . ., pp. 101–2
51 Ibid., p. 103
52 Ibid., p. 106
53 Ibid., p. 115
54 Ibid.
55 Ralph Hopkins, 'The Louisiana Leper Home', unidentified cutting from 1920, p. 251
56 CM, SCR, Sister Ursula, *The History* . . ., p. 120
57 CM, SCR, Sister Edith, Supt Carville, to Mrs Frank Deshon, Tulsa, Oklahoma, 5 May 1920

58 National Archives and Records Administration (Record Group 90), Dr I. Dyer to Dr W.C. Rucker, 17 Nov 1915
59 CM, SCR, Memo of Board of Control Meeting, 21 Jan 1919
60 National Archives and Records Administration (Record Group 90), G.W. McCoy, Chairman, Board for Selection of Site for The Federal Home for Lepers, to Surgeon General, Washington DC, 17 Nov 1915
61 'Doctor in the Lincoln Mold: A Tribute to the Memory of Dr G.W. McCoy 1876–1952', *The Star*, Sept 1952, p. 9
62 John Parascandola, 'The Gillis W. Long Hansen's Disease Center at Carville', *Public Health Reports*, Vol. 109, No. 6, Nov–Dec 1994, pp. 728–30
63 Stein, *Alone No Longer*, pp. 67–8
64 Ibid., pp. 100–1
65 National Archives and Records Administration (Record Group 90), O.E. Denney, MOC Carville, to Surgeon General, Washington DC, 18 Oct 1923
66 Ibid.
67 Cited in Kalisch, 'The Strange Case of John Early'
68 Ibid.
69 CM, SCR, newspaper cutting from *The Menace*, n.d. (but on internal evidence Aug/Sept 1924)
70 National Archives and Records Administration (Record Group 90), Rev. Benedict Stetter to O.E. Denney, MOC Carville, 5 March 1926; W. Myles Phillips to O.E. Denney, 10 April 1926
71 Ibid., John McMullen, Surgeon Director, New Orleans Quarantine Station, to Surgeon General, Washington DC, 14 April 1926
72 Ibid., John Early *et al.*, 'To Whom It May Concern', 20 May 1926
73 Ibid., Dr Denney's Statement to the Board, n.d. (1926)
74 Ibid., Wm. S. Terriberry, Asst Surgeon General (R), to Surgeon General, Washington DC, 7 June 1926
75 Ibid.
76 Cited in Stein, *Alone No Longer*, p. 183
77 National Archives and Records Administration (Record Group 90), O.E. Denney, MOC Carville, to Surgeon General, Washington DC, 18 Jan 1928
78 Ibid., O.E. Denney, MOC Carville, to Dr F.C. Smith, Asst Surgeon General, Washington DC, 27 Aug 1928
79 Stein, *Alone No Longer*, p. 183
80 Kalisch, 'The Strange Case of John Early'
81 Stein, *Alone No Longer*, p. 184
82 National Archives and Records Administration (Record Group 90), T.H. Pruett *et al.*, Carville, to W.M. Danner, New York, 10 June 1935
83 Kalisch, 'The Strange Case of John Early'
84 Stein, *Alone No Longer*, p. 185

9 Sir Leonard Rogers and BELRA

1 Sir Leonard Rogers, *Happy Toil: 55 Years of Tropical Medicine* (Muller, London 1950), Foreword by Maj-Gen. Sir John W.D. Megaw, p. xii
2 Ibid., pp. 4–5
3 Ibid., pp. 6, 8, 15
4 Helen J. Power, *Sir Leonard Rogers FRS (1868–1962): Tropical Medicine in the Indian Medical Service* (Univ. of London PhD thesis, 1993), p. 22
5 Rogers, *Happy Toil*, pp. 10, 19, 59–60
6 Power, *Sir Leonard Rogers*, p. 143
7 The Mission to Lepers, *Report of a Conference of Leper Asylum Superintendents and Others on the Leper Problems of India* (Cuttack, India 1920), p. 7
8 Ibid., pp. 77, 18

9 Ibid., p. 63
10 Ibid.
11 The Leprosy Mission International Archives, W.H.P. Anderson, 'The Problem Created by the Existence of a Dual Policy with Regard to the Housing of the Sexes at Different Asylums Connected with The Mission to Lepers; and Suggestions for its Solution', 8 Sept 1924
12 Cited in Sister Mary Stella, *Makogai: Image of Hope* (Lepers' Trust Board, New Zealand 1978), p. 56
13 Wellcome Contemporary Medical Archive Collections, L. Rogers papers, PP/ROG/C.13, Leonard Rogers to H.W. Wade, London 30 Jan 1924
14 George Thompson Brown, *Mission to Korea* (Board of World Missions, US 1962), pp. 146–7
15 Richard S. Buker, 'Leper Colonization in Kengtung State, Burma', *International Journal of Leprosy*, Vol. 8, No. 2, April–June 1940, pp. 167–78
16 A.T.W. Simeons, *The Mask of a Lion* (Gollancz, London 1952); all subsequent quotations in this section come from this novel
17 The Leprosy Mission International Archives, Dr H.W. Wade, Culion, to A. Donald Miller, The Mission to Lepers, 13 Jan 1953; Miller to Wade, 12 Feb 1953
18 Wellcome CMAC, L. Rogers papers, PP/ROG/C.13, 'For Private Circulation Only', BELRA 1923, p. 4
19 Maj-Gen. Sir Leonard Rogers, 'Progress in the Control of Leprosy in the British Empire', *Journal of the Royal Society of Arts*, Vol. xciv, No. 4722, 19 July 1946, pp. 525–39
20 G.H. Ree, 'Pattern of Leprosy in Queensland, Australia, 1855–1990', *Leprosy Review*, Vol. 62, 1991, pp. 420–30
21 Cape of Good Hope, *Report on the General Infirmary, Robben Island, for the Year 1867* (Cape Town 1868), p. 2
22 'Lepers at the Cape: Wanted, a Father Damien', *Blackwood's Edinburgh Magazine*, Sept 1889, pp. 293–9
23 'The Lepers at Robben Island', *British Medical Journal*, 14 Sept 1889, p. 636
24 Simon A. de Villiers, *Robben Island: Out of Reach, Out of Mind* (C. Struik (Pty) Ltd, Cape Town 1971), p. 91
25 William Tebb, *The Recrudescence of Leprosy and Its Causation* (London 1893), pp. 276–8
26 De Villiers, *Robben Island*, pp. 92–3
27 Harriet Deacon, 'Outside the Profession; Nursing Staff on Robben Island, 1846–1910', in Anne Marie Rafferty, Jane Robinson and Ruth Elkan (eds), *Nursing History and the Politics of Welfare* (Routledge & Kegan Paul, London and New York 1997), pp. 95–7
28 Wellcome CMAC, L. Rogers papers, PP/ROG/C.13, Dr J. Alexander Mitchell, Sec. for Public Health and Chief Health Officer, Union of South Africa, to Sir Leonard Rogers, BELRA, 30 Jan 1924
29 Ibid., memo on 'Leprosy Measures and Expenditure' by Dr J.A. Mitchell, Dept of Public Health, SA, 23 Oct 1922
30 Ibid., Mitchell to Rogers, 15 March 1927
31 Ibid., Rogers to Mitchell, 10 Oct 1928
32 Ibid., Mitchell to Rogers, 2 Aug 1929
33 *Journal of the Medical Association of South Africa*, 22 Feb 1930
34 Sir Leonard Rogers, 'In Place of Compulsory Segregation', *Leprosy Notes*, No. 4, Jan 1929
35 Wellcome CMAC, L. Rogers papers, PP/ROG/C.13, Mitchell to Rogers, 20 Nov 1928
36 T.J. Tonkin, 'Some General and Etiological Details Concerning Leprosy in the Sudan', *Lepra*, Vol. III, Fasc. 3 (London, Leipzig and Paris 1903), p. 135
37 Charles Henry Robinson, *Hausaland: Or Fifteen Hundred Miles through the Central Soudan* (London 1896), p. 147
38 Wellcome CMAC, GC/146/1, Letters and Reports from Yaba Lunatic and Leper Asylums, Lagos, Nigeria, 1907–1912
39 G.W. St C. Ramsay, 'A Study of Leprosy in Southern Nigeria', *Transactions of the Royal Society of Tropical Medicine & Hygiene*, Vol. XXII, No. 3, Nov 1928, pp. 249–62
40 Cited in BELRA Annual Report for 1928, 'Some Questions of Empire Suffering'
41 Ramsay, 'A Study of Leprosy . . .'

42 A.B. Macdonald, 'Rehabilitation – The Industrial and Social Work of a Leper Colony', *Leprosy Review*, Vol. XIX, No. 2, Apr 1948, pp. 45–55
43 Ibid.
44 J.A. Kinnear Brown, 'The Role of Leprosaria and Treatment Villages in Mass Campaigns in Tropical Africa', *International Journal of Leprosy*, Vol. 29, No. 1, Jan–March 1960, pp. 1–11
45 T. Frank Davey, 'Uzuakoli Leper Colony', *Leprosy Review*, Vol. X, No. 3, July 1939, pp. 171–85
46 Electra Dory, *Leper Country* (Muller, London 1963), pp. 46–7
47 Ibid., pp. 107–8
48 Eric Silla, *People Are Not the Same: Leprosy and Identity in Twentieth-century Mali* (Heinemann, Portsmouth, NH/James Currey, Oxford 1998), pp. 66–7, 134
49 Ibid., p. 129
50 Cited in BELRA Annual Report for 1930
51 See Megan Vaughan, *Curing Their Ills: Colonial Power and African Illness* (Polity Press, Cambridge 1991), p. 93
52 The Leprosy Mission International Archives, Confidential 'Memorandum for the Consideration of the General Secretary of The Mission to Lepers and the Medical Secretary of the British Empire Leprosy Relief Association', undated and anonymous: BELRA Annual Report for 1933, introducing 'Tubby', Rev. P.B. Clayton MC, Founder Padre of Toc H
53 BELRA Annual Reports for 1931 and 1945
54 The Leprosy Mission International Archives, Frank Oldrieve, 'Can We Rid Africa of Leprosy?', text of radio broadcast from Johannesburg, 9.00 p.m., 27 Feb 1948
55 'The Late Mr. Oldrieve', *The Times of Swaziland*, 25 March 1948
56 Rogers, *Happy Toil*, p. 246
57 BELRA Annual Report for 1963
58 'Happy Birthday, Sir Leonard Rogers', *The Star*, Jan–Feb 1960, p. 11

10 Stanley Stein and the Miracle at Carville

1 Stanley Stein (with Lawrence G. Blockman), *Alone No Longer* (*The Star*, Carville, La 1974; 1st pubd 1963), pp. 3–4
2 Ibid., p. 21
3 Ibid., p. 11
4 Ibid., pp. 36–7
5 Ibid.
6 Ibid., pp. 14–15
7 Ibid., pp. 47, 49
8 Ibid., p. 51
9 *The Sixty-six Star*, Vol. II, No. 2, 28 May 1932
10 Ibid., Vol. II, No. 15, 27 Aug 1932, 'Looking Out from Within'
11 Stein, *Alone No Longer*, p. 136
12 *The Sixty-six Star*, Vol. 3, No. 10, 15 Oct 1933, 'Without the Camp'
13 Ibid., Vol. 4, No. 3, Aug 1934, 'That Word – Leper'
14 Stein, *Alone No Longer*, p. 160
15 Ibid., p. 81
16 Ibid., pp. 118, 122
17 Ibid., p. 106
18 Betty Martin (ed. Evelyn Wells), *Miracle at Carville* (Doubleday, New York 1950), pp. 89–90
19 Stein, *Alone No Longer*, p. 107
20 Ibid., p. 129
21 Ibid., pp. 175, 177–8, 191, 198–9
22 National Archives and Records Administration (Record Group 90), H.E. Hasseltine, MOC Carville, to Surgeon General, Washington DC, 18 Sept 1939
23 Stein, *Alone No Longer*, p. 171

24 National Archives and Records Administration (Record Group 90), Hasseltine to Surgeon General, 18 Sept 1939
25 Stein, *Alone No Longer*, pp. 175–6
26 National Archives and Records Administration (Record Group 90), G.W. McCoy, Medical Director, US Public Health Service, to Surgeon General, Washington DC, 18 Sept 1939; H.E. Hasseltine, MOC Carville, 'First Indorsement'
27 Clarence A. Mills, *Climate Makes the Man* (Harper, New York 1942), pp. 128–9
28 National Archives and Records Administration (Record Group 90), S.L. Christian, Asst Surgeon General, Hospital Division, Washington DC, to E.D. Lewison, Chairman, Executive Cttee, Patients' Federation, Carville, 20 Sept 1938
29 Stein, *Alone No Longer*, pp. 203–5
30 Ibid., pp. 206–7
31 National Archives and Records Administration (Record Group 90), H.E. Hasseltine, MOC Carville, to S.L. Christian, Asst Surgeon General, Washington DC, 29 Feb 1940
32 Stein, *Alone No Longer*, pp. 215–16, 220–1
33 Ibid., pp. 218–19
34 Johnny P. Harmon, *King of the Microbes* (privately printed, fifth printing 1999), pp. 25–7
35 Martin, *Miracle at Carville*, pp. 36–7
36 Ibid., pp. 37, 61, 81, 101–2, 105
37 Ibid., p. 121
38 Stein, *Alone No Longer*, p. 200
39 Martin, *Miracle at Carville*, p. 128
40 Ibid., pp. 128–31
41 Ibid., pp. 45, 136
42 Ibid., pp. 138–9, 142
43 Ibid., pp. 143–51
44 Ibid., pp. 167–70, 174, 180, 187
45 Ibid., pp. 180–1, 188–9, 194–5
46 Ibid., pp. 187, 202, 205
47 Ibid., p. 189
48 Stein, *Alone No Longer*, pp. 210–11
49 Martin, *Miracle at Carville*, p. 223
50 Ibid., pp. 222–30
51 Ibid., pp. 232–5
52 Stein, *Alone No Longer*, pp. 231–3
53 Ibid., pp. 233–4
54 Ibid., pp. 247–8; Martin, *Miracle at Carville*, pp. 249–50
55 Harmon, *King of the Microbes*, p. 86
56 Stein, *Alone No Longer*, p. 251
57 Ibid., pp. 239, 222–3
58 Martin, *Miracle at Carville*, pp. 285–6
59 Stein, *Alone No Longer*, pp. 240–3; cited in Zachary Gussow, *Leprosy, Racism and Public Health* (Westview Press, Col. 1989), p. 167
60 Gussow, *Leprosy . . .*, pp. 161–2; Stein, *Alone No Longer*, p. 224; Martin, *Miracle at Carville*, pp. 267–8; *The Star*, Sept–Oct 1961, pp. 17–22, 'Two Decades of Carville'
61 *The Star*, Sept–Oct 1961, pp. 18–19
62 Cited in Gussow, *Leprosy . . .*, p. 162
63 National Library of Medicine, History of Medicine Division, Public Health Service Hospitals Historical Collections, MS C471: R.C. Williams, Asst Surgeon General, Washington DC, to Stanley Stein, Editor, *The Star*, Carville, 30 Oct 1947
64 Eugene R. Kellersberger, 'The Social Stigma of Leprosy', *Annals of the New York Academy of Sciences*, Vol. 54, Art. 1, March 1951, pp. 126–33
65 National Library of Medicine, HMD, PHSHHC, MS C471: Stanley Stein to Theodore Hayes, Federal Economic Security Commission, Washington DC, 11 Oct 1949
66 Ibid., unsigned, undated report on 'The STAR'

67 Ibid.
68 Ibid.
69 Ibid.
70 Ibid., P. Hall, Liverpool, England, to Stanley Stein, Carville, 12 July 1949
71 Stein, *Alone No Longer*, p. 282
72 Ibid., pp. 283–1
73 Ibid., pp. 294–7
74 *The Star*, 'Two Decades of Carville'
75 Harmon, *King of the Microbes*, p. 92
76 *The Star*, 'Two Decades of Carville'; Stein, *Alone No Longer*, pp. 307–8
77 National Library of Medicine, HMD, PHSHHC, MSC471, J. Stewart Hunter to Leonard A. Scheele, Surgeon General, Washington DC, 6 July 1956
78 Stein, *Alone No Longer*, pp. 309, 314
79 Ibid., p. 311
80 Ibid., pp. 312–13
81 Betty Martin (ed. Evelyn Wells), *No One Must Ever Know* (Doubleday, New York 1959), p. 202
82 Gussow, *Leprosy* . . ., pp. 176–7
83 Ibid., pp. 185–6
84 Jim Duncan, 'Twenty-one Months at Carville', *The Star*, Sept–Oct 1965, pp. 2, 16
85 Gussow, *Leprosy* . . ., p. 177
86 Ibid., pp. 185–6
87 Ibid.
88 Zachary Gussow and George S. Tracy, 'Stigma and the Leprosy Phenomenon: The Social History of a Disease in the 19th and 20th Centuries', *Bulletin of the History of Medicine*, Vol. 44, No. 5, Sept–Oct 1970, pp. 425–49
89 Z. Gussow and G. Tracy, 'Status, Ideology and Adaptation to Stigmatized Illness: A Study of Leprosy', *Human Organization*, 1968, No. 27, pp. 316–25, cited in Nancy E. Waxler, 'Learning to Be a Leper: A Case Study in the Social Construction of Illness' in Elliot G. Mischler *et al.*, *Social Contexts of Health, Illness, and Patient Care* (Cambridge University Press, Cambridge, 1981), pp. 182–3
90 'Comments on Betty Martin's New Book', A. M. Davison, Chief, Rehabilitation Branch, *et al.*, *The Star*, May–June 1959, p. 18
91 Martin, *No One* . . ., p. 231
92 Stein, *Alone No Longer*, pp. 329–30
93 Martin, *No One* . . ., pp. 199–200
94 'Cast Away: Betty Martin's Fearful Illness Meant a Sentence of Exile', *People*, 24 May 1999

11 Peter Greave and the Homes of St Giles

1 Peter Greave, *The Second Miracle* (Chatto & Windus, London 1955), p. 4 [all other page refs below are to the Henry Holt, New York 1955 edition, which cut this particular sentence]
2 Ibid., pp. 15–20
3 Ibid., pp. 17–23
4 Ibid., pp. 28–9
5 Ibid., p. 31
6 Peter Greave, *The Seventh Gate* (Temple-Smith, London 1976; Penguin, London 1978), p. 46 [all page refs are to the Penguin paperback edition]
7 Ibid., p. 17; Peter Greave, *The Painted Leopard* (Eyre & Spottiswoode, London 1960), p. 20
8 Greave, *The Seventh Gate*, pp. 18–19
9 Ibid., pp. 22–3; Greave, *The Second Miracle*, p. 44
10 Greave, *The Seventh Gate*, pp. 24–5
11 Ibid., pp. 30, 76–116
12 Ibid., p. 139

13 Ibid., pp. 140–1
14 Ibid., pp. 149–52
15 Greave, *The Seventh Gate*, p. 153; Greave, *The Painted Leopard*, p. 70; Greave, *The Seventh Gate*, p. 154
16 Greave, *The Seventh Gate*, p. 155; Greave, *The Painted Leopard*, pp. 144–5, 69
17 Peter Greave, *Young Man in the Sun* (Eyre & Spottiswoode, London 1958), pp. 229, 211; Greave, *The Painted Leopard*, pp. 69–70, 171, 169
18 Greave, *The Seventh Gate*, p. 169
19 Greave, *The Painted Leopard*, pp. 135–6; Greave, *The Seventh Gate*, pp. 170, 158–60
20 Greave, *The Second Miracle*, p. 138
21 Greave, *The Seventh Gate*, pp. 173–5
22 Gen. Sir Francis Tuker, *While Memory Serves* (Cassell, London 1950)
23 Greave, *The Seventh Gate*, pp. 175–6
24 Richard Greene (ed.), *Selected Letters of Edith Sitwell* (Virago, London 1997), p. 411; Elizabeth Salter, *The Last Years of a Rebel: A Memoir of Edith Sitwell* (The Bodley Head, London 1967), pp. 73–5
25 Salter, *The Last Years* . . .
26 Public Record Office, MH55/554. Confidential memo from Sir Arthur Downes (Senior Medical Inspector for Poor Law purposes), 'Provision for Lepers in the British Isles', June 1914
27 Ibid.
28 John Bhoyroo, *The British Leper: A Study of Leprosy in Britain 1867–1951* (Wellcome Institute for the History of Medicine dissertation, 1997), pp. 77–9
29 Downes, as note 26
30 Stanley G. Browne, *Leprosy in England – Yesterday and Today* (Leprosy Study Centre, Kettering, Northants 1977), p. 37
31 Ibid.; Downes, as note 26
32 Browne, *Leprosy in England*, p. 37
33 Ibid., p. 40
34 The Leprosy Mission International Archives, John Jackson, Sec. to the Mission to Lepers, to Wellesley C. Bailey, Edinburgh, 25 Jan 1916; 7 Hon. G. Scott, Danbury, Essex, to Wellesley C. Bailey, 2 March 1916
35 The Leprosy Mission International Archives, Scott to Bailey, 2 March 1916
36 J.M.H. MacLeod, 'Contact Cases of Leprosy in the British Isles', *Leprosy Review*, Vol. 3, No. 1, Jan–March 1935 (condensed version of an article originally published in the *BMJ* in 1925); MH55/509, Minute by Col. James for Sir George Buchanan, Chief Medical Officer, 20 Dec 1924; MH55/515, Arthur Downes, 'Strathcona Trust: Notes of a Visit of Inspection to Moor House, East Hanningfield, Essex, by the Trustees on 3 Oct 1924', 14 April 1926
37 Public Record Office, MH55/509, Memo from J.A. Glover to Sir George Buchanan, CMO, 3 Jan 1925; MH55/324, Dr Ralph M.F. Picken, Cardiff Public Health Dept, to Howell E. James, Welsh Board of Health, 12 June 1933
38 Public Record Office, AIR10/4562, Memo from W.V. Shaw, Ministry of Health, Whitehall, to SMO, Med. 1, 'Cardiff County Borough. Leprosy – Joseph Attard', 31 Aug 1933; Ivor Pirrie, Maldon, Essex, to Dr W.V. Shaw, 8 Oct 1934
39 Public Record Office, AIR10/4562, Ministry of Health minute, 12 Oct 1934: MH55/1800, 'Leprosy, General File, 1947–1953'
40 Greave, *The Second Miracle*, pp. 140–1
41 Ibid., pp. 145–7
42 Ibid., p. 254
43 Ibid., pp. 86–7
44 BELRA, *Annual Report for 1948*, p. 1
45 BELRA, *Annual Report for 1949*, pp. 12–13
46 Stanley Stein, 'Gordon Ryrie – He Honored His Pledge', *The Star*, Sept 1953, p. 15
47 Ibid.; obit. of Gordon Ryrie in *The Lancet*, 21 March 1953, citing article in *Leprosy Review*, Jan 1947
48 Public Record Office, MH55/1800, Dr Melville D. Mackenzie, Ministry of Health, to Dr H.A.

Raeburn, Principal Regional Medical Officer, Liverpool, 8 Jan 1947; Dr Raeburn to Dr Mackenzie, 22 Jan 1947

49 Public Record Office, MH55/1800, Sir William Jameson, Ministry of Health, to Rt Hon. Walter Elliot MP, 2 Jan 1947; H.H. George, Ministry of Health, to E. Hale, Treasury, 3 March 1947

50 Public Record Office, MH55/1800, Miss H.M. Hedley, private sec. to Sir William Douglas, Ministry of Health, to Rt Hon. Walter Elliot MP, 3 Sept 1948

51 Public Record Office, MH55/1800, Memo from Dr. E.L. Sturdee, Ministry of Health, to CMO, 7 March 1947

52 American Leprosy Mission Archives, Peter Hall, 'Dreams Do Come True', *Leprosy Mission Digest*, n.d. (but on internal evidence 1947), pp. 25–7

53 Ibid.

54 Public Record Office, MH55/1803, Peter Hall, Melling, Liverpool, to Rt Hon. Aneurin Bevan, Secretary of State for Health, 3 July 1949; Peter Hall, 'Prisoners of Ancient Fears', undated, unpublished typescript memoir

55 Public Record Office, T164/481, Staff Welfare Report on 'Peter Hall – Retired', by E. Robinson, Chief Welfare Officer, Ministry of Aviation, 1 Sept 1964; Hall, 'Prisoners of Ancient Fears'

56 Hall, 'Prisoners of Ancient Fears' – from which the following several unreferenced quotations also come

57 Public Record Office, MH55/1803, Hall to Bevan, 3 July 1949

58 Public Record Office, MH55/1804, Gordon Ryrie, BELRA, to Dr. G.E. Godber, Ministry of Health, 7 April 1949

59 Public Record Office, MH55/1804, G.A. Ryrie, 'Note on Carville Leprosarium, USA'

60 'Notification of Leprosy', *British Medical Journal*, 23 June 1951

61 'Hansen's Disease Now Notifiable in Britain', *The Star*, July–Aug 1951, pp. 7–8

62 Public Record Office, MH55/1804, Minutes of a Meeting at the Ministry of Health, 28 Dec 1951

63 William H. Jopling, 'Recollections and Reflections', *The Star*, March–April 1992, pp. 5–10

64 Ibid.; obit. of William Henry Jopling by G.C. Cook in *BMJ*, 22 Nov 1997

65 Author interviews with ex-patients of the Jordan Hospital, Reigate, conducted Jan 2001

66 Author interview with Patrick M, 5 Oct 2000; his medical notes

67 Ibid.

68 Patrick M's medical notes

69 Ibid.

70 Author interview with Patrick M; his medical notes

71 Jopling, 'Recollections and Reflections'

72 Ibid.

73 Mavourneen B. Morriss, 'A Visit to the Homes of St Giles – England', *The Star*, Jan–Feb 1968, pp. 8–9

74 Author interview with Les Parker, 17 Sept 2001

75 Ibid.

76 G. Les Parker, 'Progress or Abandonment?' *The Star*, Oct–Dec 1998, pp. 1–2

77 Greave, *The Seventh Gate*, p. 171

12 'Saint Paul' Brand and 'Mr Leprosy' Browne

1 Paul Brand, with Philip Yancey, *Pain: The Gift Nobody Wants* (Marshall Pickering, London 1994), p. 12

2 'Mr A. Donald Miller answers *The Times*', *Without the Camp* (quarterly journal of The Leprosy Mission), No. 289, Jan–March 1969, p. 6

3 S.G. Browne, 'Leprosy: The Christian Attitude', *The Expository Times*, Vol. lxxiii, No. 8 (1962), pp. 242–5

4 Brand, *Pain*, p. 15
5 Ibid., p. 26
6 Ibid., pp. 21–2
7 Ibid.
8 Ibid., p. 23
9 Ibid., pp. 28–9
10 Ibid., pp. 30–1, 72; Dorothy Clarke Wilson, *Ten Fingers for God: The Life and Work of Paul Brand* (first published 1965; Paul Brand Publishing, Seattle 1989), p. 67
11 Brand, *Pain*, pp. 73, 80
12 Paul Brand's obit. of Robert Greenhill Cochrane, 1899–1985, *International Journal of Leprosy*, Vol. 54, No. 1, March 1986, pp. 112–13; Brand, *Pain*, pp. 88–92
13 Brand, *Pain*, pp. 88–92
14 L.M. Bechelli, 'Advances in Leprosy Control in the Last 100 Years', *International Journal of Leprosy*, Vol. 41, No. 3, July–Sept 1973, pp. 285–97
15 Brand, *Pain*, pp. 94–5
16 Ibid., pp. 104, 9–11
17 Ibid., pp. 96–102
18 Ibid., pp. 104, 113, 126
19 Ibid., pp. 127–8
20 Ibid., pp. 118, 130
21 Daniel C. Riordan, 'Vision of Hope', *The Star*, March 1951, p. 4
22 Brand, *Pain*, pp. 135–7
23 Paul Brand's obit. of Prof. T.N. Jagadisan, 1909–91, *The Star*, Jan–Feb 1992, pp. 2, 16; T.N. Jagadisan, *Fulfilment Through Leprosy* (Tamil Nadu, India 1988), pp. 1, 4, 8, 13–15, 28
24 Jagadisan, *Fulfilment Through Leprosy*, pp. 66–7
25 Ibid., pp. 71–73, 104
26 Ibid., pp. 79–81, 84
27 Ibid., pp. 329, 130, 90
28 T.N. Jagadisan, 'Chairman's Statement on Social Aspects', *Transactions of the VIIth International Congress of Leprology* (Tokyo 1959), pp. 417–24
29 Ibid.
30 Brand's obit. of Prof. T.N. Jagadisan
31 Ibid.
32 Brand, *Pain*, pp. 140–5
33 Ibid., pp. 150–3
34 Ibid., pp. 155–6
35 Ibid., pp. 148, 158–9
36 Ibid., p. 161
37 Ibid., pp. 162–5
38 Ibid., pp. 165, 182, 188, 205
39 Ibid., p. 251
40 'Brands' Farewell to Carville', *The Star*, Jan–Feb 1988, p. 13
41 P.W. Brand, 'The Beginning of ALERT', *Leprosy Review*, Vol. 57, Suppl. 1, pp. 1–8
42 Phyllis Thompson, *Mister Leprosy: Dr Stanley Browne's Fight against Leprosy* (Hodder & Stoughton, London 1980–1), pp. 197–8
43 Brand, 'The Beginning of ALERT'
44 Thompson, *Mister Leprosy*, pp. 5–53
45 S.G. Browne, 'Some Pages from My African Diary', *Medical History*, Vol. XVII, No. 4, Oct 1973, pp. 405–10
46 Ibid.; see also Tony Gould, *In Limbo: The Story of Stanley's Rear Column* (Hamish Hamilton, London 1979)
47 Thompson, *Mister Leprosy*, p. 56; Browne, 'Some Pages . . .'
48 Thompson, *Mister Leprosy*, pp. 92–5
49 Ibid., pp. 128–9
50 Ibid., pp. 138, 154, 159

51 Ibid., pp. 161–3
52 Ibid., pp. 165–6
53 Ibid., pp. 168–9
54 Ibid., p. 173
55 Wellcome Contemporary Medical Archive Collections, Stanley G. Browne papers. Mali Browne, 'How "The Nun's Story" Came to Yalisombo', typescript (1959), pp. 1–2, 6
56 Ibid., pp. 7, 14–15
57 Prof. Michel F. Lechat, 'Remembering Graham Greene', *The Bulletin*, 18 April 1991, pp. 14–16
58 Ibid.
59 Graham Greene, *In Search of Characters: Two African Journals* (Bodley Head, London 1961), pp. 24–60
60 'Dr Cochrane Reviews Graham Greene's New Book for THE STAR', *The Star*, March–April 1961, p. 10
61 Lechat, 'Remembering Graham Greene'
62 Greene, *In Search of Characters*, p. 65
63 Thompson, *Mister Leprosy*, p. 212
64 Dr S.G. Browne, 'Report on B663', *The Star*, Nov–Dec 1969, pp. 5, 14
65 James Brabazon, *Albert Schweitzer: A Biography* (Gollancz, London 1976), p. 456
66 Ibid., pp. 393–4
67 'Dr Schweitzer Will Use Nobel Peace Prize to Build HD Village', *The Star*, Jan 1954, p. 5
68 Wellcome CMAC, Stanley G. Browne papers. S.G. Browne, 'Leprosy – The Prime Disabler', 1966 lecture typescript
69 P. Brand, '14th International Leprosy Congress (Keynote Address)', *The Star*, Sept–Oct 1993, pp. 2–5
70 Ibid.
71 Ibid.

13 Leprosy in One Country . . . and Beyond

1 S.G. Browne, 'The Integration of Leprosy into the General Health Services', *Leprosy Review*, Vol. 43, 1972, pp. 16–20
2 Tony Gould, *Imperial Warriors: Britain and the Gurkhas* (Granta Books, London 1999), p. 334
3 Stephen Neill, *A History of Christian Missions* (Penguin, London 1964; 2nd edn rev. by Owen Chadwick 1986), p. 424
4 The Leprosy Mission International Archives, report entitled 'Nepal Prospect, Oct. 2–17, 1955'
5 Grace Nies Fletcher, *The Fabulous Flemings of Kathmandu* (Dutton, New York 1964), pp. 16–17, 29, 71–2
6 'Nepal Prospect'; author interview with Eileen Lodge, 17 March 2001
7 'Nepal Prospect'; 'Dr [I.] B. Mali Returns to Nepal', *The Star*, March–April 1966, p. 5
8 'Nepal Prospect'
9 Ibid.
10 The Leprosy Mission International Archives, A. Donald Miller to Dr J.C. Pedley, 22 Nov 1956; Cecil Pedley to ADM, 8 Dec 1956; ADM to JCP, 22 Jan 1957
11 The Leprosy Mission International Archives, Dr Fraser's confidential report on his visit to Kathmandu 21 Feb–4 March 1960; N.D. Fraser, 'Leprosy in Nepal', *Leprosy Review*, Vol. 31, No. 4, Oct 1960, pp. 286–9
12 The Leprosy Mission International Archives, Cecil Pedley's newsletters of 27 May 1961 and 1 April 1962
13 The Leprosy Mission International Archives, Pedley's newsletters of 1 April and 28 Aug 1962
14 The Leprosy Mission International Archives, Pedley's newsletters of 14 Aug and 20 Oct 1963
15 Ibid.
16 Ibid.
17 Ibid.

18 'Dr [I.]B. Mali Returns to Nepal'
19 The Leprosy Mission International Archives, J.C. Pedley's newsletter of 22 March 1967
20 The Leprosy Mission International Archives, JCP's newsletter of Feb 1969
21 The Leprosy Mission International Archives, Dr Stanley G. Browne's Report to the Leprosy Mission, 'Visit of Medical Consultant to Nepal', n.d.
22 The Leprosy Mission International Archives, Browne's Report
23 Ibid.
24 Ibid.
25 The Leprosy Mission International Archives, JCP's newsletter of 4 Nov 1969
26 The Leprosy Mission International Archives, Johs G. Andersen, Adviser to NELRA, 'Project Report', 1 Sept 1970
27 Ibid.
28 Ibid.
29 The Leprosy Mission International Archives, Johs G. Andersen to Stanley G. Browne, 18 May 1970
30 The Leprosy Mission International Archives, Andersen to Browne, 19 May 1970
31 The Leprosy Mission International Archives, Andersen, 'Project Report'
32 Author interview with Eileen Lodge, Kathmandu, 17 March 2001
33 Ibid.
34 Ibid.
35 Ibid.
36 Patrick Lynch, 'A New Face for an Old Disease: Some Reflections on the Role of the Media in Nepal's First National Leprosy Elimination Campaign', *Leprosy Review*, Vol. 71, No. 1, March 2000, pp. 62–70
37 Ibid.
38 Ibid.
39 Author interviews with Hugh Cross, Lalgadh, 5 and 6 March 2001
40 Ibid.
41 Ibid.
42 Ibid.
43 Hugh Cross, 'A Bundle of Rags', unpublished typescript
44 D.H. de Stigter, L. de Geus and M.L. Heynders, 'Leprosy: Between Acceptance and Segregation. Community Behaviour Towards Persons Affected by Leprosy in Eastern Nepal', *Leprosy Review* (2000), Vol. 71, pp. 492–8
45 Linda M. Robertson, Peter G. Nichols and Ruth Butlin, 'Delay in Presentation and Start of Treatment in Leprosy: Experience in an Outpatient Clinic in Nepal', *Leprosy Review* (2000), Vol. 71, pp. 511–16
46 S.G. Browne, 'The Integration of Leprosy into General Health Services', *Leprosy Review* (1972), Vol. 43, pp. 16–20
47 Ibid.
48 Michel F. Lechat, 'The International Leprosy Association at 50 Years', *International Journal of Leprosy*, Vol. 49, No. 1, March 1981, pp. 60–4
49 Stanley G. Browne, 'Caring Still Counts', *The Star*, Nov–Dec 1982, pp. 2–3
50 Emanuel Faria, 'Life after MDT', *The Star*, March–April 1994, pp. 8–10
51 Alison Anderson, 'Towards Leprosy Eradication in Nepal', n.d.
52 Ibid.
53 Kommer L. Braber, 'WHO Leprosy Elimination Campaign – Beyond 2005', *Leprosy Review* (2000), Vol. 71, pp. 389–91
54 Ibid.
55 Diana N.J. Lockwood, 'Leprosy Elimination – A Virtual Phenomenon or a Reality?', *British Medical Journal*, Vol. 324, 22 June 2002, pp. 1516–18
56 Ibid.
57 Ibid.

14 A Kind of Closure

1 Govt of India, Ministry of Health and Family Welfare, 'National Public Health Act – 2002', final draft, 149 (1) 'Persons found to be suffering from an infective stage of leprosy may be directed to remain in isolation at home to the extent possible . . . '; 152 (1) 'Government or local health authority shall have the power to regulate that no infectious patient of leprosy be allowed to work in establishments like school, food establishments etc. where they are likely to come in contact with healthy population. (2) Government or local health authorities shall have the power to restrict the movement of infectious patients of leprosy in crowded places, in public conveyance etc.'
2 Fujio Ohtani, *The Walls Crumble: The Emancipation of Persons Affected by Hansen's Disease in Japan* (n.p., Tokyo 1998), various pages
3 Ibid., pp. xvii, 107, 73, 66, 83–4
4 Ibid., p. 107
5 Ibid., p. 38
6 Ibid., p. 211
7 Ibid., pp. 109–14
8 Ibid., p. 139
9 Shigetaka Takashima, 'New Orientation in the Control of Leprosy in Japan', *International Journal of Leprosy*, Vol. 33, No. 1, Jan–March 1965, pp. 1–17
10 Ohtani, *The Walls Crumble*, pp. 133–6
11 Ibid., pp. 148–54
12 Ibid., pp. 153–5
13 Ibid., p. 161
14 Ibid., p. 167
15 Ibid., pp. 215–16, 230
16 Ibid., p. xiii
17 Anwei Skinsnes Law, 'Japan – A Recovery of Rights', *The Star*, Sept 1996
18 Doug Struck and Akiko Yamamoto, 'Japan Confronts Leprosy's Legacy', *The Washington Post*, 12 May 2001, p. A01
19 Ibid.
20 'State Blamed for Leprosy Misery', *Mainichi Daily News*, 12 May 2001
21 'Man Reclaims Name after 61 Years', *The Daily Yomiuri* (Tokyo), 12 May 2001, p. 2
22 Personal information from Kay Yamaguchi of the Sasakawa Memorial Health Foundation, Tokyo
23 'Q & A about the Assisted Living Allowance for Residents of the Gillis W. Long HD Center', July 1998
24 Author interview with Tom K., Carville, 25 May 2001
25 Ibid.; Matthew Teague, 'A Hard Way Home', *The Times-Picayune* (New Orleans), 4 Feb 2001, pp. E-1, E-4–5
26 Author interview with Tom K.
27 'First Annual International Day of Dignity and Respect', *The Star*, Jan–March 1999, pp. 2–3
28 Author interview with Dr. Robert R. Jacobson, Baton Rouge, 22 May 2001
29 Author interview with Mary Ruth Daigle, Carville, 28 May 2001
30 Ibid.
31 Gilla Kaplan, 'Leprosy (Hansen's Disease)' in L. Goodman and J.C. Bennett (ed.), *Cecil Textbook of Medicine* (21st edn, 1999), pp. 1733–8
32 C.K. Job, 'Leprosy – the Source of Infection and its Mode of Transmission', *Leprosy Review* (1981) 52, Suppl. 1. pp. 69–76
33 The Leprosy Mission International Archives, S.G. Browne's confidential memorandum to members of the Leprosy Mission's executive committee, 'Has the causative organism of leprosy been grown in an artificial cell-free culture medium?'
34 Ibid.
35 Meny Bergel, *Leprosy as a Metabolic Disease* (n.p., Buenos Aires 1988); Michael G. Corcos, ' "Leprosy Can Be Cured!": New Wine in an Old Bottle?', *The Star*, March–April 1988, pp. 3–6

36 Bergel, *Leprosy as a Metabolic Disease*, pp. 1–4
37 Corcos, '"*Leprosy Can Be Cured!*"'
38 Bergel, *Leprosy as a Metabolic Disease*, p. 6
39 Laszlo Kato, 'Reflections of the Reflections of Hansen', in G. Armauer Hansen, *Memories and Reflections* (1st English edn, 1976), p. 3
40 Author interview with Dr Diana Lockwood, 30 July 2003
41 Kaplan, 'Leprosy (Hansen's Disease)'
42 Diana N.J. Lockwood, 'Leprosy Elimination – a Virtual Phenomenon or a Reality?', *British Medical Journal*, 22 June 2002, pp. 1516–18
43 Hermann Feldmeier, 'The Tortuous Path of the Leprosy Bacilli: Questioning an Old Paradigm', *ESCMID* [European Society of Clinical Microbiology and Infectious Diseases] *News*, No. 1, 2001, pp. 26–7
44 Ibid.
45 Dr G. Armauer Hansen and Dr Carl Looft, *Leprosy: In its Clinical & Pathological Aspects* (Bristol 1895), p. 6

SELECT BIBLIOGRAPHY

The following is a selection of books and articles consulted during the writing of this book. Details of public and private papers cited are to be found in the chapter notes and references. The main documentary sources in England include the British Library, Oriental and India Office Collections (BL – OIOC), the Leprosy Mission International (TLMI), LEPRA (the British Leprosy Relief Association), the Public Record Office (PRO), the Royal Geographical Society (RGS) and the Wellcome Trust Contemporary Medical Archive Collections (CMAC). In the United States they include the American Leprosy Mission (ALM), Carville Museum (CM), the National Archives and Records Administration (NARA) and the National Library of Medicine (NLM). Newspapers and journals most frequently consulted include *The Times*, the *British Medical Journal* (*BMJ*), *The Lancet*, the *Bulletin of the History of Medicine* (*Bull. Hist. Med.*), the *International Journal of Leprosy* (*Int. J. Lepr.*) and *Leprosy Review* (*Lepr. Rev.*); also, and most invaluably, the journal of the patient activists at Carville, *The Star*.

Anon., 'Lepers at the Cape: Wanted, a Father Damien', *Blackwood's Edinburgh Magazine*, Sept 1889, pp. 293–9

Bailey, Paul, *Hawaii's Royal Prime Minister: The Life and Times of Walter Murray Gibson* (Hastings House, New York 1980)

Bechelli, L.M., 'Advances in Leprosy Control in the Last 100 Years', *Int. J. Lepr.*, Vol. 41, No. 3, July–Sept 1973, pp. 285–97

Bergel, Meny, *Leprosy as a Metabolic Disease* (n.p., Buenos Aires 1988)

Bhoyroo, John, *The British Leper: A Study of Leprosy in Britain 1867–1951* (Wellcome Institute for the History of Medicine dissertation 1997)

Blom, Knut, 'Armauer Hansen and Human Leprosy Transmission: Medical Ethics and Legal Rights', *Int. J. Lepr.*, Vol. 41, No. 2, 1973, pp. 199–203

Boyd, Julia, *Hannah Riddell: An Englishwoman in Japan* (Charles E. Tuttle, Rutland 1996)

Brabazon, James, *Albert Schweitzer: A Biography* (Gollancz, London 1976)

Braber, Kommer L., 'WHO Leprosy Elimination Campaign – Beyond 2005', *Lepr. Rev.*, Vol. 71, 2000, pp. 389–91

Brand, P.W., 'The Beginning of ALERT', *Lepr. Rev.*, Vol. 57, Suppl. 1, pp. 1–8

Brand, Paul, with Philip Yancey, *Pain: The Gift Nobody Wants* (Marshall Pickering, London 1994)

Brown, George Thompson, *Mission to Korea* (Board of World Missions, US 1962)

Browne, S.G., 'Leprosy: The Christian Attitude', *The Expository Times*, Vol. lxxiii, No. 8, 1962, pp. 242–5

————, 'The Integration of Leprosy into the General Health Services', *Lepr. Rev.*, Vol. 43, 1972, pp. 16–20

————, 'Some Pages from My African Diary', *Medical History*, Vol. XVII, No. 4, Oct 1973, pp. 405–10

————, 'The Leprosy Mission: A Century of Service', *Lepr. Rev.*, Vol. 45, 1974, pp. 166–9

————, *Leprosy in England – Yesterday and Today* (Leprosy Study Centre, Kettering, Northants 1977)

————, 'Caring Still Counts', *The Star*, Nov–Dec 1982, pp. 2–3

Buker, Richard S., 'Leper Colonization in Kengtung State, Burma', *Int. J. Lepr.*, Vol. 8, No. 2, 1940, pp. 167–78

Burgess, Perry, *Who Walk Alone* (Holt, New York 1940)

————, *Born of Those Years: An Autobiography* (Dent, London 1952)

Cape of Good Hope, *Report on the General Infirmary, Robben Island, for the Year 1867* (Cape Town 1868)

Carter, Henry Vandyke, *On Leprosy and Elephantiasis* (London 1874)

————, *Report on Leprosy and Leper-Asylums in Norway: With References to India* (London 1874)

Chapman, Ronald Fettes, *Leonard Wood and Leprosy in the Philippines: The Culion Leper Colony, 1921–1927* (University Press of America 1982)

Clifford, Edward, 'The First-Born Son of Death', *The Nineteenth Century*, Aug 1888, pp. 576–8

————, *Father Damien: A Journey from Cashmere to His Home in Hawaii* (London 1889)

Corcos, Michael G., '"Leprosy Can Be Cured!": New Wine in an Old Bottle?' *The Star*, March–April 1988, pp. 3–6

Creighton, Charles, *A History of Epidemics in Britain* (London 1894)

Cust, Robert Needham, *Memoirs of Past Years of a Septuagenarian* (Privately printed 1899)

————, *Linguistic and Oriental Essays: Third Series* (London 1891)

Davey, Cyril, *Caring Comes First: The Leprosy Mission Story* (Marshall Pickering, London 1987)

Davey, T. Frank, 'Uzuakoli Leper Colony', *Lepr. Rev.*, Vol. X, No. 3, July 1939, pp. 171–85

Daws, Gavan, *Holy Man: Father Damien of Molokai* (Univ. of Hawaii Press, Honolulu 1973)

Deacon, Harriet, 'Outside the Profession; Nursing Staff on Robben Island, 1846–1910', in Rafferty, Anne Marie, Robinson, Jane, and Elkan, Ruth (ed.), *Nursing History and the Politics of Welfare* (Routledge & Kegan Paul, London and New York 1997), pp. 95–7

De Stigter, D.H., de Geus, L., and Heynders, M.L., 'Leprosy: Between Acceptance and Segregation. Community Behaviour Towards Persons Affected by Leprosy in Eastern Nepal', *Lepr. Rev.*, Vol. 71, 2000, pp. 492–8

De Villiers, Simon A., *Robben Island: Out of Reach, Out of Mind* (C. Struik (pty) Ltd, Cape Town 1971)

Dharmendra, 'Leprosy in Ancient Indian Medicine', *Int. J. Lepr.*, Vol. 15, No. 4, Oct–Dec 1947, pp. 424–30

Dory, Electra, *Leper Country* (Muller, London 1963)

Duncan, Jim, 'Twenty-one Months at Carville', *The Star*, Sept–Oct 1965, pp. 2, 16

Dutton, Charles J., *The Samaritans of Molokai: The Lives of Father Damien and Brother Dutton Among the Lepers* (London 1934)

Dyer, Isadore, 'The Sociological Aspects of Leprosy and the Question of Segregation', *Journal of Cutaneous Diseases, Including Syphilis*, May 1911

Eynikel, Hilde, *Molokai: The Story of Father Damien* (Hodder & Stoughton, London 1999)

Faria, Emanuel, 'Life after MDT', *The Star*, March–April 1994, pp. 8–10

Farrow, John, *Damien the Leper* (New York 1937)

Feeny, Patrick, *The Fight Against Leprosy* (Elek Books, London 1964)

Feldmeier, Hermann, 'The Tortuous Path of the Leprosy Bacilli: Questioning an Old Paradigm', *ESCMID* [European Society of Clinical Microbiology and Infectious Diseases] *News*, No. 1, 2001, pp. 26–7
Fletcher, Grace Nies, *The Fabulous Flemings of Kathmandu* (Dutton, New York 1964)
Fraser, N.D., 'Leprosy in Nepal', *Lepr. Rev.*, Vol. 31, No. 4, Oct 1960, pp. 286–9
Gerould, Katharine Fullerton, 'Kalaupapa: The Leper Settlement on Molokai', *Scribner's Magazine*, Vol. LX, No. 1, July 1916, pp. 1–18
Greave, Peter, *The Second Miracle* (Chatto & Windus, London/Henry Holt, New York 1955)
———, *Young Man in the Sun* (Eyre & Spottiswoode, London 1958)
———, *The Painted Leopard* (Eyre & Spottiswoode, London 1960)
———, *The Seventh Gate* (Temple-Smith, London 1976; Penguin, London 1978)
Greene, Graham, *A Burnt-Out Case* (Bodley Head, London 1961)
———, *In Search of Characters: Two African Journals* (Bodley Head, London 1961)
Greene, Linda W., *Exile in Paradise: The Isolation of Hawaii's Leprosy Victims and Development of Kalaupapa Settlement, 1865 to the Present* (National Park Service, Denver, Col., Sept 1985)
Gussow, Zachary, *Leprosy, Racism and Public Health: Social Policy in Chronic Disease Control* (Westview Press, Boulder, Col. 1989)
Gussow, Zachary, and Tracy, George S., 'Status, Ideology, and Adaptation to Stigmatized Illness: A Study of Leprosy', *Human Organization*, No. 27, 1968, pp. 316–25
———, 'Stigma and the Leprosy Phenomenon: The Social History of a Disease in the 19th and 20th Centuries', *Bull. Hist. Med.*, Vol. 44, No. 5, Sept–Oct 1970, pp. 425–49
Hamilton-Paterson, James, *America's Boy* (Granta Books, London 1998)
Hanley, Sister Mary Laurence OSF, and Bushnell, O.A. *A Song of Pilgrimage and Exile: The Life and Spirit of Mother Marianne of Molokai* (Franciscan Herald Press, Chicago 1980)
Hansen, G. Armauer, 'On the Report of the Leprosy Commission in India, 1890–91: A Criticism', *The Lancet*, 30 Dec 1893, pp. 1053–4
———, *Memories & Reflections* (German Leprosy Relief Association, Würzburg, Germany 1976)
Hansen, G. Armauer, and Looft, Carl, *Leprosy: In its Clinical and Pathological Aspects* (Bristol 1895)
Harboe, Morton, 'Armauer Hansen – The Man and His Work', *Int. J. Lepr.*, Vol. 41, No. 4, 1973, pp. 417–24
Harmon, Johnny P., *King of the Microbes* (privately printed, 5th printing 1999)
Heiser, Victor, *A Doctor's Odyssey* (London 1936)
Hutchinson, Jonathan, *On Leprosy and Fish-Eating* (London 1906)
Irgens, Lorentz M., 'Leprosy in Norway: An Interplay of Research and Public Health Work', *Int. J. Lepr.*, Vol. 41, No. 2, 1973, pp. 189–98
———, *Leprosy in Norway: An Epidemiological Study Based on a National Patient Register*, *Lepr. Rev.*, Vol. 51, Supp. 1, March 1980)
———, 'Hansen, 150 Years After His Birth, the Context of a Medical Discovery', *Int. J. Lepr.*, Vol. 60, No. 3, Sept. 1992, pp. 466–9
Jackson, John, *In Leper-Land* (London 1901)
Jagadisan, T.N., 'Chairman's Statement on Social Aspects', *Transactions of the VIIth International Congress of Leprology* (Tokyo 1959), pp. 417–24
———, *Fulfilment Through Leprosy* (Tamil Nadu, India 1988)
Job, C.K., 'Leprosy – the Source of Infection and its Mode of Transmission', *Lepr. Rev.*, Vol. 52, Suppl. 1, 1981, pp. 69–76
Johnson, Henry, *The Life of Kate Marsden* (London 1895, 2nd edn)
Johnson, Thomas M., 'Joey's Quiet War', *Reader's Digest*, 1964
Kalisch, Philip A., 'Tracadie and Penikese Leprosaria: A Comparative Analysis of Societal Response to Leprosy in New Brunswick, 1844–1880, and Massachusetts, 1904–1921', *Bull. Hist. Med.*, Vol. XLVII, 1973, pp. 480–512
———, 'The Strange Case of John Early: A Study of the Stigma of Leprosy', *Int. J. Lepr.*, Vol. 40, No. 3, 1972, pp. 291–305
Kaplan, Gilla, 'Leprosy (Hansen's Disease)', in L. Goodman and J.C. Bennett (ed.), *Cecil Textbook of Medicine* (21st edn 1999)

Karlen, Arno, *Plague's Progress* (Gollancz, London 1995)
Kendall, John Smith, 'Little Known Chapter in the History of Carville', *The Star*, Nov 1952, pp. 1–2
Kellersberger, Eugene R., 'The Social Stigma of Leprosy', *Annals of the New York Academy of Sciences*, Vol. 54, Art. 1, March 1951, pp. 126–33
Kinnear Brown, J.A., 'The Role of Leprosaria and Treatment Villages in Mass Campaigns in Tropical Africa', *Int. J. Lepr.*, Vol. 29, No. 1, Jan–March 1960, pp. 1–11
Knight, Alanna (ed.), *Robert Louis Stevenson in the South Seas* (Mainstream Publishing, Edinburgh 1986)
Lambert, Agnes, 'Leprosy: Present and Past. 1, Present', *The Nineteenth Century*, Aug 1884, pp. 210–27
Law, Anwei Skinsnes, 'Japan – A Recovery of Rights', *The Star*, Sept 1996
Lechat, Michel F., 'The International Leprosy Association at 50 Years', *Int. J. Lepr.*, Vol. 49, No. 1, March 1981, pp. 60–4
————, 'Remembering Graham Greene', *The Bulletin*, 18 April 1991, pp. 14–16
————, 'The Paleoepidemiology of Leprosy: An Overview', *Int. J. Lepr.*, Vol. 67, No. 4, Dec 1999, pp. 460–70
Leprosy in Foreign Countries (Honolulu 1886)
Leprosy in Hawaii: Extracts from Reports (Honolulu 1886)
Leprosy in India: Report of the Leprosy Commission in India 1890–91 (Calcutta 1892)
Lewis, T.R., and Cunningham, D.D., *Leprosy in India: A Report* (Calcutta 1887)
Lie, H.P., 'Report of the Leper Hospital . . . in Bergen for the 3 Years 1899–1901', *Lepra*, Vol. IV, Fasc. 1
————, 'Why Is Leprosy Decreasing in Norway?' *Int. J. Lepr.*, Vol. 1, No. 2, 1933, pp. 205–16
Lockwood, Diana N.J., 'Leprosy Elimination – a Virtual Phenomenon or a Reality?' *BMJ*, Vol. 324, 22 June 2002, pp. 1516–18
London, Jack, *Tales of Hawaii* (Press Pacifica, Hawaii 1984)
Losier, M.J., *Children of Lazarus: The Story of the Lazaretto at Tracadie* (n.p., New Brunswick 1984)
Lowe, J., 'A Curious Chapter of the History of Leprosy in India, the Indian Leprosy Commission of 1890', *Leprosy in India*, July 1939, pp. 82–6
Lynch, Patrick, 'A New Face for an Old Disease: Some Reflections on the Role of the Media in Nepal's First National Leprosy Elimination Campaign', *Lepr. Rev.*, Vol. 71, No. 1, March 2000, pp. 62–70
Macdonald, A.B., 'Rehabilitation – The Industrial and Social Work of a Leper Colony', *Lepr. Rev.*, Vol. XIX, No. 2, April 1948, pp. 45–55
MacLeod, J.M.H., 'Contact Cases of Leprosy in the British Isles', *Lepr. Rev.*, Vol. 3, No. 1, Jan–March 1935
Manchester, Keith, 'Leprosy: The Origin and Development of the Disease in Antiquity', in Gourevitch, Danielle (ed.) *Maladie et Maladies* (Librairie Droz, Geneva 1992)
Marsden, Kate, *On Sledge and Horseback to Outcast Siberian Lepers* (London 1883)
————, *My Mission in Siberia: A Vindication* (London 1921)
Martin, Betty (ed. Evelyn Wells), *Miracle at Carville* (Doubleday, New York 1950)
————, *No One Must Ever Know* (Doubleday, New York 1959)
Mayo, Katherine, *The Isles of Fear: The Truth about the Philippines* (London 1925)
Mercier, Charles A., *Leper Houses and Mediaeval Hospitals* (London 1915)
Merwin, W.S., *The Folding Cliffs: A Narrative of 19th-Century Hawaii* (Knopf, New York 1998)
Middleton, Dorothy, *Victorian Lady Travellers* (Routledge & Kegan Paul, London 1965)
Millinship, William, 'Heroine of Russia Cast Out into the Cold', *The Times*, 15 Aug 1994
Miller, A. Donald, *An Inn Called Welcome: The Story of the Mission to Lepers 1874–1917* (Mission to Lepers, London 1964)
Mills, Clarence A., *Climate Makes the Man* (Harper, New York 1942)
Mission to Lepers, The, *Report of a Conference of Leper Asylum Superintendents and Others on the Leper Problems of India* (Cuttack, India 1920)
Monaghan, Father Forbes, 'The Story of Billy', *The Star*, Feb 1948
Mouritz, A.A. St M., *'The Path of the Destroyer': A History of Leprosy in the Hawaiian Islands* (Honolulu 1916)

———, *A Brief World History of Leprosy* (Honolulu, rev. edn 1943)
———, 'Human Inoculation Experiments in Hawaii Including Notes of Those of Arning and Fitch' (condensed, arranged and annotated by H.W. Wade), *Int. J. Lepr.*, Vol. 19, No. 2, April–June 1951, pp. 203–15
Muir, Ernest, *Manual of Leprosy* (E. & S. Livingstone, Edinburgh 1948)
Munro, W., *Leprosy* (Manchester 1879, reprinted from the *Edinburgh Medical Journal*, Sept 1876–Nov 1879)
Neill, Stephen, *A History of Christian Missions* (Penguin, London 1964; 2nd edn rev. by Owen Chadwick 1986, repr. 1990)
Newman, George, *On the History of the Decline and Final Extinction of Leprosy as an Endemic Disease in the British Isles* (London 1895)
Ohtani, Fujio, *The Walls Crumble: The Emancipation of Persons Affected by Hansen's Disease in Japan* (n.p., Tokyo 1998)
Oldrieve, Frank, *India's Lepers: How to Rid India of Leprosy* (London 1924)
Pamphile, Father (ed.), *Life and Letters of Father Damien* (London 1889)
Pandya, Shubhada S., 'Anti-Contagionism in Leprosy, 1844–1897', *Int. J. Lepr.*, Vol. 66, No. 3, Sept 1998, pp. 374–84
———, '"Very Savage Rites": Suicide and the Leprosy Sufferer in Nineteenth Century India', *Indian Journal of Leprosy*, Vol. 73, No. 1, 2001, pp. 27–36
Parascandola, John, 'The Gillis W. Long Hansen's Disease Center at Carville', *Public Health Reports*, Vol. 109, No. 6, Nov–Dec 1994, pp. 728–30
Power, Helen, *Sir Leonard Rogers FRS (1868–1962): Tropical Medicine in the Indian Medical Service* (University of London PhD thesis, 1993)
Pyle, Ernie, *Home Country* (William Sloane Associates, New York 1947)
Ramsay, G.W. St. C., 'A Study of Leprosy in Southern Nigeria', *Transactions of the Royal Society of Tropical Medicine & Hygiene*, Vol. XXII, No. 3, Nov 1928, pp. 249–62
Rankin, Nicholas, *Dead Man's Chest: Travels After Robert Louis Stevenson* (Faber, London 1987)
Rawcliffe, Carole, 'Learning to Love the Leper: Aspects of Institutional Charity in Anglo Norman England', *Anglo-Norman Studies XXIII*, 2000, pp. 231–50
———, *Medicine and Society in Later Medieval England* (Sutton Publishing, Stroud 1995)
Ree, G.H., 'Pattern of leprosy in Queensland, Australia, 1855–1990', *Lepr. Rev.*, Vol. 62, 1991, pp. 420–30
Report on Leprosy by the Royal College of Physicians (London 1867)
Richards, Peter, 'Leprosy in Scandinavia', *Centaurus*, Vol. 7, No. 1, 1960, pp. 101–33
Robertson, Linda M., Nichols, Peter G., and Butlin, Ruth, 'Delay in Presentation and Start of Treatment in Leprosy: Experience in an Outpatient Clinic in Nepal', *Lepr. Rev.*, Vol. 71, 2000, pp. 511–16
Robinson, Charles Henry, *Hausaland: Or Fifteen Hundred Miles through the Central Soudan* (London 1896)
Rogers, Sir Leonard, *Happy Toil: 55 Years of Tropical Medicine* (Muller, London 1950)
Rokstad, Ingvald, 'Gerhard Henrich Armauer Hansen', *Int. J. Lepr.*, Vol. 32, No. 1, Jan–March 1964, pp. 64–70
Ryrie, G. A., 'The Psychology of Leprosy', *Lepr. Rev.*, Vol. 22, Nos 1 and 2, 1951, pp. 13–24
Silla, Eric, *People Are Not the Same: Leprosy and Identity in Twentieth-Century Mali* (Heinemann, Portsmouth, NH/James Currey, Oxford 1998)
Simeons, A.T.W. *The Mask of a Lion* (Gollancz, London 1952)
Simpson, James Y., 'Antiquarian Notes of Leprosy and Leper Hospitals in England and Scotland', *Edinburgh Medical & Surgical Journal*, Vols 56 and 57, 1841–2, pp. 301–30, 394–429
Stanley, Laurie C.C., *Unclean! Unclean! Leprosy in New Brunswick 1844–1880* (Les Editions d'Acadie, New Brunswick 1982)
Stanley-Blackwell, Laurie C.C., 'A Singular Obsession: New Brunswick's Leprosy Doctor', *Int. J. Lepr.*, Vol. 61, No. 4, Dec 1993, pp. 619–27
[Stead, W.T.], 'The Quest for the Holy Grail: An English Lady among the Lepers of Siberia', *The Review of Reviews*, Vol. 6, July–Dec 1892, pp. 185–8
Stein, Stanley, *Alone No Longer* (*The Star*, Carville, La, 1974; 1st pubd 1963)

Stella, Sister Mary, *Makogai: Image of Hope* (Lepers' Trust Board, New Zealand 1978)
Stevenson, Robert Louis, *An Open Letter to the Rev. Dr Hyde of Honolulu* (Ave Maria Press, Notre Dame, Ind., 1927 edn)
Stoddart, Charles Warren, *The Lepers of Molokai* (Ave Maria Press, Notre Dame, Ind. 1893 edn.)
Takashima, Shigetaka, 'New Orientation in the Control of Leprosy in Japan', *Int. J. Lepr.*, Vol. 33, No. 1, Jan–March 1965, pp. 1–17
Tebb, William, *The Recrudescence of Leprosy and Its Causation* (London 1893)
Thangaraj, R.H., and Yawalkar, S.J., *Leprosy for Medical Practitioners and Paramedical Workers* (Ciba-Geigy Ltd, Basle, Switzerland, 4th edn 1989)
Thompson, Phyllis, *Mister Leprosy: Dr Stanley Browne's Fight against Leprosy* (Hodder & Stoughton, London 1980–1)
Tonkin, T.J., 'Some General and Etiological Details Concerning Leprosy in the Sudan', *Lepra*, Vol. III, Fasc. 3, 1903, p. 135
Updike, John, *Problems and Other Stories* (Knopf, New York 1979)
Vaughan, Megan, *Curing Their Ills: Colonial Power and African Illness* (Polity Press, Cambridge 1991)
Vogelsang, Th. M., 'The Old Leprosy Hospitals in Bergen', *Int. J. Lepr.*, Vol. 32, No. 3, July–Sept 1964, pp. 306–9
————, 'Leprosy in Norway', *Medical History*, Vol. 9, Jan 1965, pp. 29–35
————, 'Gerhard Henrik Armauer Hansen 1841–1912', *Int. J. Lepr.*, Vol. 46, No. 3, July–Sept 1978, pp. 257–323
Wade, H. Windsor, 'High Lights of Wartime Culion', *The Star*, Oct 1946, pp. 1–3
Waxler, Nancy E., 'Learning to Be a Leper: A Case Study in the Social Construction of Illness', in Elliot G. Mischler *et al.*, *Social Contexts of Health, Illness, and Patient Care* (Cambridge Univ. Press, Cambridge 1981)
Weymouth, Anthony, *Through the Leper-Squint: A Study of Leprosy from pre-Christian Times to the Present Day* (London 1938)
Wilson, Dorothy Clarke, *Ten Fingers for God: The Life and Work of Paul Brand* (1965; Paul Brand Publishing, Seattle 1989)
Wright, H.P., *Leprosy: An Imperial Danger* (London 1889)

INDEX